P9-CFP-816

# Population Mobility and Infectious Disease

# Population Mobility and Infectious Disease

Edited by
## Yorghos Apostolopoulos

*Cyprus International Institute for the Environment and Public Health*
*in association with Harvard School of Public Health*
*Nicosia, Cyprus*

*Emory University School of Medicine*
*Atlanta, Georgia, USA*

and
## Sevil Sönmez

*Cyprus College*
*Nicosia, Cyprus*

*Emory University School of Medicine*
*Atlanta, Georgia, USA*

Foreword by
Janet Hatcher Roberts

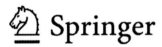 Springer

Yorghos Apostolopoulos, Ph.D.
Visiting Professor of Social
　Epidemiology
Cyprus International Institute for the
　Environment and Public Health in
　association with Harvard School of
　Public Health
5 Iroon Street
Nicosia 1105, Cyprus
E-mail: yapostol@cyprusinstitute.org

Associate Clinical Professor of Social
　Epidemiology
Emory University School of Medicine
Department of Medicine, Division of
　Infectious Diseases
Atlanta, GA 30303, USA
E-mail: yaposto@emory.edu

Sevil Sönmez, Ph.D.
Associate Professor
Cyprus College
6 Diogenes Street
Nicosia 1516, Cyprus
E-mail: sonmez@cycollege.ac.cy

Assistant Professor of Medicine
Emory University School of Medicine
Department of Medicine, Division of
　Infectious Diseases
Atlanta, GA 30303, USA
E-mail: ssonmez@emory.edu

Library of Congress Control Number: 2006940353

ISBN-10: 0-387-47667-9          eISBN-10: 0-387-49711-0
ISBN-13: 978-0-387-47667-4      eISBN-13: 978-0-387-49711-2

© 2007 Springer Science+Business Media, LLC
All rights reserved. This work may not be translated or copied in whole or in part without the
written permission of the publisher (Springer Science+Business Media, LLC, 233 Spring Street,
New York, NY 10013, USA), except for brief excerpts in connection with reviews or scholarly
analysis. Use in connection with any form of information storage and retrieval, electronic
adaptation, computer software, or by similar or dissimilar methodology now known or hereafter
developed is forbidden.
The use in this publication of trade names, trademarks, service marks and similar terms, even if
they are not identified as such, is not to be taken as an expression of opinion as to whether or
not they are subject to proprietary rights.

9 8 7 6 5 4 3 2 1

springer.com

We dedicate this book
to the sweet memory of Müzehher Sönmez

077 256600

# Foreword

Globalization has created new challenges to our paradigm of population movement, health and disease, challenges which call us to find new approaches, models and perspectives to address global inequities and the impact these inequities have on migrant populations. Governments, intergovernmental organizations and other stakeholders have increasingly recognized the influence of mobility on the disease burden of populations, identifying factors at different stages of the migration process.

Population mobility and the health of those who move are increasingly a concern for public health professionals around the world. Public health professionals, policy makers and governments alike are finding that they are not only addressing the traditional diseases, including infectious diseases, but also new and emerging diseases. Within such contexts, the critical links to the significant determinants of health such as poverty, equity literacy and environment can not be overlooked.

Much has been accomplished, yet more can be done. Appropriate application of public health tools and research can be used to strengthen national health systems to address issues relating to migrants' health. This groundbreaking book, *Population Mobility and Infectious Disease,* delves into several variations of population mobility (e.g. labour migration, forced migration, internal migration, disasters, trafficking, military, and tourists) and discusses their effects on the health of migrants and receiving countries. Readers who are not familiar with migration issues will find this book an excellent resource. In addition, this volume can be particularly helpful in the identification of public health interventions for mobile populations.

Contributors to this fine volume include some of the most distinguished scholars in the field. Throughout the book, the work of governments, international organizations, academe, research institutions and individual researchers are highlighted. This is of particular significance as global intersectoral collaboration is critical to building effective, sustainable and evidence-based solutions for future management of migration health.

At a point of history where the only constant is the endless and growing movement of populations, in both frequency and numbers, *Population Mobility and Infectious Disease* brings to the fore a long-overdue comprehensive work of prime value for students, researchers, and practitioners. This book has the added potential to become a catalyst for additional and more authoritative works on the state of health, dynamics, and management of mobile populations around the globe.

Janet Hatcher Roberts
*Director, Migration Health Department*
*International Organization for Migration*
*Geneva, Switzerland*
*February 2007*

# Preface

In an increasingly globalized world, humans and materials—transported by automobiles, cargo ships and airplanes in a matter of hours—are the most effective vectors of infectious pathogens. Over the course of human history, some of the deadliest disease outbreaks have been traced back to one type or another mobile population or to transport routes. In this context, our own intimate research involvement with several mobile populations in the U.S. such as vacation travelers, long-haul truck drivers, and floating Latin farmworkers as well as thrilling fieldwork with pastoralists (nomads) in southern Ethiopia brought into light the critical role of the complex spectrum of population mobility and infectious disease.

This book is long overdue and is intended to fill a serious gap in the international public health literature. It is the first transdisciplinary volume that provides a comprehensive overview of what happens to the health of people when they migrate from countrysides to cities, from one city to another, or from one country to another, regardless of the voluntary or forced nature of that movement. One of the major strengths of this book lies in its transdisciplinary approach—spanning across anthropological, demographic, economic, epidemiological, geographical, historical, legal, mathematical, political, psychological, sociological perspectives.

In the over two years that it has taken to complete this book, it has overcome several hurdles and gone through numerous phases. This book would never have materialized without the collective support of all individuals and organizations involved. It was a great challenge to locate, commission, and coordinate high-caliber international scholars and practitioners in various facets of public health. However, the quality of their work made the review and revision process highly enjoyable tasks.

We would like to extend our thanks to Bill Tucker at Springer publishers for his encouragement, guidance, and especially his immense patience, understanding and support during this process. We would also like to thank our colleagues Rich Rothenberg, Jennie Kronenfeld, Dale Stratford, Mario Bronfman, Rebecca Clark, Vivian Levy, Shabbir Ismail, Johan Helland, Tadesse Wuhib, Aklilu Kidanu, Keith Bletzer, Hailom Banteyerga, and

Lucia McLendon for their valuable advice and assistance during various phases of the project. Last, but certainly not least, we extend our heartfelt thanks to all the U.S. truckers, Latin migrant farmworkers, Ethiopian pastoralists, and U.S. spring-breakers who taught us so much.

Yorghos Apostolopoulos
Sevil Sönmez
Nicosia, Cyprus

# Contents

**Part IV**
**Leisure Migration and Health Concerns: A Paradox or Inevitability?**

**Chapter 11**
**Casual Sex in the Sun Makes the Holiday: Young Tourists' Perspectives**
EUGENIA WICKENS AND SEVIL SÖNMEZ . . . . . . . . . . . . . . . . . . . . . . . .  199

**Chapter 12**
**In Search of the Exotic: Sex Tourism and Disease Risks**
SEVIL SÖNMEZ, EUGENIA WICKENS,
AND YORGHOS APOSTOLOPOULOS . . . . . . . . . . . . . . . . . . . . . . . . . . . . .  215

**Epilogue**
**New Directions in Migration Health and Medicine**

**Chapter 13**
**Mapping and Modeling Disease Risk Among Mobile Populations**
HENRY G. MWAMBI AND KHANGELANI ZUMA . . . . . . . . . . . . . . . . . . . .  245

**Chapter 14**
**Ethical and Legal Issues Impacting Migrant Health**
SANA LOUE . . . . . . . . . . . . . . . . . . . . . . . . . . . . . . . . . . . . . . . . . . . . . . . .  267

# Contributors

**Yorghos Apostolopoulos, Ph.D.**
Visiting Professor of Social Epidemiology
Cyprus International Institute for the Environment
   and Public Health in association with Harvard School
   of Public Health
5 Iroon Street
Nicosia 1105, Cyprus

Associate Clinical Professor of Social Epidemiology
Emory University School of Medicine
Department of Medicine, Division of
   Infectious Diseases
49 Jesse Hill Jr. Drive, S.E.
Atlanta, GA 30303, USA

**Frederick M. Burkle, Jr., M.D., M.P.H.**
Professor and Director
Asia-Pacific Center for Biosecurity, Disaster
   & Conflict Research
John A. Burns School of Medicine
University of Hawaii
Honolulu, HI, USA

Senior Fellow
Harvard Humanitarian Initiative
Harvard School of Public Health
Boston, MA, USA

**Brian D. Gushulak, B.Sc., M.D.**
Migration Health Consultants, Inc.
Vienna, Austria

**Elizabeth Ioannidi-Kapolou, Ph.D.**
Senior Research Scientist
Department of Sociology
National School of Public Health
196 Alexandra's Avenue
Athens 11521, Greece

**Stuart J. Kingma, M.D.**
Director
Civil-Military Alliance to Combat HIV & AIDS,
    Switzerland
20, route de l'Hôpital
CH-1180 Rolle, Switzerland

**Anthony P. Lombardo, M.A., Ph.D. Candidate**
Community Health (Health and Behavioural Sciences)
Department of Public Health Sciences
Faculty of Medicine
University of Toronto
155 College St., 5th Floor
Toronto, ON M5T 3M7, Canada

**Sana Loue, J.D., Ph.D., M.P.H.**
Professor
Director, Center for Minority Public Health
Case Western Reserve University
School of Medicine
Department of Epidemiology and Biostatistics
10900 Euclid Avenue
Cleveland, OH 44106-4945,USA

**Mark N. Lurie, Ph.D.**
Research Assistant Professor of Community Health
Brown University Medical School and the International
    Health Institute
Box G-S 2 / 169 Angell Street
Providence, RI 02912, USA

**Douglas W. MacPherson, M.D., M.Sc.(CTM), F.R.C.P.C.**
Associate Professor, Faculty of Health Sciences
McMaster University
Hamilton, ON L8N 3Z5, Canada

Migration Health Consultants, Inc.
Cheltenham, ON L7C 1Y4, Canada

**Jonathan D. Mayer, Ph.D.**
Professor of Epidemiology
International Health, and Geography
Adjunct Professor of Medicine (Infectious Diseases),
Family Medicine, and Health Services
Clinical Consultant
Travel and Tropical Medicine Service
University of Washington Medical Center
University of Washington, Box 353550
Seattle, WA 98195, USA

**Lynn McDonald, Ph.D.**
Professor, Faculty of Social Work
Director, Institute for Life Course and Aging
University of Toronto
222 College Street, Suite 106
Toronto, ON M5T 3J1, Canada

**Henry G. Mwambi, Ph.D.**
Senior Lecturer of Statistics
School of Statistics and Actuarial Science
University of KwaZulu-Natal, South Africa
Private Bag X01 Scottsville, Pietermaritzburg, South Africa

**Sevil Sönmez, Ph.D.**
Associate Professor
Cyprus College
6 Diogenes Street
Nicosia 1516, Cyprus

Assistant Professor of Medicine
Emory University School of Medicine
Department of Medicine, Division of Infectious Diseases
49 Jesse Hill Jr. Drive, S.E.
Atlanta, GA 30303, USA

**Varda Soskolne, Ph.D.**
Senior Lecturer
School of Social Work
Bar-Ilan University
Ramat-Gan 52900, Israel

Research Scientist
Braun School of Public Health
Hadassah - Hebrew University Medical Center
Jerusalem, Israel

**Natalya Timoshkina, M.S.W., Ph.D. Candidate**
Research Coordinator
Faculty of Social Work and
Institute for Life Course and Aging
University of Toronto
222 College Street
Toronto, ON M5T 3J1, Canada

**Eugenia Wickens, Ph.D.**
Buckinghamshire Chilterns
University College
Faculty of Leisure and Tourism
Wellesbourne Campus, Kingshill Road
High Wycombe, Buckinghamshire, HP13 5BB UK

**Mary E. Wilson, M.D., F.A.C.P.**
Associate Clinical Professor of Medicine
Harvard Medical School

Associate Professor of Population and International Health
Harvard School of Public Health
Boston, MA, USA

**Rodger D. Yeager, Ph.D.**
Associate Director
Civil-Military Alliance to Combat HIV & AIDS
369 Horseshoe Road
Morgantown, WV 26508-910, USA

**Khangelani Zuma, Ph.D.**
Chief Research Specialist
Social Aspects of HIV/AIDS and Health Research Program
Human Sciences Research Council
Private Bag X41, Pretoria  0001, South Africa

# List of Abbreviations

| | |
|---|---|
| ACHR | American Convention on Human Rights |
| AFRIMS | Armed Forces Research Institute of Medical Sciences (Thailand) |
| AIDS | Acquired Immunodeficiency Syndrome |
| ARVs | Antiretroviral Drugs |
| ASEAN | Association of Southeast Asian Nations |
| BBIs | Bloodborne Infections |
| BICE | Bureau of Immigration and Customs Enforcement (USA) |
| BTS | Bureau of Transportation Statistics (USA) |
| CAREC | Caribbean Regional Epidemiological Centre |
| CARICOM | Caribbean Community |
| CATW | Coalition Against Trafficking in Women |
| CB | Citizens Band |
| CDC | Centers for Disease Control and Prevention (USA) |
| CD4 cells | Term that refers to sub-group of lymphocytes (type of white blood cell or leukocyte) that plays cornerstone role in establishing and maximizing capabilities of immune system–testing for numbers of circulating CD4 cells offers measure of current functional capacity of immune system. |
| CE | Complex Emergencies |
| CHD | Coronary Heart Disease |
| CIA | U.S. Central Intelligence Agency (USA) |
| CMA | Civil-Military Alliance to Combat HIV & AIDS (Switzerland, USA) |
| CSIR | Council for Scientific and Industrial Research (South Africa) |
| CSIS | Center for Strategic and International Studies (USA) |
| CSWs | Commercial Sexworkers |
| DCI | Director of Central Intelligence |
| DFID | British Department for International Development (UK) |
| DHS | Department of Homeland Security (USA) |
| DPKO | Department of Peacekeeping Operations (UN) |
| DSA | Demographic Surveillance Area |

| | |
|---|---|
| ECHR | European Convention on Human Rights and Fundamental Freedoms |
| ECOMOG | Economic Community of West African States Ceasefire Monitoring Group |
| ECPAT | End Child Prostitution/Pornography and Trafficking |
| ECRE | European Council on Refugees and Exiles (Belgium, UK) |
| EE/CA | Eastern Europe and Central Asia |
| ENSO | El Niño Southern Oscillation |
| EOT | Hellenic National Tourism Authority (Greece) |
| ETM | Enhanced Thematic Mapper |
| EU | European Union |
| EUROHIV | European Centre for the Epidemiological Monitoring of AIDS (UK) |
| EUROPAP | European Network for HIV-STD Prevention in Prostitution (UK) |
| EWRRS | Early Warning Rapid Response System |
| FHI | Family Health International (USA) |
| FSU | Former Soviet Union |
| GBGM | General Board of Global Ministries of the United Methodist Church (USA) |
| GDP | Gross Domestic Product |
| GHC | Global Health Council (USA) |
| GIS | Geographic Information Systems |
| GLM | Generalized Linear Model |
| GLMMs | Generalized Linear Mixed Models |
| GOARN | Global Outbreak Alert and Response Network |
| GPHIN | Global Public health Information Network |
| HAART | Highly Active Antiretroviral Therapy |
| HBV | Hepatitis B Virus |
| HCV | Hepatitis C Virus |
| HHD | High Human Development |
| HIS | Health Information System |
| HIV | Human Immunodeficiency Virus |
| HIV2 | A second strain of HIV found in West Africa |
| HPA | Hypothalamic-Pituitary-Adrenal |
| IAS | International AIDS Society (Switzerland) |
| ICCPR | International Covenant on Civil and Political Rights |
| ICESCR | International Covenant on Economic, Social and Cultural Rights |
| IDPs | Internally Displaced Persons |
| IDUs | Injecting/Intravenous Drug Users |
| IHR | International Health Regulations |
| IIRAIRA | Illegal Immigration Reform and Immigrant Responsibility Act |
| ILO | International Labor Office |
| ILO | International Labor Organization (Switzerland) |

| | |
|---|---|
| INAA | Immigration and Nationality Act Amendments |
| INS | Immigration and Naturalization Service (USA) |
| IOM | International Organization for Migration (Switzerland) |
| IPCC | Intergovernmental Panel on Climate Change (Switzerland) |
| IPEC | International Program on the Elimination of Child Labor |
| LHD | Low Human Development |
| LSD | Lysergic Acid Diethylamide (hallucinogenic drug) |
| MCMC | Markov Chain Monte-Carlo |
| MDRTB | Multiple Drug Resistant Tuberculosis |
| MRF | Markov Random Field |
| MSM | Men who Have Sex with Men |
| NASA | National Aeronautics and Space Administration (USA) |
| NATHNAC | National Travel Health Network and Centre (UK) |
| NATSO | National Association of Truckstop Operators (USA) |
| NDVI | Normalized Difference Vegetation Index |
| NGOs | Non-Governmental Organizations |
| NIC | U.S. National Intelligence Council (USA) |
| OCHA | Office of the Coordinator for Humanitarian Affairs (UN) |
| PAHO | Pan American Health Organization (WHO) |
| PCR | Polymerase Chain Reaction |
| PEM | Protein Energy Malnutrition |
| PHASE | Prevention of HIV/AIDS and STIs among Women in Europe |
| PHLS | Public Health Laboratory Service (UK) |
| PHS | Public Health Service (USA) |
| PLWHA | People Living with HIV/AIDS |
| PRWORA | Personal Responsibility and Work Opportunity Reform Act (USA) |
| PTSD | Post-Traumatic Stress Disorder |
| RCMP | Royal Canadian Mounted Police (Canada) |
| RR | Relative Risk |
| RSV | Respiratory Synctial Virus |
| RTA | Royal Thai Army (Thailand) |
| SARDI | South Asian Research and Development Initiative |
| SARS | Severe Acute Respiratory Syndrome |
| SC | State Capacity |
| SEA | Southeast Asia |
| SEIR | Susceptible-Exposed-Infected-Recovered Model |
| SEQIJR | Susceptible-Exposed-Quarantined-Infected-Isolated Recovered Model |
| SIR | Susceptible-Infected-Recovered and Immune Model |
| SIS | Susceptible-Infected-Susceptible Model |
| SMR | Standardized Mortality Ratio |
| SMRC | South African Medical Research Council (South Africa) |
| SOSTRIS | Social Strategies in Risk Societies |
| SSA | Sub-Saharan Africa |

| | |
|---|---|
| STD | Sexually Transmitted Disease |
| STI | Sexually Transmitted Infection |
| TAMPEP | Transnational AIDS/STD Prevention Among Migrant Prostitutes in Europe Project (The Netherlands) |
| TB | Tuberculosis |
| UN | United Nations |
| UNAIDS | The Joint United Nations Programme on HIV/AIDS |
| UNDP | United Nations Development Programme |
| UNEP | United Nations Environment Program |
| UNESCAP | United Nations Economic and Social Commission for Asia and the Pacific |
| UNESCO | United Nations Educational, Social, and Cultural Organization |
| UNHCR | United Nations High Commissioner for Refugees |
| UNICEF | United Nations Children's Fund |
| US | United States of America |
| USAID | United States Agency for International Development (USA) |
| USDHHS | United States Department of Health and Human Services (USA) |
| USDOJ | United States Department of Justice (USA) |
| USDOS | United States Department of State (USA) |
| USDOT | United States Department of Transportation (USA) |
| USGS | United States Geological Survey (USA) |
| USSR | Union of Soviet Socialist Republics |
| VCT | Voluntary Counseling and Testing |
| VFRs | Visiting Friends or Relatives |
| WHA | World Health Assembly (WHO) |
| WHO | World Health Organization |
| WNV | West Nile Virus |
| WPRO | Western Pacific Regional Organization (WHO) |
| WTO | World Tourism Organization |

# Prologue
## Bridging the Divide:
## Population Mobility and the
## Emergence of Disease

# Chapter 1

## Demographic and Epidemiological Perspectives of Human Movement

YORGHOS APOSTOLOPOULOS, PH.D. AND
SEVIL SÖNMEZ, PH.D.

### Globalization, Mobility, and Population Health

When in the aftermath of the telegraph and radio, humans viewed the globe as "a single large village" (McLuhan, 1964), they would have never been able to even imagine the unprecedented consequences of a rapidly integrating world as a result of globalization[1] in the latter part of the 20th century and onwards. Population mobility and migration as integral parts of globalization are some of its most visible and significant dimensions. Crossborder migrants searching for employment in more affluent economies with less stringent immigration policies or internal migrants moving to different parts of a country following the relocation of a transnational manufacturing corporation in pursuit of cheaper labor illustrate the intertwined links between globalization and migration.

Over the course of human history, myths and legends of our ancestors were based on nomadic heroes such as Gilgamesh, Hercules, and Ulysses, as well as on great traveler-lecturers like Herodotus and the Arabian Ibn Battutah. In more recent history, diverse types of population mobility in the forms of exploration and survival, pilgrimage, warfare and exploitation, innate curiosity, colonization, as well as emigration and immigration have dramatically shifted following the dramatic events of two world wars, decolonization, ethnic cleansing and expulsion, collapse of the USSR, catastrophic natural disasters, and globalization (Huynen, Martens, & Hilderink, 2005; Lee, 2003). As we live in the early 21st century, we experience a world with constant movement characterized by skyrocketing flows of refugees, asylum seekers, economic immigrants, business travelers, armies, mass tourists, transport personnel, and seamen, among others. Such movement brings people from

---

[1] Globalization is defined as a process of closer interaction of human activity within economic, political, cultural, social, and other spheres and along spatial, temporal, and cognitive dimensions (Lee, 2003).

tropical, subtropical, and mostly isolated environments into close proximity and contact with the people of industrialized nations.

This global human diaspora in its diverse forms holds a plethora of socio-cultural, political, economic, and health implications for all involved. Among others, population mobility is a potent force in disease emergence and spread and its consequences extend beyond the traveler to the populations visited and the ecosystems involved (Wilson, 1995). The collateral movement of infectious disease pathogens as a result of mobile segments of human societies has had profound effects on the course of human history. Population mobility has become the bridge between epidemiologically disparate and socially and spatially isolated regions and peoples. As a result, human mobility has been linked to disease outbreaks, epidemics, and even pandemics over the course of history: from the plague pandemic of the 14th century, the syphilis outbreak of the 15th century, the measles and smallpox spread during European colonization of the Americas in the 15th century, the human influenza epidemic in the early 20th century, the global spread of HIV/AIDS from the early 1980s onward, the West Nile virus outbreak in New York in 1999, the SARS outbreak first identified in China in late 2002, to the early signs of a potential avian influenza outbreak of the early 21st century (Weitz, 2007).

## Population Mobility and Migration: An Overview

When I (first author) teach introductory demography courses, in my effort to clearly define migration and also relax my students a bit, I use the elementary but nevertheless effective example of Adam and Eve who became the world's first migrants upon leaving the Garden of Eden and explain further that, since that time, men and women have been moving around the globe, bringing disparate cultures into contact with each other. While humans have been migrating through the ages, the advent of relatively inexpensive and fast forms of ground, water, and air transportation has given migration new dimensions. Furthermore, the simultaneously occurring phenomena of rapidly declining mortality and accelerated population growth have also contributed to migration. Paradoxically, although the unprecedented migration flows of the past two decades constitute an integral part of globalization, discussions of globalization focus primarily on trade, investment, and capital flows while the movement of people is inexplicably ignored. While long-standing migratory patterns continue in new forms, new flows develop in response to economic changes, political strife, and violent conflicts. Yet, despite their diversity, there exist certain tendencies that are likely to play a major role. Foremost among these are the globalization, acceleration, differentiation, feminization, and growing politicization of migration (Castles & Miller, 2003).

Within this context, migration[2] can be seen as the process of any permanent or semi-permanent change of residence involving "detachment from the organization of activities at one place and the movement of the total round of social activities to another" (Goldscheider, 1971). Thus the most important aspect of migration is spatial by definition. In its most general form, spatial movement can be understood as a transfer from one place to another, from one social or political unit to another. This concept rests upon the understanding of space as a sort of container for a socially, politically, and economically relevant construct.

For a newcomer to social demography, population mobility and migration remain a baffling puzzle and eventually bring many questions to mind. Who is the migrant? Why do people choose to migrate? Why are there so many migrants out of such few places? Where do people migrate to? What are those forces that sustain migration? While concrete answers to several of these questions are not always possible (nor within the scope of this essay), and despite the rapid evolution of crossborder migration and population mobility, there are some concepts that many agree upon. For example, we all agree in the differentiation between forced and voluntary, temporary and permanent movements, and legal and illegal/irregular migration. These distinctions all fall under this umbrella term we include oftentimes as diverse terms and categories of migrants such as displaced persons, refugees, asylum seekers, migrant laborers, immigrants, tourists, student travelers, business travelers, military personnel, smuggled and trafficked persons, temporary visitors, pilgrims, transport personnel, and long-term temporary residents abroad (expatriates, missionaries, humanitarian workers).

In the early 21st century, the numbers of people on the move looked impressive. There were about 191 million international migrants in 2005 while over 105 million people worked legally or illegally in other countries (UN, 2006), further, there were 130 million migrant workers and 10 to 15 million undocumented migrants (ILO, 2000). The annual total of refugees reached 20.8 million in 2005 (UNHCR, 2006) and nearly four million victims of international trafficking were recorded annually (USAID, 2004). International tourist flows reached 806 million in 2006, and are expected to exceed 1.6 billion by 2020 (WTO, 2006). If this "nation of migrants and travelers" was merged into a single country, it would be the world's 10th largest nation-state (Faist, 2000).

At least half of those who migrate move from one developing country to another but not to developed countries (Faist, 2000). South-South migration flows are numerically more significant that South-North streams, and this is

---

[2] While there are conceptual distinctions between migration and immigration, we use the term migration somewhat loosely to refer to international migration, generally the emphasis of most essays in this volume. Further, we use the terms migration, travel, and mobility interchangeably.

even true for refugee flows, albeit for somewhat different reasons with about 96% of the world's refugees remaining in developing countries. In 1996, over half of the world's refugees and asylum seekers lived in the Middle East and South Asia—Palestinians and Afghanis constitute over 40% of the world's refuges and asylum seekers—while the top five countries from which they came (adding Iraq, Liberia, and Bosnia-Herzegovina to the aforementioned) accounted for over 60% of the total (Faist, 2000). It is also noteworthy to mention the direction of migration: six of the world's wealthiest countries—France, Germany, Italy, Japan, UK, and USA—receive about one third of the world's migrants (Faist, 2000).

A plethora of scholarship and theories and models have conceptualized and attempted to delineate the "nuts-and-bolts" of migration. In the premodern world, migration rates were comparatively very low just as birth and death rates were generally very high. The demographic transition has contributed significantly to the unleashing of migration activity, and it is reasonable to assert that a migration transition has occurred in concert with fertility and mortality transitions (Weeks, 2002). Within this context, the push-pull theory (Ravenstein, 1889) from the end of the 19th century was the pioneering effort to analyze migration, using data from the census of England. Since then, a series of major theories have offered to explain international migration, such as the neoclassical economic approach, the new household economics of migration, the dual labor market theory, world-systems theory, network theory, institutional theory, and theory of cumulative causation (Hirschman, Kasinitz, & De Wind, 1999; Massey, Arango, Hugo, Kouaouci, Pellegrino, & Taylor, 1993, 1994). A comprehensive review of this literature reveals the absence of a unifying universal theoretical approach to the study of migration. While macro and micro perspectives and levels of analysis provide answers to some of the fundamental questions, a comprehensive meso link is urgently needed to deal with the question of migration dynamics (Faist, 2000).

## Population Movement and Disease Risks

While through the ages only a handful of infectious (or communicable) diseases have afflicted mankind such as influenza or the plague, in the contemporary world, a total of only six diseases—diarrhoeal diseases, HIV/AIDS, malaria, tuberculosis (TB), respiratory infections, and measles—constitute the cause of over 90% of infectious-disease related deaths (WHO, 2005). Although according to the epidemiological transition school of thought, infectious diseases were believed to be retreating, we see that not only are they making a deadly comeback but also new, killer diseases are emerging (WHO, 2005).

Most infectious diseases are preventable but their aetiology oftentimes lies outside the control of the health sector. Top among their key determining factors are: urbanization, bad housing, and poor environment; smoke from wood and other fuels; global warming; deforestation; agricultural development;

dams and irrigation schemes; poverty, malnutrition, and immunosuppression; and transportation, travel, migration, and population displacement (Olshansky, Carnes, Rogers, & Smith, 1997). Communicable diseases spread most quickly in conditions of poverty, powerlessness, and social instability. For a series of interrelated reasons—oftentimes difficult to articulate, define, and ultimately measure—demographers appear to have a greater understanding for the fertility and mortality aspects of population than they have for migration, which represents one third of the components of population change.

Even chronic diseases once thought to be unrelated to infectious diseases are now known to be the result of chronic infections. Cervical cancer, one of the most common cancers among women in the developing world, is now known to be associated with human papillomavirus infection. Both chronic and infectious HBV and HCV can cause liver cancer, and it is estimated that over 6% of the world's population is at risk, while bladder cancer can result from chronic infection with schistosomiasis. The distribution of the (aforementioned six) most lethal infections of our time is unevenly concentrated around the globe with the developing regions paying the heaviest toll (e.g., nearly 80% of people infected worldwide with HIV live in Sub-Saharan Africa). Of the global burden of disease in disability-adjusted life years (in 1999), communicable diseases account for 48.2% of all recorded cases (WHO, 2005).

As globalization poses a challenge to traditional concepts of health determinants against the contextual background of emerging and re-emerging infections, the relationship between diverse forms of population mobility in different geographies and the global spread of disease is noted by social and health scientists as well as historians (Williams, Gouws, Lurie, & Crush, 2002). Historically, transient groups of traders, sailors, laborers, refugees, sexworkers, and long-haul truckers, among others, have been recognized as a pathway for dissemination of infectious diseases (Caldwell, Caldwell, Anarfi, Ntozi, Orubuloye, Marck, Cosford, Colombo & Hollings, 1999). Trade routes between Asia and Europe brought rats carrying bubonic plague to Europe during the Middle Ages. Slave ships from West Africa to the Americas transported smallpox as well as yellow fever-carrying mosquitoes in the 16th and 17th centuries (Hays, 2000). Cholera spread from its most likely origin of India to the rest of the world through travel and trade. Epidemics of infectious disease have influenced the outcome of exploration, military expeditions, colonization, and industrial development.

Today trade routes encompass the entire globe and automobiles, cargo ships, and airplanes are much more effective transport vectors than the slow-moving caravans and sailing ships of the past. Living and non-living agents and materials capable of carrying infectious agents are inadvertently transported across vast distances in a mere matter of hours. For example, tons of fresh seafood cross international borders daily and rapidly end up on kitchen countertops, in refrigerators, in ovens, and eventually in the bodies of humans living thousands of miles away from the fishing boats, docks, and seas, rivers, lakes, or fish farms where fish are caught.

Livelihood and survival mobility are oftentimes outcomes of uneven socio-economic development[3]. The epidemiologically most critical types of migration in developing regions, which are predominantly poverty-driven—labor migration, forced migration, and survival sexwork—place men and women in particularly high-risk situations. Migrating populations are oftentimes faced with further poverty, discrimination and exploitation, alienation and a sense of anonymity, limited access to social and health services, separation from families and partners, and separation from the sociocultural norms that guide behavior in stable communities. Many of the underlying factors sustaining mobility, such as an unbalanced distribution of resources, unemployment, socioeconomic instability, and political unrest, are also determinants of the increased risk of migrants and their families to infectious diseases.

## Organization and Themes of the Book

Although the connections between population mobility and disease are well documented, the social and behavioral mechanisms underlying this relationship remain poorly understood. There exists an inexplicable lacuna in contemporary interdisciplinary scholarship in the delineation of those contexts in which mobile populations are not only more vulnerable to disease but they can also exacerbate its spread. The international literature is rich with journal articles as well as research and policy reports bringing together prevalent issues of population, migration, and associated risks for acquisition and dissemination of infectious diseases. There exist three relevant books that make invaluable scholarly and applied contributions—*Crossing Borders: Migration, Ethnicity and AIDS* (Haour-Knipe & Rector, 1996), *Sexual Cultures and Migration in the Era of AIDS* (Herdt, 1997), and *Migration Medicine and Health* (Gushulak & MacPherson, 2006)—but with very specific scope, focus, and perspective. While all discuss the magnitude of the relationship between migration and disease, there remains a gap in efforts to provide a comprehensive umbrella to explain human migration and public health. This is what the present volume attempts to do.

For this volume, high-caliber scholars with anthropological, demographic, economic, epidemiological, geographical, historical, legal, mathematical, political, psychological, and sociological backgrounds were commissioned to author chapters on issues that cross disciplines and audiences. As a result, the book is organized along six broad but interdependent thematic units.

---

[3] In this essay, development goes beyond traditional, purely economic concepts; among others, key themes include economy and poverty, institutions and infrastructure, health and disease, the environment, demography, and issues regarding women and children.

The Prologue includes only Chapter 1 and delves in the broad topics under investigation—the nexus of human mobility and disease—and points to the central demographic and epidemiological themes of the book. Part I includes three chapters that address central themes pertaining to migration, health, and disease. In Chapter 2, Wilson discusses the role of human migration in shaping infectious disease distribution and patterns. She explains that humans not only carry their own collection of microbial flora but also cause the movement of other species and biological material through extensive travel and trading networks and by entering new areas and affecting environmental change with the potential to trigger new microbial threats. Wilson also touches upon social, economic, political, climatic, technological, and environmental patterns that influence microbial threats to health and their consequences. Further, she explains that infectious diseases are global in their distribution with broad ramifications involving numerous species and populations. In her conclusions, Wilson writes that the global community should identify high-risk populations and situations and improve surveillance, laboratory support and communication networks, and should work to reduce the burden of infectious diseases as well as the vulnerability to the spread of new microbial threats by beginning with basic interventions. In Chapter 3, Ioannidi-Kapolou highlights factors that contribute to migrants' poor health and limited access to health care, which in turn become barriers for their integration into the host country. Social isolation and marginalization result from the formation of distinct ethnic minorities in countries due to increasing ethnic heterogeneity. The author touches upon issues that exacerbate inequalities affecting migrant and refugee populations such as race/ethnicity, poverty, illiteracy, gender, and class—which in turn leave migrants (women in particular) vulnerable to health risks. Ioannidi-Kapolou places particular emphasis on female migrants and contends that migrant women are "triply disadvantaged" by race/ethnicity, status as a non-national, and gender inequalities and as a result, encounter higher health risks including STIs/HIV due to their vulnerability to sexual abuse and rape. The author also suggests that migration itself places women at greater risk because they may have to practice survival sex or to establish sexual partnerships in transit or at destination countries for protection or resources, or because they are trafficked into the sex sector. The author concludes by calling for greater sensitivity on the part of public-health practitioners, policy makers, educators, and researchers to the challenges that migrants and refugees experience, which are rooted in the interrelated issues of racism, xenophobia, social exclusion, poverty, and health risks. In Chapter 4, Soskolne contends that HIV/STI prevalences among migrants are shaped by interactions between the pathogen, individual behaviors, and the prevention efforts that are developed to limit impacts. She highlights the importance of social environment to migrants' adjustment and integration as well as in determining health outcomes. She adds that the value orientation and belief systems that shape behavioral patterns (including those concerning health) founded on one's social environments can break down when humans leave their own social networks. According to Soskolne, migration should be viewed as an ongoing social process spanning space and time in which networks are developed between places of origin and destination as the microstructures are at its core. Such networks provide migration information, support and assistance at the destination country, and especially shape health behaviors. To this end, Soskolne reviews a series of theoretical and empirical perspectives to delineate the role of social networks, support, and capital in HIV/AIDS among migrants, and presents a conceptual framework of pathways that link migration, social networks, and HIV risk. This framework—anchored in epidemiological models that view emerging infectious diseases as resulting from changes in the equilibrium between agent (HIV), host (the individual), and environment—considers social networks as a central link between migration and other structural, community and individual factors, and HIV infection. The chapter stresses the importance of understanding network structures at both population and individual levels in order to characterize migrant populations, to understand disease transmission, to identify risk factors and individual risk, and to target prevention strategies effectively.

In Part II the focus turns toward labor-induced population mobility and the ways it affects health and disease diffusion. In Chapter 5, Lurie brings to the fore the importance of superstructural, structural, and environmental determinants of labor migration in migrants' elevated health susceptibility. Superstructural forces, as macrosocial, economic, and political in nature, shape the distribution of resources and opportunities. Labor migration emerges from and creates systems of economic inequality, political oppression, marginalization, and social fragmentation, all of which can render migrants at greater risk for sexual coercion, unhealthy working and living conditions, and exploitation and violence. Structural factors enforce and perpetuate systems of inequality and oppression. In fact, few governments have instituted policies protecting the legal rights of migrants and providing them with health education and services and in places where government policies formally protect the health rights of migrants, such policies are often inadequate or may not be properly implemented. Finally, the environmental conditions in which migrant laborers move, work, and live are shaped by systems of social and economic inequality and lack of legal protection precipitate overall unhealthy conditions. Migrants are subject to poor working conditions and are vulnerable to sexual exploitation, coercion, and violence from employers, host communities, and other migrants. Within this framework, Lurie presents two case studies to explore the complex association between migrant labor and health vulnerability. The first study focuses on the relationship between migration and TB in Norway and the second on the role of labor migration in the spread of HIV/AIDS in South Africa. Finally, Lurie underlines the critical importance of regional and national interventions that include the proper assessment of the health impacts of migration and greater understanding of the mechanisms behind the spread of disease through migration. In Chapter 6, Kingma and Yeager examine how and whether military personnel are vulnerable to STIs/HIV. Overall, deployed military personnel find themselves in biological environments hostile to their immune systems, in adverse physical conditions of weather, climate, and human nutrition, and in disrupted social settings that serve as ideal breeding grounds for infectious bacteria, viruses, and parasitic organisms. Within this context, the authors examine policy and operational issues that impact the health of military personnel. Policy issues include the military workplace, which imposes heightened vulnerability to HIV infection via a transmission dynamic similar to that seen in long-distance transport workers and migrants employed in the mining sector with military installations that attract sexworkers. Command and control structures, while they include a well-developed span of control and chain of command hierarchies capable of influencing a wide range of behaviors, are difficult to affect sexual behaviors particularly during off-duty periods. The authors suggest potential adverse and accelerated impacts of military training and service on the immune system, in relation to either the susceptibility to or progression of HIV infection. Deployment and combat in HIV-endemic areas may be associated with HIV infection risks, although supported by limited empirical evidence. During complex humanitarian emergencies and peacekeeping operations, infectious diseases can thrive almost unchallenged in the emergencies created and sustained by socioeconomic and political disintegration, communal strife, and armed conflict. HIV risks are extremely important factors to consider when peacekeeping forces are sent in to sustain the peace between contending parties and to help restore public order. Troops can bring the virus home with them and they can transmit it to comrades-in-arms and civilians in the field. The authors offer a number of preventive strategies ranging from education, condom promotion and provision, STI/HIV testing and counseling to treatment, care and support. In Chapter 7, Timoshkina, Lombardo, and McDonald address the links of mobile sexwork and associated STI/HIV risks. The authors discuss the extent of trafficking and mobile sexwork and highlight data on STI/HIV prevalence rates among sexworkers and continue with a discussion on responses to STI/HIV among sexworkers that have been undertaken thus far, and what others are required. The chapter provides an overview of the changing nature of trafficking and mobile sexwork, while it elaborates on the ways mobile sexworkers are impacted by STIs/HIV. Links between growing mobility patterns and STI/HIV prevalence rates increase vulnerability of mobile sexworkers to health problems. The authors conclude with a call for urgent interventions specifically aimed at mobile sexworkers to protect not only sexworkers themselves but to help stem STI/HIV transmission to their sex contacts. Recommendations for preventive measures include confidential, culturally sensitive, and non-judgmental programs and services to address the unique needs of mobile sexworkers in STI/HIV prevention, distribution of condoms and safe sex information materials in relevant languages, substance abuse treatment and harm-reduction programs for IDU sexworkers, and general health services with an emphasis on outreach in all workplaces of migrant sexworkers. In Chapter 8, Apostolopoulos and

Sönmez place the transport sector firmly within the discourse of epidemiology, demography, sociology, and anthropology and critically review its far-reaching role in the acquisition and diffusion of communicable diseases. The primary emphasis of their review is on STIs and BBIs, including HIV, while a secondary emphasis is placed on TB, SARS, avian influenza, and malaria. The authors provide an overview of all transport modes with a particular emphasis on the role of trucking and maritime sectors in developing regions as well as of trucking in North America. This combined movement of humans and goods and services among different geographic points has an ultimate impact on the juxtaposition of various species of disparate ecosystems, which often accelerates and even facilitates disease movement from one area to another.

Part III includes two chapters that examine diverse dimensions and the ramifications of forced migration. In Chapter 9, Burkle addresses ways in which increasing global conflict, war, refugee influxes, population migration, and the political and developmental inequities of these factors influence risk to infectious diseases. He suggests that many parallel factors occur globally, which may adversely affect the capacity of public health systems to respond and protect the populations they serve. Burkle goes on to provide examples of political violence, civil war, ethnic and religious strife, and in particular, the generation of millions of refugees by forced migration—which alter the natural balance between human beings and microorganisms. Burkle argues that public health can no longer be narrowly confined to aspects of preventive healthcare but that it is increasingly understood in the context of multidisciplinary and multisectoral capacities of governance and political will, economics, judiciary, public safety, quality of public-health utilities, health security, agriculture, communication, transportation, education and training, and other capacities that allow states to functionally protect their citizens. The author further suggests that current wars, internal conflict, refugees, migration, and the consequential apprehension over the spread of infectious diseases have become a catalyst to what might be feared as the prelude to a downward trend or eventual worldwide collapse of public health as we know it. The author reminds us of those lessons that should be learned from the SARS epidemic, which must serve as the sentinel alarm for a stronger WHO with clear guidelines for improved local, national, and regional capacity to deal with disease investigation and control, particularly for migrant populations and nation-states regardless of peace, war, or conflict. In Chapter 10, Mayer examines the human ecology of disease and how the environment affects human health through examples of natural disasters and global climate change. Mayer suggests that behavior, culture, population, environment, and biology interact in a "web of causation." For example, to understand the aetiology of malaria occurrence in a particular place at a particular time, one must not only understand the vector biology, but also the distribution of population, anopheline habitats, and human behaviors that bring people into contact with the vector. Further, behaviors and the cultural underpinnings that underlie peoples' daily travel patterns, which dictate movement that makes populations susceptible to anopheline feeding behavior, must be understood as well as political decisions that impact population behaviors. Mayer refers to the recent example of Hurricane Katrina and its implications for local and regional health conditions and notes the significance of disaster epidemiology in understanding health effects of natural disasters. With population displacement, migration may occur over long or short distances and result in large numbers of people concentrated in refugee camps, which in turn creates appropriate ecological conditions for disease transmission. The chapter continues with a discussion of the potential effects of climate change and sea-level rise on populations and touches upon some climate change scenarios that predict more significant increases in sea-level in the future—which are likely to create environmental refugees—particularly in countries below or close to sea level in developing regions. The author points out that although health effects of natural disasters are significant, health effects of planned displacement in anticipation of a "natural" event with decades of warning and planned mitigation, as well as individual psychological and collective adaptive responses are unpredictable. The author concludes by attributing resulting public-health effects from both natural hazards and global climate change to human activities themselves. More specifically, the political ecology of global climate change is related to the human modification of the earth, which indirectly causes increases in vectorborne disease in addition to sea-level rise.

Part IV includes two chapters and examines the paradox of how leisure (pleasure) travel might render human populations vulnerable to disease risks. In Chapter 11, Wickens and Sönmez present young travelers' health risk behaviors through a critical review of literature followed by examples from authors' own research studies. According to the WTO, young people (16-24 years-old) comprise the fastest growing segment of travelers, and according to CDC, 96% of all STIs occur between the ages of 15-29. Furthermore, the fastest growth rate in cases of HIV infection is found among young people traveling and on holiday. Cross-cultural research indicates that young tourists from Western countries travel farther from home than ever before, they prefer sun-and-beach holidays, and frequently include casual sex in their travel experiences. Research is presented in the chapter that suggests that hedonistic holidays are designed to stress the availability of alcohol and sex and are instrumental in influencing travelers' decisions in the selection of 'sun-and-fun' destinations. A number of studies corroborate themes of casual sex, alcohol bingeing, and how touristic spaces (e.g., beach resorts) provide young people with the ideal conditions for suspending social codes of behavior. In a study of American organized youth-travelers in Florida, significant numbers expressed intentions to get drunk, experiment sexually, and have sex with someone they met on vacation and upon returning home, about a third reported engaging in casual sex, while a majority reported irregular condom use. In another study of British travelers to Northern Greece, young tourists expressed getting a suntan, having sex, and getting drunk as common motives, strengthened by expectations of anonymity and relative freedom from social constraints. The authors conclude that young tourists not only represent a significant risk group in terms of sexual health, but must be targeted by effective preventive strategies to positively impact their sexual choices and behaviors and to control the spread of STIs/HIV, stressing the need for an increased focus on situational and social contexts. In Chapter 12, Sönmez, Wickens, and Apostolopoulos examine sex tourism, discuss types of locations where sex tourism flourishes, and provide case studies of sex tourism destinations where STIs/HIV have become particularly problematic. Sexual interactions that carry STI/HIV risks occur between travellers and locals or other travellers; however, "sex tourism" in particular is an important vector for STI/HIV transmission and has potentially explosive ramifications for public health. By virtue of their behavioral interactions with a "core group" of efficient transmitters of STIs/HIV (sexworkers) and sex partners back in their home environments, sex tourists are particularly vulnerable for both acquiring and transmitting STIs/HIV. Consequently, sex tourists themselves become an STI/HIV core group, along with sexworkers and similar to seafarers and truckers (discussed in chapter 8). The authors discuss the growth of international tourism and present links between tourism and issues of human trafficking for purposes of sexual exploitation, *femmigration*, and child prostitution. Simultaneous globalization of tourism as leisure migration and sexual exploitation (via trafficking, sex sector, survival sex, and child prostitution) converge to fuel the growth of sex tourism. The chapter examines the sex tourist typology, the wide and free marketing of sex tourism, and also the locations where the activity is most prevalent. Further, factors that fuel the growth of child sex tourism are presented as well as international efforts to curb the activity. The health costs of sexual exploitation are presented within the context of leisure migration. Critical public health issues (e.g., global STI/HIV/AIDS rates) are linked to the relationship of transactional sex between those involved in the commercial sex industry and sex tourists. The authors conclude by presenting intervention strategies that include international efforts to combat problems of trafficking and sexual exploitation of vulnerable populations, the eradication of child sex tourism, the recognition of the abusive circumstances in which sexworkers live and work, a more concentrated focus on structural issues that cause poverty and that facilitate and support the sex sector, and the examination of the health effects of sexwork in terms of both sexworkers and clients.

The Epilogue points toward new directions in migration medicine and health. In Chapter 13, Mwambi and Zuma discuss the importance and process of examining mobility patterns and their distribution to explain the spread of existing, emerging, or re-emerging diseases via mathematical and statistical modeling and mapping. The SIR model is presented as the basic epidemic model upon which further extensions and modifications can be implemented to capture more complex disease processes. HIV/AIDS risks of migrant workers are discussed with an example from a study conducted on the effects of migration in the HIV transmission dynamics to which a mathematical model is applied in order to estimate the relative risk of infection for migrant and non-migrant men and women from their spouse and from extramarital partners. Fitting the model to the data shows that both men and women are more likely to be infected from outside the relationship than to be infected by their spouse, whether or not the man is a migrant. Disease mapping is discussed in the context of GIS and mapping/clustering technology, which improves decision-making processes in disease surveillance and control activities. GIS is used to visualize spatial patterns in the geographical distribution of disease, usually for explorative and descriptive purposes, as well as to provide information for further studies. Three case studies are presented to illustrate the use of GIS techniques in disease mapping and control among migrants. The chapter stresses the need to develop statistical methods to enable the estimation of key parameters of a disease process and to be able to evaluate the significance of some key factors that drive epidemics such as HIV. In Chapter 14 Loue discusses international legal measures to curtail globalization of disease, particularly in light of the speed and ease with which disease can spread as a result of the increased mobility of individuals for trade, tourism, and other forms of migration. The international community has made efforts to address the risk of contagion that may be associated with migration between nations. The WHO was created under the UN system as one of the first specialized agencies to develop international rules relating to the control of infectious disease. Through a series of actions, the IHR were adopted to "ensure the maximum security against the international spread of diseases." Efforts to achieve this objective have led to the establishment of a global surveillance system for various infectious diseases, requirements for health-related capabilities at ports and airports, and have set forth provisions related to a number of diseases such as the use of isolation of suspected disease carriers at border entries. The author explains that although earlier measures to control disease transmission have decreased in favor of epidemiological surveillance and improvement of basic health services, IHR measures appear to have little effect on the global control of infectious disease. Despite increased emphasis on surveillance to curtail disease globalization, many countries have adopted exclusionary provisions that deny individuals the ability to legally cross through and into their borders. Loue discusses disagreement among commentators regarding the legality of these measures under international law and the possible violation of human rights. The chapter covers issues of international protections and restrictions related to immigrants and health as well as refugees and their access to care. In conclusion, the author advises greater cooperation across countries to prevent crossborder disease transmission. In the concluding Chapter 15, Gushulak and MacPherson examine emerging and re-emerging diseases and public-health interventions in the context of migration. Public-health interventions follow a recurrent pattern of stimulus and response, which is the result of two main factors that influence the perception of threat and the subsequent conversion to a measurable and managed risk. Two major factors that link migration and disease threat and risk are: uncertainty due to limited knowledge, experience, and understanding of the disease and real and perceived disease outcomes such as loss of livelihoods, population displacements, security considerations, economic impacts, and death. The chapter examines more closely, the roles of disease uncertainty and outcome in developing response strategies and the current nature of mobility and interventions designed to control international disease. The discussion of migration health is broken down into "five Ps" of population mobility, prevalence gaps, process, population health, and perceptions of risk, and furthered by an examination of how the five components converge. The authors continue with a discussion of the challenges and consequences of migrant health that result from globalization and state simply that population mobility globalizes disease risk. The authors point out that in the case of HIV/AIDS, in spite of significant concern and rhetoric, actual interventions have neither affected the globalization of the disease nor significantly affected global migration. Gushulak and MacPherson suggest that as mobility continues to bridge regions with different disease prevalences, public-health endeavors or plans to mitigate or manage the risks of emerging diseases must factor in the role of population mobility. The authors conclude with a discussion of necessary health interventions, implications of public-health problems on health systems, and needed international cooperation and suggest that for future health interventions and policy development, efforts need to be multi-dimensional and resources more focused at migrant source areas than simply at new arrivals (upon their arrival).

## Postscript

As a multitude of factors affect the patterns and distribution of disease, the connectedness and movement of populations undoubtedly facilitates the emergence of infectious diseases and shapes the frequency, patterns, and distribution of global infectious diseases. As population mobility and the evolution of microbes continue, so will new infections continue to emerge, and known infections to change in distribution, severity and frequency. Population migration will continue to be a potent factor in disease emergence. The combination of human mobility at unprecedented levels and profound changes in the physical environment can lead to unprecedented disease spread via multiple channels. In many instances, the use of containment or quarantine is not feasible. Research and surveillance can map the global movement and evolution of microbes and guide interventions. Interdisciplinary integration of knowledge and skills from the social, biological, and physical sciences remains an imperative need, while the focus should be system analysis and the ecosystem instead of a disease, microbe, or host.

## *References*

Caldwell, J.C., Caldwell, P., Anarfi, J.K., Ntozi, J., Orubuloye, I.O., Marck, J., Cosford, W., Colombo, R., & Hollings, E. (Eds.) (1999). *Resistances to Behavioral*

*Change to Reduce HIV/AIDS Infection in Predominantly Heterosexual Epidemics in Third World Countries.* Canberra: Australian National University.

Castles, S. & Miller, M.J. (2003). *The Age of Migration.* New York, NY: Guilford Press.

Collin, J. & Lee, K. (2002). *Globalization and Public Health.* London School of Hygiene and Tropical Medicine: Unpublished Report.

Collins, J. & Rau, B. (2000). *AIDS in the Context of Development.* UNAIDS.

Faist, T. (2000). *The Volume and Dynamics of International Migration and Transnational Social Spaces.* New York, NY: Oxford.

Goldscheider, C. (1971). *Population, Modernization, and Social Structure.* Boston, MA: Little, Brown.

Hays, J.N. (2000). *The Burdens of Disease.* New Brunswick, NJ: Rutgers University Press.

Hirschman, C., Kasinitz, P., & De Wind, J. (1999). *The Handbook of International Migration: The American Experience.* New York, NY: Russell Sage Foundation.

Haour-Knipe, M. and Rector, R. (Eds.) (1996). *Crossing Borders: Migration, Ethnicity, and AIDS.* London, UK: Taylor and Francis.

Herdt, G. (Ed.) (1997). *Sexual Cultures and Migration in the Era of AIDS.* New York, NY: Oxford.

ILO (2006). *Facts of Migrant Labor.* Geneva: International Labor Organization.

Huynen, M., Martens, P., & Hilderink, H. (2005). The health impacts of globalization: A conceptual framework. *Globalization and Health*, 1, 1-14.

Lee, K. (Ed.) (2003). *Health Impacts of Globalization.* New York: Palgrave Macmillan.

Massey, D., Arango, J., Hugo, G., Kouaouci, A., Pellegrino, A., & Taylor, J.E. (1993). Theories of international migration: A review and appraisal. *Population and Development Review*, 19(3), 431-466.

Massey, D., Arango, J., Hugo, G., Kouaouci, A., Pellegrino, A., & Taylor, J.E. (1994). An evaluation of international migration theory: The North American case. *Population and Development Review*, 20(4), 669-751.

McLuhan, M. (1964). *Understanding Media: The Extensions of Man.* New York, NY: Signet.

Olshansky, S.J., Carnes, B., Rogers, R.G., & Smith, L. (1997). *Infectious Diseases—New and Ancient Threats to World Health.* Washington, D.C.: Population Reference Bureau.

Ravenstein, E. (1889). The laws of migration. *Journal of the Royal Statistical Society*, 52, 241-301.

UN (2006). *International Migration.* New York, NY: United Nations.

UNDP (2004). Development, spatial mobility, and HIV/AIDS.

UNHCR (2006). *State of the World's Refugees.* New York, NY: United Nations High Commissioner for Refugees.

USAID (2004). *Trafficking in Persons: USAID's Response.* Washington, D.C.: United States Agency of International Development.

WHO (2005). *Infectious Diseases.* Geneva: World Health Organization.

Weeks, J.R. (2002). *Population.* New York, NY: Wadsworth.

Weitz, R. (2007). *The Sociology of Health, Illness, and Health Care.* New York: Wadsworth.

Williams, B., Gouws, E., Lurie, M., & Crush, J. (2002). *Spaces of Vulnerability: Migration and HIV/AIDS in South Africa.* Kingston: Queen's University.

Wilson, M. (1995). Travel and the emergence of infectious diseases. *Emerging Infectious Diseases*, 1, 39-46.

World Tourism Organization (2006). *Tourism Highlights 2006 Edition.* Madrid Spain: World Tourism Organization. www.world-tourism.org

# Part I
## Key Themes Pertinent to Migration, Health, and Disease

# Chapter 2

## Population Mobility and the Geography of Microbial Threats

MARY E. WILSON, M.D., F.A.C.P.

## Introduction

Migration of humans shapes the distribution and patterns of infectious diseases globally (Wilson, 1995a). This has been true throughout recorded history (Berlinguer, 1992; Bruce-Chwatt, 1968; Crosby, 1989; Winkelstein, 1995). Today human travel is unprecedented in volume, reach, and speed. This massive and rapid movement is occurring in the context of global changes that favor the appearance of previously unrecognized microbial threats and a change in the distribution and burden from well known infectious diseases (Smolinski, Hamburg, & Lederberg, 2003; Wilson, Levins, & Spielman, 1994). Humans, in addition to carrying their own assemblage of microbial flora, orchestrate the movement of other species and biological material through extensive global travel and trading networks (Wilson, 2003). Humans also explore and enter new areas and change the environment in ways that place them at risk for new microbial threats (Wilson, 2000). Infectious diseases also threaten plants and animals; infections in other species have economic consequences and have direct and indirect impacts on human health and well being (Wilson, 1995b). Animals increasingly are recognized as a source of many newly recognized infectious diseases in humans. Social, economic, political, climatic, technologic, and environmental patterns influence microbial threats to health as well as their consequences and the responses to them. This chapter will review these themes and the central role of human migration in the dynamic geography of infectious diseases and context in which this is occurring (see Table 2.1).

## Migration

### Numbers and Reasons

The movement of the human population today is unprecedented in volume, reach, and speed. Data collected by the World Tourism Organization (WTO) (2006) showed that over 800 million people traveled internationally in 2005 and

TABLE 2.1. Key Concepts: Migration and microbial threats
- Human migration shapes the distribution and patterns of infectious diseases.
- Human travel today is unprecedented in volume, reach, and speed.
- The impact of migration is on the individual, on places, and on populations; consequences occur during and may persist long after travel.
- The impact of migration must be considered in the current global context of population size, density, location, vulnerability, and inequalities.
- Infectious diseases in humans, plants, and animals are dynamic; the current global milieu favors the continued changes in microbial threats.
- Animals are a source of many recently identified microbial threats.
- Human activities are potent factors driving changes in microbial threats.
- Social, economic, political, climatic, technologic, and environmental patterns influence disease emergence as well as responses and consequences.
- Addressing changing microbial threats requires a systems approach and participation from a broad range of disciplines.

of these, 45% of inbound tourists arrived by air. Although leisure, recreation, and holidays accounted for more than 50% of global travel in 2005, about 16% of global international travel was for business and professional reasons. In the 1990s, more than 5,000 airports had regularly scheduled international flights, linking urban and periurban areas throughout the world. Destinations are shifting, with increasing numbers of travelers visiting Asia and developing countries in Africa. Through adventure travel organizations using current technology (including small planes, helicopters, boats, etc.), more travelers are reaching remote areas. In the U.S., more than 44 million flights take place annually through 19,500 U.S. airports (Fischetti, 2004). More than 5,000 airplanes are simultaneously airborne at peak times. The projected number of air travelers in the U.S. in 2003 was 641 million with 117 million being international travelers.

Counting tourists captures only a fraction of mobile populations. Troops are regularly mobilized for military, humanitarian, and other support services; populations are displaced because of political, economic, ethnic reasons, or environmental changes, or catastrophic events, such as floods, hurricanes, volcanoes, earthquakes, and tsunamis. Refugees and displaced persons may live in crowded temporary facilities, often with limited access to clean water and food and sanitary facilities (Toole, 1994). Poor housing may allow exposure to mosquitoes and other disease vectors and to rodents and other animals that can be a source of infection (Connolly, Gayer, Ryan, Salama, Spiegel, & Heymann, 2004). Good medical care may be limited or absent, allowing preventable and treatable infectious diseases, such as measles and cholera, to spread in the crowded community with resulting high mortality. As of 2002, an estimated 35 million people worldwide were fleeing war or persecution, the highest number since the 1940s. In the U.S., there are 34.2 million foreign-born residents, more than half from Latin America and about a quarter from Asia (Doyle, 2005). An estimated 10.3 million of them are illegal immigrants, many of whom lack access to preventive services and medical care.

Travelers often enter environments that are riskier than their home environments. Even today tropical and developing countries are areas where travelers face the risk of diarrhea, malaria, dengue, and other tropical diseases. When a stay in a tropical area is brief and travel rapid, onset of symptoms and period of contagion for those infections that are communicable, may begin after return home, and travelers may spread infection to close contacts (Wilson, 2003). Today much can be done to reduce but not eliminate risk to travelers. In the era before vaccines and antimicrobials were available, visits to most tropical areas were substantially more dangerous. Curtin (1989), in his book, *Death by Migration,* analyzes the excess mortality in European troops stationed in various locations and quantifies what he calls "relocation costs" – comparing mortality of troops in England and France, for example, with those in various locations in Africa and Asia during the same years.

## Speed

Travel today is rapid and frequent. In 1850 a person took about a year to circumnavigate the globe. Today it is possible to reach most places on earth within 48 hours and within the incubation period of most infectious diseases. Grubler and Nakicenovic (1991) estimated the spatial mobility of the French population from 1800 to 2000 and concluded that the number of kilometers traveled daily for the average French person had increased more than 1,000-fold over the 200 year period. The rapid dispersal of Severe Acute Respiratory Syndrome (SARS) into Canada and other countries by air travelers is a recent reminder of the global interconnectedness (Peiris, Guan, & Yuen, 2004).

## Conveyances and Contact

Travel often involves multiple, sequential shared environments (e.g., bus, train, terminal, airplane, ship, underground railway) and should be seen as a loop and not just an origin and destination (Wilson, 2003). With cruise ships, the time and place of transport become the primary place of activity. Cruise ships are often massive, transporting thousands of passengers and crew in a conveyance with many shared indoor spaces. Passengers from multiple different origins travel together for a few to many days in a common environment and then disperse to multiple destinations, providing an ideal way to disseminate infections that are spread from person to person, such as influenza (Miller, Tam, Maloney, Fukuda, Cox, Hockin, Kertesz, Klimov, & Cetron, 2000) and norovirus infection. Many outbreaks have been documented on cruise ships, including rubella (CDC, 1998), Legionnaires disease (Jernigan, Hofman, Cetron, M, Genese, C, Nuorti, Pekka Fields, Benson, Carter, Edelstein, Guerro, Paul, Lipman, & Breiman, 1996) and gastrointestinal infections (Minooee & Richman, 1999). En route transmission has been documented on airplanes and trains, including potentially fatal infections such as tuberculosis (TB) (and multidrug resistant TB) (Kenyon, Valway,

Ihle, Onorato, & Castro, 1996) and SARS. On a 3-hour flight between Hong Kong and Beijing carrying 120 persons, one symptomatic passenger, who later died of SARS, spread infection to 8 of 23 persons seated in the three rows in front of him. Overall, 22 passengers on the plane became ill, 16 with laboratory-confirmed SARS, and others with illness consistent with SARS (Olsen, Chang, Cheung, Tang, Fisk, Ooi, Kuo, Jiang, Chen, Lando, Hsu, Chen, & Dowell, 2003). Transmission of influenza on a commercial aircraft has also been documented (Moser, Bender, Margolis, Noble, Kendal, & Ritter, 1979). During the loop that constitutes travel humans often have contact with a large, diverse sample of people and sometimes animals and arthropod vectors as well.

## Human as Interactive Units

Humans can be considered interactive biological units who carry an assemblage of microbial flora along with their immunological profile, shaped by previous exposures, infections, and immunizations (Wilson, 2003). The microbial community in one adult human weighs up to one kg and may include 100 trillion bacteria, the largest numbers residing in the large bowel (Nicholson, Holmes, Lindon, & Wilson, 2004). Humans not only pick up and drop off microbes during travel but interact with them immunologically influencing which strains or variants survive. Humans also carry microbial genetic material, including resistance genes (O'Brien, Pla, Mayer, Kishi, Gilleece, Syvanen, & Hopkins, 1985; Okeke & Edelman, 2001). Humans also have distinctive, individual genetic characteristics, which can make them more or less susceptible to certain infections or likely to suffer severe consequences from them. Humans may provide the vessel where microbes undergo mutation or exchange genetic material. Humans can acquire and transport potential pathogens and resistance genes in the absence of symptoms. For example, strains of *Neisseria meningitidis* W135, a cause of meningitis and sepsis, colonized the nasopharyngeal tissues of pilgrims to the Hajj in Saudi Arabia, often without causing symptoms. In some instances, after the pilgrims returned home, the bacteria spread to family members or other close contacts, leading to serious infection (Dull, Abdelwahab, & Sacchi, 2005; Hahne, Gray, Aguilera, Crowcroft, Nichols, Kaczmarski, & Ramsay, 2002; Wilder-Smith, Barkham, Earnest, & Paton, 2002). Gastrointestinal carriage of the polio virus by visitors to countries with inadequate vaccine coverage, especially if sanitation is poor, can spark new cases (Heymann & Aylward, 2004). Transmission of some human pathogens, such as hepatitis B virus and HIV, can occur in the absence of symptoms and long after the infection was acquired. TB can reactivate years after acquisition in a place far from where it was acquired.

The large number of potential contacts of a single traveler is demonstrated by a recent case of measles carried into the U.S. state of Iowa (Dayan, Orftega-Sanchez, LeBaron, Quinlisk, & the Iowa Measles Response Team, 2005). A U.S. student, unvaccinated against measles, became ill on a return trip from India, where he had been exposed to measles. His return itinerary involved connections in two busy airports. Despite a prompt diagnosis of measles and vigorous interventions, two months of containment efforts were required in Iowa at an estimated direct cost of US $142,452 to the public health infrastructure. More than 2,500 hours of personal time were expended to contact exposed passengers, set up vaccination clinics, trace over 1,000 potentially exposed contacts, among other activities.

## Other Transport

Humans, in addition to carrying their own microbiological flora, transport or facilitate the transport of other species, including live animals, animal parts, plants, seeds, arthropods (including mosquitoes and other potential vectors of infectious diseases), microbes, and microbial genetic material. The ballast water of ships can contain potential pathogens and invasive species that can contaminate waterways and change local ecology (Carlton & Geller, 1993; McCarthy & Khambaty, 1994; Ruiz, Rawlings, Dobbs, Drake, Mullady, Huq, & Colwell, 2000). Much of the fresh produce eaten in the U.S. is imported from other countries. Contamination has led to outbreaks caused by unusual pathogens, such as *Cyclospora cayetanensis* (Herwaldt, 2000), as well as more common ones. Because of mass processing and wide food distribution networks, outbreaks may involve cases in multiple different countries (Van Beneden, Keene, Strang, Werker, King, Mahonn, Hedberg, Bell, Kelly, Balan, MacKenzie, & Fleming, 1999). Today the food chain is very long and includes multiple points at which contamination or improper handling can occur.

The U.S. also imports live animals, many of them for pets. For example, in 2002, legal imports included 47,000 mammals, 379,000 birds, 2 million reptiles, 49 million amphibians, and 223 million fish (Communication from Paul Arguin, CDC). Many of them are wild caught and not screened for infection prior to shipment to the U.S. A large trade in illegal plants and animals also exists, estimated at US $3 billion per year in the U.S. In 2004 customs inspectors in Brussels seized two eagles carried in hand luggage by a Thai man on a commercial flight from Thailand via Vienna (Van Borm, Thomas, Hanquet, Lambrecht, Boschmans, Dupont, Decaestecker, Snacken, & van den Berg, 2005). Both birds were found to be infected with the influenza H5N1, the strain of avian influenza that causes high mortality in humans.

## Animals

One highly visible (and expensive) consequence of animal importations into the U.S. was a 2003 outbreak of monkeypox, an infection caused by a virus previously documented only in Africa (Guarner, Johnson, Paddock, Shieh, Goldsmith, Reynolds, Damon, Regnery, Zaki, & the Veterinary Monkeypox Virus Working Group, 2004; Reed, Melski, Graham, Regnery, Sotir, Wegner,

Kazmierczak, Stratman, Li, Fairley, Swain, Olson, Sargent, Kehl, Frace, Kline, Foldy, David, & Damon, 2004). Investigation revealed that prairie dogs (captured in the U.S. to be sold as pets) had been housed with exotic rodents imported from Ghana in Africa. The rodents had unrecognized infection with monkeypox, which spread from them to the prairie dogs, which were sold as pets and infected their human owners. The U.S. also exports animals for pets. In 2002, tularemia, an infection that can be fatal to humans, caused a die-off in wild-caught prairie dogs at a Texas animal facility (Petersen, Schriefer, Carter, Zhou, Sealy, Bawiec, Yockey, Urich, Zeidner, Svashia, Kool, Buck, Lindley, Celeda, Monteneiri, Gage, & Chu, 2004). In June and July of 2002, this facility had distributed more than 1,000 prairie dogs to be sold as pets to 10 states and seven European and Asian countries.

Animals have been the source of many of the recently appearing microbial threats (Smolinski et al., 2003). This underscores a need to have a better understanding of interspecies transmission of viruses and other pathogens (Webby, Hoffmann, & Webster, 2004). Some recently identified agents of zoonoses, in addition to monkeypox virus, include the SARS coronavirus, avian influenza, variant Creutzfeldt-Jakob, HIV, Nipah virus, West Nile virus, several newly identified hantaviruses, and *Escherichia coli* O157:H7. Travel and trade have played a pivotal role in the emergence and spread of most of these, either through movement of infected animals or their tissues or humans. Most, but not all, are viruses. Notably, multiple different modes of transmission are involved. Fortunately for humans, at present only one, HIV, has the characteristics that allow it to undergo sustained transmission from person to person, which it has done inexorably around the globe, largely via sexual transmission. There is good evidence that the AIDS pandemic originated from multiple independent introductions of simian immunodeficiency viruses from African apes and monkeys into humans and their subsequent evolution and spread (Hahn, Shaw, De Cock, & Sharp, 2000; Sharp, Bailles, Chaudhuri, Rodenburg, Santiago, & Hahn, 2001).

The threat of pandemic influenza is ever present, but the concern has been heightened recently because of the appearance of highly pathogenic avian influenza H5N1 that has caused outbreaks in avian species, initially concentrated in Southeast Asia but with recent spread via migratory birds into western China (Chen, Smith, Zhang, Qin, Wang, Li, Webster, Peiris, & Guan, 2005) and Europe. The virus has an expanded mammalian range (including cats and zoo animals, such as tigers and leopards) and has infected humans who have had close contact with avian species. To date, fewer than 200 human cases have been documented, but mortality has been high (about 50%). If the virus evolves, via mutation, recombination or reassortment, to become easily transmissible from person to person, it could cause global devastation. Recently scientists were successful in characterizing the genes of the virus causing the 1918 influenza, which was estimated to cause 40 million or more deaths globally, and found that the virus was likely derived from an avian source (Taubenberger, Reid, Lourens, Wang, Guozhong, & Fanning, 2005).

Recent studies in Africa and Asia have documented ongoing transmission of simian viruses to humans, through contact with primates as pets or with primate tissue through butchering of primates for food (Wolfe, Heneine, Carr, Garcia, Shanmugam, Tamoufe, Prosser, Torimiro, LeBreton, Mpoudi-Ngole, McCutchan, Birx, Folks, Burke, & Switzer, 2005; Wolfe, Switzer, Carr, Bhulla, Shanmugam, Tamoufe, Prosser, Torimiro, Wright, Mpoudi-Ngole, McCutchan, Birx, Folks, Burke, & Heneine, 2004). A survey in rural Cameroon found that more than 60% of local inhabitants reported contact with fresh blood or body fluids from nonhuman primates, most often through hunting and butchering chimpanzees, monkeys, or gorillas (Wolfe, Prosser, Carr, Aamoufe, Mpoudi-Ngole, Torimiro, LeBreton, McCutchan, Birs, & Burke, 2004). In Central Africa alone, the estimate for trade and local and regional consumption of wild animal meat (which includes nonhuman primates) is over 1 billion kg per year (Wilkie & Carpenter, 1999).

In general, the amount of space used by animals is strongly linked to body size; larger animals have a larger home range size (Jetz, Carbone, Fulford, & Brown, 2004). Humans are the only animal that regularly and vastly exceeds the distance that can be traveled by self locomotion. Some birds, land animals and fish migrate long distances, and occasionally animals, plants, and other material can be dispersed over long distances by being carried in water (sometimes on floating logs or debris, especially after major storms), and also via winds and dust storms. Humans stand alone as the species that has been able to inhabit or explore most areas of the earth and to change many of them.

## Arthropod Vectors

Most arthropod vectors, such as mosquitoes and ticks, can travel only limited distances, unless carried by a migrating bird or animal or assisted by humans. Mosquitoes are regularly transported by planes and boats and other conveyances of human transport and trade (Lounibos, 2002). In 1985, the mosquito, *Aedes albopictus* (Asian tiger mosquito) was introduced into North America (Texas) from Asia (Hawley, Reiter, Copeland, Pumpuni, & Craig, 1987). *Aedes* mosquito eggs are desiccation resistant and survived the trip by ship in the protected environment of used tires. The mosquito subsequently spread to at least 25 states over 12 years, its movements following interstate highways, presumably carried by human traffic and trade (Moore & Mitchell, 1997). In recent years it has been introduced into many countries in Latin America. In the past, water containers on ships provided a protected habitat for mosquitoes during travel; modern ships, especially those with container vessels, likewise have been effective in permitting the survival and introduction of mosquitoes into new areas. This is relevant to human health because *Aedes albopictus* is competent to transmit a number of viruses that are human pathogens, and it was the primary vector implicated in the dengue outbreak in Hawaii in 2001-2002 (Effler, Pang, Kitsutani, Ayers, Nakata,

Vorndam, Elm, Tom, Reiter, Rigau-Perez, Hayes, Mills, Napier, Clark, & Gubler, 2005).

Mosquitoes can survive long airplane flights. One study reported finding mosquitoes on 12 of 67 airplanes that had arrived in London from Africa. Mosquitoes, house flies, and beetles have also been shown to survive in wheel bays of airplanes on flights of 6 to 9 hours (Russell, 1987). In a quantitative risk assessment of pathways by which West Nile Virus (WNV) could reach Hawaii, investigators estimated that 7 to 70 infected mosquitoes could reach the island each year, based on number of airplane flights arriving from areas with ongoing viral circulation and the expected number of viable mosquitoes per flight. They concluded that human-transported mosquitoes and human-transported birds or other vertebrates posed the greatest risk for introduction of WNV into Hawaii (Kilpatrick, Gluzberg, Burgett, & Daszak, 2004). WNV entered the U.S. (presumably in an infected human, mosquito, or bird) in 1999 (Nash, Mostashari, Fine, Miller, O'Leary, Murray, Huant, Rosenberg, Greenberg, Sherman, Wong, & Layton, 2001) and subsequently has spread throughout the continental U.S., into Canada, Mexico, the Caribbean and Central America. Migrating birds have played an essential role in the movement of WNV in the Americas (Rappole, Derrickson, & Hubalek, 2000), a region already inhabited by several mosquito species competent to transmit it.

## Customs and Traditions

Humans also carry with them customs and traditions, including food preferences and methods of preparing foods, sexual mores, ways of dressing, and other behavioral patterns that can influence their risk of exposure to some pathogens. Activities that would not be considered risky in their home environment (e.g., swimming and wading in fresh water; receiving injections at a local clinic; sleeping in a room without screens or bednets) could potentially place them at risk for infections, such as schistosomiasis, blood-borne pathogens (e.g., hepatitis B and C, HIV), or malaria in certain locations. Immigrants and their families may prefer foods from their country of origin. In San Diego, California a review of culture-confirmed TB (1980-1997) in children under 15 years found that 34% were infected with *Mycobacterium bovis*, a type of TB that typically comes from cattle (Dankner, Waecker, Essey, Moser, Thompson, & Davis,1993) and is now rare in the U.S. Approximately 90% were of Hispanic ethnicity (but U.S. born). An important source of infection was thought to be fresh cheese made in Mexico from unpasteurized milk and brought to the U.S.A study published in 2000 found that 17% of cattle sampled at meat-processing plants in Mexico were infected with *M. bovis* (Milian, Sanchez, Toledo, Ramirez, & Santillan, 2000). In the U.S. human infection with *M. bovis* has become rare because of pasteurization of milk and disease control in cattle herds.

# Context

## Microbial World

The attributes of the microbial world must be taken into account in trying to understand microbial threats to human health. The microbial world is vast. Only a tiny fraction of microbes have been identified and characterized. Contrary to common belief, most microbes do not harm humans, and many are essential for life as we know it. Human life as it exists today would be impossible without the beneficial services performed by microbes. Microbes are abundant and also resilient, living in a broad range of habitats, and many being able to survive at extremes of heat, cold, pH, and salinity that would kill humans. They also have a short generation time, giving them capacity to undergo rapid evolution. The generation time for a staphylococcus is 20 to 30 minutes, in contrast to 20 to 30 years for humans. Microbes undergo change through mutation and other molecular maneuvers that allow them to exchange or acquire new genetic material (e.g., through recombination, conjugation, reassortment) and respond rapidly to changes in the environment. The exposure of a microbe to an antimicrobial or specific chemical represents just another change in the environment and one that microbes adapt to regularly.

## Population Factors

### Size

The movement of humans and other species is occurring in the context of other population factors that also influence microbial threats to health. These are population size, density, location, vulnerability, and inequality. The size of the human population is larger than ever in history. The size of the domestic animal population, driven by the need for animal protein and nutrition for the growing human population, is also larger than ever in history. Because of limited habitable space on the earth, more humans are living in close proximity to large animal populations. Figures in China illustrate the changes over a few decades. In 1968, at the time of the last influenza pandemic, the human population of China was 790 million, the pig population was 5.2 million, and the poultry population was 12.3 million. The numbers today are 1.3 billion people, 508 million pigs, and 13 billion poultry (Osterholm, 2005). Many people live in close association with poultry and pigs, a reason for concern given outbreaks of avian influenza H5N1. A larger population provides more hosts in which microbial replication can occur and the potential for the emergence of more transmissible or virulent forms.

As of 2004, there were an estimated 34.2 million foreign born persons in the U.S., accounting for 11.3% of the total population (Doyle, 2005). Half of the growth in the U.S. population is in the foreign born. Many foreign-born residents have close relatives living in other countries, whom they visit regularly. This group of travelers (designated as "visiting friends and relatives" or

VFRs) account for a disproportionate burden of travel-related infections, such as malaria and typhoid fever (Bacaner, Stauffer, Boulware, Walker & Keystone, 2004) in the U.S. and other developed countries (e.g., 45% of imported malaria cases in the U.S. in 2002 and 77% of imported typhoid fever cases. The countries contributing the largest number of foreign born have shifted over the last decades and now include Mexico, China, the Philippines, India, Vietnam, Cuba, and South Korea (Doyle, 2005).

Density

More people are living in urban areas than ever in history (2.9 billion in 2000 and projected to reach 5 billion by 2030), and the mass relocation of rural populations to urban areas that began in the latter half of the twentieth century continues, with cities growing at four times the rate of rural populations (UN Population Division, 2002). Most new megacities (defined as urban areas with a population of 10 million or more) are in developing countries at low latitudes. Many cities are surrounded by vast periurban slums, where access to clean water, sanitation, and health care is limited. Many of those who have migrated to urban areas have families in rural areas, so connections with rural areas persist. Today about half of people globally live in urban areas, but the urban to rural ratio varies greatly by region. In Latin America and the Caribbean about 75% of the population is urban, in contrast to Africa and Asia where only about 37% of the population lived in urban areas in 2000 (UN Population Division, 2002). Many people also live and work in large buildings with shared indoor spaces. The trend in urbanization is expected to continue. The combination of mobility, size, and density of the population means that people are having contact with large numbers of people, including some from distant countries. This is relevant given the importance of person-to-person spread in many infectious diseases. Urban populations also may share water supplies; focal contamination can lead to large outbreaks.

Location

Population growth is most rapid in low latitude areas, many of the countries characterized by tropical and subtropical climates and large low-income populations. At least 40% of urban growth is from migration. Circulation of some viruses is linked to population size, as the virus must continue to find susceptibles to survive. The maintenance of a dengue virus serotype (an infection transmitted by mosquitoes), for example, requires a population of somewhere between 150,000 and one million (Wilson, 2004). More and more urban areas in subtropical regions are reaching a critical population size that will permit sustained circulation of dengue virus and increase the risk of severe and complicated forms of dengue fever (hemorrhagic fever and dengue shock syndrome). Outbreaks of dengue fever have increased in geographic reach and severity. A contributing factor is the global movement of dengue viruses carried by human travelers. Some dengue viruses are more virulent than others as measured by the level of viremia they produce and their potential to cause hemorrhagic infection (which is more likely to be fatal). Recent studies give evidence that more virulent dengue viruses (Southeast Asian genotype) can "out compete" viruses that cause milder infection and can be expected to displace the less virulent viruses. Mosquitoes may also participate in the selection process. In general, mosquitoes are more likely to become infected with a virus that causes higher level and more sustained viremia in humans (Cologna, Armstrong, & Rico-Hesse, 2005).

Malaria continues to kill an estimated million people each year, predominantly children in Africa. Projections for the global population at risk for malaria show an increase from about 3 billion exposed in 2002 to 3.4 billion exposed in 2010 based on expected population growth in malarious areas (Hay, Guerra, Tatem, Noor, & Snow, 2004). Despite the reduction by half of the land area supporting malaria during the last century, the total population exposed to malaria risk has increased by 2 billion because of population growth in endemic areas.

Greater biodiversity is found near the equator; the number of marine and terrestrial species declines with distance from the equator, the so-called latitudinal species diversity gradient. Guernier and colleagues looked at the relationship between parasitic and infectious disease species richness and latitude and found that the number of pathogen species also increases near the equator (Guernier, Hockberg, & Guegan, 2004). They reviewed 332 human pathogens across 224 countries and found that, on average, tropical areas had more species diversity than temperate areas. Rainfall was the climatic variable most strongly correlated with species diversity. That the areas of the earth with greatest population growth and with largest poor populations are also those with greatest pathogen diversity suggests that these regions will continue to be those where infectious diseases will thrive and cause a disproportionate burden of disease.

## Vulnerability

Three areas of vulnerability that may contribute to the burden from infectious diseases are especially noteworthy and will be mentioned briefly. The continued spread of HIV/AIDS exacts a huge toll on the global population. HIV also kills through other infections, by far the most important one being TB. In some countries in East and southern Africa, rates of reported cases of TB have increased five-fold or more because of the concurrent epidemic of HIV infection (WHO, 2005). Approximately one third of the human population is infected with *Mycobacterium tuberculosis*. The interaction between HIV and TB is bidirectional, with each making the other worse.

The elderly population is growing rapidly. In many countries the most rapidly growing segment of the population is the over 80 year-old group (Kinsella & Velkoff, 2001). In 2000, less than 10% of the global population was older than 60 years (but was almost 20% in Europe). This is expected to exceed 20% by 2050 (and reach 35% in Europe). The elderly are more susceptible to infections because of waning cell-mediated immunity and impaired host defenses but also because of chronic diseases and use of drugs and treatments that may be immunosuppressive. The elderly also respond less well to immunizations.

Poor nutrition and micronutrient deficiencies increase the risk of many infections (including diarrhea, malaria, measles, and pneumonia) and death from them. A study by Ezzati and colleagues identified undernutrition as a leading global cause of loss of health (Ezzati, Lopez, Rodgers, Hoorn, Murray, & the Comparative Risk Assessment Collaborating Group, 2002). They found that globally 9.5% of the disease burden, as measured by disability adjusted life years, could be attributed to childhood and maternal underweight and 6.2% to deficiencies of iron, vitamin A, zinc or iodine.

# Technology

## Medical

Technologic changes provide many ways to improve lives but also provide the means to amplify the dispersal of microbes that occurs naturally. Injections of medication used to treat schistosomiasis in mass treatment campaigns in Egypt probably contributed to the spread of hepatitis C in the population because the needles were inadequately sterilized between reuse (Frank, Mohamed, Strickland, Lavanchy, Arthur, Magder, Khoby, Abdel-Wahab, Ohn, Anwar, & Saliam, 2000). After WNV entered the U.S., blood transfusions, dialysis, organ and tissue transplantation led to infection in patients who had not been exposed through the usual route, the bite of an infective mosquito (Pealer, Marfin, Petersen, Lanciotti, Page, Stramer, Stobierski, Signs, Newman, Kapoor, Goodman, & Chamberland, for the West Nile Virus Transmission Investigation Team, 2003). Because of good medical diagnostic laboratories, transmission of WNV through breastfeeding, a previously unproven route of transmission, was also identified as a risk. Transmission of Chagas disease (caused by a protozoan parasite that can persist for decades in the human host) in the U.S. was documented after transplantation of organs from a person who had previously lived in endemic areas in Latin America (CDC, 2002).

Antimicrobials are lifesaving for a number of infections, yet their wide use and misuse has contributed to the emergence of resistant microbes, not just for a few minor pathogens, but for major killers including parasites (e.g., malaria), viruses (e.g., HIV, influenza), bacteria (e.g., Staphylococcus aureus, Streptococcus pneumoniae, Mycobacterium tuberculosis), and even some fungi. Sometimes alternative forms of treatment exist, but they may be more toxic or more expensive or in short supply, making them operationally unavailable for many, particularly poor populations. Travel of humans has contributed to the movement of resistance genes and pathogens (Aires de Sousa, Santos Sanches, Ferro, Vaz, Saraiva, Tendeiro, Serra & de Lencastre, 1998). Resistance that develops in an individual patient can potentially affect a larger population if the infection is transmissible, such as is the case with TB, HIV, and many other infections.

## Habitats and Land Use

Humans have made profound changes in the biophysical environment by clearing lands, building dams, creating large urban areas, and building roads. Clearing lands may change the ecology for arthropod vectors (that can transmit human infections) and for reservoir and intermediate hosts, such as rodents. Humans may intrude on environments inhabited by potentially pathogenic microbes that were previously unrecognized. Roads provide paths for travel but also breach biophysical barriers and fragment habitats. They provide a path for the movement of other species, in addition to humans. Two examples show how roads may have contributed to the spread of HIV. In Africa logging roads have facilitated the trade in bushmen (Laurent, Bourgeois, Mpoudi, Butei, Peeters, Mpoudi-Ngole, & Delaporte, 2004; Nisbett & Monath, 2001). In Asia and elsewhere HIV spread along trucking routes, traveled by men away from home for long periods.

Geographic areas and populations vary in their receptivity to the introduction and establishment of new pathogens (Wilson, 2004). Infections that can be spread from person-to-person, such as TB, HIV, and influenza, can be carried by travelers to any part of the earth. Some infections require a specific arthropod vector or intermediate host, so may not be easily transplanted into a new geographic area. Many other factors may influence receptivity and spread. These include housing, sanitation, and living conditions. Good nutrition and immunity through vaccination or past infection may blunt the impact of an infection. Education and change in behavior may be able to stop the spread. Good surveillance, solid public health infrastructure, and access to care can also stem the spread and burden from infection. Stigma and concern about economic consequences have sometimes inhibited free sharing information about outbreaks (Cash & Narasimhan, 2000), a problem that persists today.

Although the continental southern U.S. had massive outbreaks of dengue fever in the past and is inhabited by competent vectors (*Ae. aegypti* and *Ae. albopictus*), few locally acquired infections have been documented in recent years. In a seroepidemiological study, investigators surveyed 622 randomly selected households in Laredo (Texas, U.S.A.) and Nuevo Laredo (Mexico), cities separated by the Rio Grande River but with similar climate and extensive cross-border traffic. They collected blood samples and assessed housing conditions. Residents of Nuevo Laredo were more likely to test positive for dengue IgM and IgG (16% and 48%, respectively) than residents of Laredo (1.3%; 23%) were. In a multivariate analysis, air conditioning was significantly associated with positive dengue serology. Dwellings without air conditioning were 2.6-fold more likely to have dengue positive occupant (Reiter, Lathrop, Bunning, Biggerstaff, Singer, Tiwari, Baber, Amador, Thirion, Hayes,

Seca, Mendez, Ramirez, Robinson, Fawlings, Vorndam, Waterman, Gubler, Clark, & Hayes, 2003). This is one of multiple ways that economic factors can influence risk of exposure to infection.

## Conclusions

The changes in infectious diseases that are occurring today are global in distribution. The impact has been broad, involving many species, populations, and disciplines. Many of the events have played out rapidly (e.g., SARS); the consequences are potentially long-lasting and may be irreversible. West Nile Virus, for example, is now clearly established in North America. Given its ecology, the virus cannot be eliminated with currently available approaches. Perhaps the best option is to protect humans through vaccination, though bird and other animal populations also are affected. The changes in infectious diseases are ongoing and can be expected to continue. The unprecedented rate of change in infectious diseases does not reflect a temporary period of instability. Given the global circumstances today, the global community should work to identify high risk populations and situations and improve surveillance, laboratory support, and communication networks. Many basic interventions, such as clean water, sanitary control of waste, good housing, good nutrition (and provision of micronutrients), handwashing, vaccinations, and education (including safe sex practices) could reduce the burden from infectious diseases and reduce the vulnerability to the spread of new microbial threats.

## References

Aires de Sousa, M., Santos Sanches, I., Ferro, M.L., Vaz, J.M., Saraiva, Z., Tendeiro, T., Serra, J., & de Lencastre, H. (1998). Intercontinental spread of a multidrug-resistant methicillin-resistant, *Staphylococcus aureus* clone. *Journal of Clinical Microbiology,* 36, 2590-2596.

Bacaner, N., Stauffer, B., Boulware, D.R., Walker, P.F., & Keystone, J.S. (2004). Travel medicine considerations for North American immigrants visiting friends and relatives. *Journal of the American Medical Association,* 291, 2856-2864.

Berlinguer, G. (1992). The interchange of disease and health between the old and new worlds. *American Journal of Public Health,* 82(10), 1407-1413.

Bruce-Chwatt, L.J. (1968). Movements of populations in relation to communicable disease in Africa. *East African Medical Journal,* 45(5), 266-275.

Carlton, J.T. & Geller, J.B. (1993). Ecological roulette: The global transport of non-indigenous marine organisms. *Science,* 261, 78-82.

Cash, R.A. & Narasimhan, V. (2000). Impediments to global surveillance of infectious diseases: consequences of open reporting in a global economy. *Bulletin of the World Health Organization,* 78, 1358-1367.

CDC (1998). Rubella among crew members of commercial cruise ships—Florida, 1997. *Morbidity Mortality Weekly Report,* 46(52), 1247-1250.

CDC (2002). Chagas disease after organ transplantation—United States, 2001. *Morbidity Mortality Weekly Report,* 51(10), 210-212.

Chen, H., Smith, G.J.D., Zhang, S. Y., Qin, K., Wang, J., Li, K.S., Webster, R.G., Peiris, J.S.M., & Guan, Y. (2005). H5N1 virus outbreak in migratory waterfowl. *Nature,* 436, 191-192.

Cologna, R., Armstrong, P.M., & Rico-Hesse, R. (2005). Selection for virulent dengue viruses occurs in humans and mosquitoes. *Journal of Virology,* 79(2), 853-859.

Crosby, A.W. Jr. (1972). *The Columbian Exchange.* Westport, CT: Greenwood Press.

Connolly, M.A., Gayer, M., Ryan, M.J., Salama, P., Spiegel, P., & Heymann, D.L. (2004). Communicable diseases in complex emergencies: impact and challenges. *Lancet,* 364, 1974-1983.

Curtin, P.D. (1989.) *Death by Migration: Europe's Encounter with the Tropical World in the Nineteenth Century.* Cambridge, UK: Cambridge University Press.

Dankner, W.M., Waecker, N.J., Essey, M.A., Moser, K., Thompson, M., & Davis, C.E. (1993). *Mycobacterium bovis* infections in San Diego: A clinicoepidemiologic study of 73 patients and a historical review of a forgotten pathogen. *Medicine,* 72, 11-37.

Dayan, G.H., Orftega-Sanchez, O., LeBaron, C.W., Quinlisk, M.P., & the Iowa Measles Response Team (2005). The cost of containing one case of measles: the economic impact on the public health infrastructure-Iowa, 2004. *Pediatrics,* 116, e1-e4.

Doyle, R. (2005). Coming to America. *Scientific American,* August, 25.

Dull, P.M., Abdelwahab, J., & Sacchi, C.T. (2005). *Neisseria meningitidis* serogroup W-135 carriage among US travelers to the 2001 Hajj. *Journal of Infectious Diseases,* 191, 33-39.

Effler, P., Pang, L., Kitsutani, P., Ayers, T., Nakata, M., Vorndam, V., Elm, J., Tom, T., Reiter, P., Rigau-Perez, J., Hayes, J.M., Mills, K., Napier, M., Clark, G., & Gubler, D. for the Hawaii Dengue Outbreak Investigation Team (2005). Dengue fever outbreak in Hawaii—2001-2. *Emerging Infectious Diseases,* 11(May), 742-749.

Ezzati, M., Lopez, A.D., Rodgers, A., Hoorn, S., Murray, C.J.L., & the Comparative Risk Assessment Collaborating Group (2002). Selected major risk factors and global and regional burden of diseases. *Lancet,* 360, 1347-1360.

Fischetti, M. (2004). Air traffic control: crowded skies. *Scientific American,* December, 106-107.

Frank, C., Mohamed, M.K., Strickland, G.T., Lavanchy, D., Arthur, R.R., Magder, L.S., Khoby, T.E., Abdel-Wahab, Y., Ohn, E.S.A., Anwar, W., & Saliam, I. (2000). The role of parenteral antischistosomal therapy in the spread of hepatitis C virus in Egypt. *Lancet,* 355(March 11), 887-891.

Grubler, A. & Nakicenovic, N. (1991). *Evolution of Transport Systems.* Laxenburg, Vienna: ILASA.

Guarner, J., Johnson, B.J., Paddock, C.D., Shieh, W-J., Goldsmith, C.S., Reynolds, M.G., Camon, I.K., Regnery, R.L., Zaki, S.R., & the Veterinary Monkeypox Virus Working Group. (2004). Monkeypox transmission and pathogenesis in prairie dogs. *Emerging Infectious Diseases,* 10, 426-431.

Guernier, V., Hockberg, M.E., & Guegan, F.-F. (2004). Ecology drives the worldwide distribution of human diseases. *Public Library of Science Biology,* 2(6), 740-746.

Hahn, B.H., Shaw, G.M., De Cock, K.M., & Sharp, P.M. (2000). AIDS as a zoonosis: scientific and public health implications. *Science,* 287, 607-614.

Hahne, S.J.M., Gray, S.J., Aguilera, J-F., Crowcroft, N., Nichols, T., Kaczmarski, E.B., & Ramsay, M.E. (2002) W135 meningococcal disease in England and Wales associated with Hajj 2000 and 2001. *Lancet, 359*, 582-583.

Hawley, W.A., Reiter, P., Copeland, R.S., Pumpuni, C.B., & Craig, G.B. Jr. (1987). *Aedes albopictus* in North America: Probable introduction in used tires from northern Asia. *Science,* 236(4805), 1114-1116.

Hay, S.I., Guerra, C.A., Tatem, A.J., Noor, A.M., & Snow, R.W. (2004). The global distribution and population at risk of malaria: past, present, and future. *Lancet Infectious Diseases,* 4, 327-336.

Herwaldt, B.L. (2000). *Cyclospora cayetanensis*: a review, focusing on the outbreaks of cyclosporiasis in the 1990s. *Clinical Infectious Diseases,* 31(4), 1040-1057.

Heymann, D.L. & Aylward, R.B. (2004). Eradicating polio. *New England Journal of Medicine,* 351, 1275-1277.

Jernigan, D.B., Hofman, J., Cetron, M.S., Genese, C.A., Nuorti, J., Pekka Fields, B.S., Benson, F.R., Carter, R.J., Edelstein, P.H., Guerro, I.C., Paul, S.M., Lipman, H.B., & Breiman, R.F. (1996). Outbreak of legionnaires' disease among cruise passengers exposed to a contaminated whirlpool spa. *Lancet,* 347, 494-499.

Jetz, W., Carbone, C., Fulford, J., & Brown, J.H. (2004). The scaling of animal space use. *Science,* 306, 266-268.

Kenyon, T.A., Valway, S.E., Ihle, W.W., Onorato, I.M., & Castro, K.G. (1996). Transmission of multidrug-resistant *Mycobacterium tuberculosis* during a long airplane flight. *New England Journal of Medicine,* 334, 933-938.

Kilpatrick, A.M., Gluzberg, Y., Burgett, J., & Daszak, P. (2004). Quantitative risk assessment of the pathways by which West Nile virus could reach Hawaii. *EcoHealth,* 1, 205-209.

Kinsella, K. & Velkoff, V.A. (2002). An aging world: 2001. U.S. Census Bureau, Series P95/01-1. Washington, D.C.: U.S. Government Printing Office.

Laurent, C., Bourgeois, A., Mpoudi, M., Butei, C., Peeters, M., Mpoudi-Ngole, E., & Delaporte, E. (2004). Commercial logging and HIV epidemic, rural equatorial Africa. *Emerging Infectious Diseases,* 10(11), 1953-1956.

Lounibos, L.P. (2002). Invasions by insect vectors of human diseases. *Annual Review of Entomology,* 47, 233-266.

McCarthy, S.A. & Khambaty, F.M. (1994). International dissemination of epidemic Vibrio cholerae by cargo ship ballast and other nonpotable waters. *Applied Environmental Microbiology,* 60, 2597-2601.

Milian, F., Sanchez, L.M., Toledo, R., Ramirez, C., & Santillan, M.A. (2000). Descriptive study of human and bovine tuberculosis in Queretato, Mexico. *Review Latinoam Microbiologica,* 42, 13-19.

Miller, J.E., Tam, T.W.S., Maloney, S., Fukuda, K., Cox, N., Hockin, J., Kertesz, D., Klimov, A., & Cetron, M. (2000). Cruise ships: High-risk passengers and the global spread of new influenza viruses. *Clinical Infectious Diseases,* 31, 433-438.

Minooee, A. & Richman, L. (1999). Infectious diseases on cruise ships. *Clinical Infectious Diseases,* 29, 737-744.

Moore, C.G. & Mitchell, D.J. (1997). *Aedes albopictus* in the United States: Ten-year presence and public health implications. *Emerging Infectious Diseases,* 3(3), 329-334.

Moser, M.R., Bender, T.R., Margolis, H.S., Noble, G.R., Kendal, A.P., & Ritter, D.G. (1979). An outbreak of influenza aboard a commercial airliner. *American Journal of Epidemiology,* 110, 1-6.

Nash, D., Mostashari, F., Fine, A., Miller, J., O'Leary, D., Murray, K., Huant, A., Rosenberg, A., Greenberg, A., Sherman, M., Wong, S., & Layton, M. for the 1999 West Nile Outbreak Response Working Group (2001). The outbreak of West Nile virus infection in the New York City area in 1999. *New England Journal of Medicine,* 344, 1807-1814.

Nisbett, R.A. & Monath, T.P. (2001). Viral traffic, transnational companies and logging in Liberia, West Africa. *Global Change & Human Health,* 2(1), 18-19.

O'Brien, T., Pla, M.P., Mayer, K.W., Kishi, H., Gilleece, E., Syvanen, M., & Hopkins, J.D. (1985). Intercontinental spread of a new antibiotic resistance gene on an epidemic plasmid. *Science,* 230, 87-88.

Okeke, I.N. & Edelman, R. (2001). Dissemination of antibiotic-resistant bacteria across geographic borders. *Clinical Infectious Diseases,* 33, 364-369.

Olsen, S.J., Chang, H.L., Cheung, T.Y.Y., Tang, A.F.Y., Fisk, T.L., Ooi, S.P.L., Kuo, H.W., Jiang, D.D.S., Chen, K.T., Lando, J., Hsu, K.H., Chen, T.J., & Dowell, S.F. (2003). Transmission of the severe acute respiratory syndrome on aircraft. *New England Journal of Medicine,* 349, 2416-2422.

Osterholm, M. (2005). Preparing for the next pandemic. *New England Journal of Medicine,* 352, 1839-1842.

Pealer, L.N., Marfin, A.A., Petersen, L.R., Lanciotti, R.S., Page, P.L., Stramer, S.L., Stobierski, M.G., Signs, K., Newman, B., Kapoor, H., Goodman, J.L., & Chamberland M.E., for the West Nile Virus Transmission Investigation Team (2003). Transmission of West Nile virus through blood transfusion in the United States in 2002. *New England Journal of Medicine,* 349, 1236-1245.

Peiris, J.S.M., Guan, Y., & Yuen, K.Y. (2004). Severe acute respiratory syndrome. *Nature Medicine* Supplement, 10(12), S88-S97.

Petersen, J.M., Schriefer, M.E., Carter, L.G., Zhou, Y., Sealy, T., Bawiec, D., Yockey, B., Urich, S., Zeidner, N.S., Svashia, S., Kool, J.L., Buck, J., Lindley, C., Celeda, L., Monteneiri, J.A., Gage, L.K., & Chu, M.C. (2004). Laboratory analysis of tularemia in wild-trapped, commercially traded prairie dogs, Texas, 2002. *Emerging Infectious Diseases,* 10(3), 419-425.

Rappole, J.H., Derrickson, S.R., & Hubalek, Z. (2000). Migratory birds and spread of West Nile virus in the Western Hemisphere. *Emerging Infectious Diseases,* 6(4), 319-328.

Reed, K.D., Melski, J.W., Graham, M.B., Regnery, R.L., Sotir, J.M., Wegner, J.V., Kazmierczak, J.J., Stratman, E.J., Li, Y., Fairley, J.A., Swain, G.R., Olson, V.A., Sargent, E.K., Kehl, S.C., Frace, J.A., Kline, R., Foldy, S.L., David, J.P., & Damon, I.K. (2004). The detection of monkeypox in humans in the Western Hemisphere. *New England Journal of Medicine,* 350, 342-50.

Reiter, P., Lathrop, S., Bunning, M., Biggerstaff, B., Singer, D., Tiwari, T., Baber, L., Amador, M., Thirion, J., Hayes, J., Seca, C., Mendez, J., Ramirez, B., Robinson, J., Fawlings, J., Vorndam, V., Waterman, S., Gubler, D., Clark, G., & Hayes, E. (2003). Texas lifestyle limits transmission of dengue virus. *Emerging Infectious Diseases,* 9(1), 86-89.

Ruiz, G.M., Rawlings, T.K., Dobbs, F.C., Drake, L.A., Mullady, T., Huq, A., & Colwell, R.R. (2000). Invasion biology: Global spread of microorganisms by ships. *Nature,* 408, 49-50.

Russell, R.C. (1987). Survival of insects in the wheel bays of a Boeing 747B aircraft on flights between tropical and temperate airports. *Bulletin of the World Health Organization,* 65, 659-662.

Sharp, P.M., Bailles, E., Chaudhuri, R.R., Rodenburg, C.M., Santiago, M.O., & Hahn, B.H. (2001). The origins of AIDS viruses; where and when? *Philosophical Transactions of the Royal Society of London Series B, 356,* 867-876.

Smolinski, M.S., Hamburg, M.A., & Lederberg, J., (Eds.) (2003). *Microbial Threats to Health: Emergence, Detection, and Response.* Institute of Medicine of the National Academies. Washington, DC: The National Academy Press.

Taubenberger, J.K., Reid, A.H., Lourens, R.M., Wang, R., Guozhong, J., & Fanning, T.G. (2005). Charactereization of the 1918 influenza virus polymerase genes. *Nature,* 437, 889-893.

Toole, M.J. (1994). The rapid assessment of health problems in refugee and displaced populations. *Medicine and Global Survival,* 1, 200-207.

UN Population Division. (2002). World Urbanization Prospects: The 2001 Revision. ESA//WP.173. New York, NY: United Nations Populations Division, Department of Economic and Social Affairs.

Van Beneden, C.A., Keene, W.E., Strang, R.A., Werker, D.H., King, A.S., Mahonn, B., Hedberg, K., Bell, A., Kelly, M., Balan, V.K., MacKenzie, W.R., & Fleming, D. (1999). Multinational outbreak of *Salmonella enterica* serotype Newport infections due to contaminated alfalfa sprouts. *Journal of the American Medical Association,* 281(2), 158-162.

Van Borm, S., Thomas, I., Hanquet, G., Lambrecht, B., Boschmans, M., Dupont, G., Decaestecker, M., Snacken, R., & van den Berg, T. (2005). Highly pathogenic H1N1 influenza virus in smuggled Thai eagles, Belgium. *Emerging Infectious Disease,* 11, 702-705.

Webby, R., Hoffmann, E., & Webster, R. (2004). Molecular constraints to interspecies transmission of viral pathogens. *Nature Medicine,* Supplement 10(12), S77-S81.

Wilder-Smith, A., Barkham, T.M.S., Earnest, A., & Paton, N.I. (2002). Acquisition of W135 meningococcal carriage in Hajj pilgrims and transmission to house contacts: prospective study. *British Medical Journal,* 325, 365-366.

Wilkie, D.S. & Carpenter, J.F. (1999). Bushmeat hunting in the Congo Basin: an assessment of impacts and options for mitigation. *Biodiversity and Conservation,* 8, 927-955.

Wilson, M.E. (1995a). Travel and the emergence of infectious diseases. *Emerging Infectious Diseases,* 1, 39-45.

Wilson, M.E. (1995b). Infectious diseases: An ecological perspective. *British Medical Journal,* 311, 1681-1684.

Wilson, M.E. (2000). Environmental change and infectious diseases. *Ecosystem Health* 6(1), 7-12.

Wilson, M.E. (2003) The traveler and emerging infections: Sentinel, courier, transmitter. *Journal of Applied Microbiology,* 94, 1S-11S.

Wilson, M.E. (2004). Geography of infectious diseases. In (J. Cohen & W.G. Powderly, Eds.), *Infectious diseases,* second edition, (pp. 1419-1427). New York, NY: Mosby.

Wilson, M.E. (2005). Ecological disturbances and emerging infections: travel, dams, shipment of goods, and vectors. In (C. Power & R. Johnson, Eds.), *Emerging neurological infections.* (pp. 35-57). Boca Raton, FL: Taylor & Francis Group.

Wilson, M.E., Levins, R., & Spielman, A. (Eds.) (1994). *Disease in Evolution: Global Changes and Emergence of Infectious Diseases.* New York, NY: New York Academy of Sciences.

Winkelstein, W., Jr. (1995). A new perspective on John Snow-s communicable disease theory. *American Journal of Epidemiology,* S3-S9. (Citing Snow J. On the mode of communication of cholera. London, UK: John Churchill, 1849.)

Wolfe, N.D., Prosser, A.T., Carr, J.K., Aamoufe, U., Mpoudi-Ngole, E., Torimiro, J.N., LeBreton, M., McCutchan, F.E., Birs, D.L., & Burke, D.S. (2004). Exposure to nonhuman primates in rural Cameroon. *Emerging Infectious Diseases,* 10(12), 2094-2099.

Wolfe, N.D., Switzer, W.M., Carr, J.K., Bhulla, V.B., Shanmugam, V., Tamoufe, U., Prosser, A.T., Torimiro, J.N., Wright, A., Mpoudi-Ngole, E., McCutchan, F.E., Birx, D.L., Folks, T.M., Burke, D.S., & Heneine, W. (2004). Naturally acquired simian retrovirus infections in central African hunters. *Lancet,* 363, 932-937.

Wolfe, N.D., Heneine, W., Carr, J.K., Garcia, A.D., Shanmugam, V., Tamoufe, U., Torimiro, J.N., Prosser, A.T., LeBreton, M., Mpoudi-Ngole, E., McCutchan, F.E., Birx, D.L., Folks, T.M., Burke, D.S., & Switzer, W.M. (2005). Emergence of unique primate T-lymphotropic viruses among central African bushmeat hunters. *Proceedings of the National Academy of Sciences,* 102(22), 7994-7999.

WHO (2005). *World Health Organization Global Tuberculosis Control Surveillance, Planning, and Financing.* Geneva: World Health Organization.

WTO (2006). *Tourism Highlights, 2006 Edition.* Madrid, Spain: World Tourism Organization (http://www.world-tourism.org).

# Chapter 3

# Health Barriers and Inequities for Migrants

ELIZABETH IOANNIDI-KAPOLOU, PH.D.

## Introduction

As the world becomes more ethnically heterogeneous than ever, the sense of belonging to one culture or another differentiates ethnic groups from one another and forms distinct ethnic minorities that are often disadvantaged and socially isolated from the larger community (Giddens, 1997). Persons who are part of excluded and marginalized minorities are often comprised of recent migrants (Cohen & Kennedy, 2000). In fact, it is estimated that there are 5,000-ethnocultural groups worldwide, often living uncomfortably within the existing approximately 200 national states and at least 175 million people living outside their country of origin (UNDP, 2004).

Although, Western societies fight for cultural diversity and the right to be different while they simultaneously struggle for equal opportunity, categorization on the basis of cultural identity still leads to racist and discriminatory behavior towards the 'other' or the 'different.' Thus, the process of integration becomes quite difficult for those who wish to adapt to the new culture where they have either decided to or are forced to live in (in the case of refugees).

In many countries, migrant and refugee populations constitute a marginalized sector of the population because they are impacted by factors that cause inequalities in numerous dimensions of social life such as race/ethnicity, poverty, illiteracy, gender and class. Migrants, refugees, and women in particular are often considered vulnerable because of their exposure to risk factors. In fact, "the greatest risk factors are rooted in those activities undertaken during the process of migration–rather than simply being a migrant" (UNAIDS, 2001b).

The focus of this chapter is to highlight those factors that contribute to migrants' and refugees' poor health and limited access to health care which in turn become barriers for their integration into the host country.

## Factors Contributing to Inequalities in Health

According to Cohen and Kennedy (2000), structured inequalities operate along the main axes of gender, race/ethnicity, and class. Sociological studies have documented the impact of these factors on the widening of inequalities in health as they have indicated the social patterning of health and illness and the mechanism for examining social inequalities (Agrafiotis, 2003; Bury, 1997). More specifically, social scientists have developed a number of theories to explain the relationship between class and health inequalities (Fox & Coldblatt, 1982; Illsley, 1986; Le Grand, 1986; Nettleton, 1995; Stern, 1983; Townsend & Davidson, 1982). Although, theorists claim that 'class' no longer exists as a concept (Pakulski & Waters, 1996), sociologists of health and illness cannot refer to inequalities in health without taking 'class' into consideration. Sometimes, they focus on other axes of inequality such as consumption and lifestyle, which do not align with class as it has been traditionally conceived by sociologists. These factors must be considered in order to explain why some people are healthier than others (Annandale, 1999).

Gender has also been studied and documented as a factor contributing to health inequalities (Arber, 1990; Bury, 1997; Nettleton, 1995) although it is a more complex issue that involves accounting for the structural position of women. Women suffer in greater numbers than men from poverty—and often depend on the male head of household or hold low income jobs—and illiteracy, both of which impact their health status. While the consequences of poverty on health inequalities are more apparent, illiteracy is also strongly related to health problems. For example, the patient may not comply with the doctor's orders due to the inability to understand or misinterpretation of medical instructions (Davis, Meldrum, Tippy, Weiss, & Williams, 1996). Furthermore there is evidence of a negative relationship between illiterate patients and health facilities; more specifically, patients receive ineffective help due to problems of comprehension and completion of forms, inability to understand advocated treatments, and unwillingness to discuss personal health problems with physicians due to the perceived shame of revealing illiteracy (Baker, Parker, Williams, Clark, & Nurss, 1997).

Further, growing literature demonstrates an association between racism and mortality and morbidity (Ahmad, 1993; Brown, 1996; Bunton, Nettleton, & Burrows, 1995; Bury, 1997; Cruikshank & Beeves, 1989; Freeman, 1993; Nettleton, 1995; Smaje, 1995). In an era characterized globally by culturally heterogeneous social configurations, sociologists of health and illness have initiated lengthy debates and have highlighted the crucial importance of the relationship between racism and the experience of health and illness (Annandale, 1998). It is fair to say that virtually all migrants, refugees, or members of ethnic minorities have confronted racism on the basis of coming from a different culture and remaining different from their communities. A European report on access to health care with a focus on migration and HIV vulnerability notes that attitudes in society towards migrants and ethnic minorities are part of a wider political climate, to which various factors contribute, including the economy, unemployment rates, and global events and developments. However, most of the European countries that contributed to the report, mentioned discrimination in society at large and in the practice of health service provision as a major problem that migrants face (Bröring, Canter, Schinaia, & Teixeira, 2003).

Arguably, the issue of migrant health is a complex one that is related to different determinants such as: lifestyle/behavior, biological/genetic factors, environmental factors (physical, economic, social, and cultural) and the availability, accessibility and quality of health care (Janssens, Bosmans, & Temmerman, 2005). It has been documented that disease patterns of migrants are influenced by the environments of source and destination countries and by the process of immigration itself. For example, studies of cardiovascular mortality have shown that migrant groups do not have a disadvantaged profile and cancer mortality studies have attributed variations in health status to genetic and/or environmental factors. Thus many factors affect the process of migration and migrants' mortality and morbidity rates (McKay, Macintyre, & Ellaway, 2003). Migration exposes people to vulnerable situations and health risks related to discrimination, loss of status, and abusive working conditions at host countries (Piper, 2005).

## 'Otherness' as a Health Barrier: Experiences of Migrants and Refugees

Human history offers many examples of the constant attempt of people to distinguish the 'different' or the 'other' on the basis of ethnicity, race, religion, class, and gender. Groups of people by virtue of shared characteristics, separate from others who they usually consider inferior and use stereotypical thinking to blame them for things that are not their fault. As a result, those perceived as 'others' are discriminated against and are deprived of many advantages enjoyed by the majority (Ioannidi & Mestheneos, 2003).

It is difficult to understand health barriers for migrants and refugees if they are examined independently from discrimination in various sectors of social life that hinder their integration process. Personal experiences of migrants and refugees are presented below in the context of the dominant society's stance towards them and the barriers to vehicles of integration such as employment, education, and health. Their experiences with racism and discrimination are also reported as evidence of national policies and ideologies of cultural pluralism in practice.

Textual data presented below are from two studies that have implemented the biographical–interpretive method and that have aimed to investigate migrants' and refugees' experiences of social exclusion and social integration in the host country. The first study (SOSTRIS or social strategies in risk societies) was conducted in seven European countries (Britain, France,

Germany, Greece, Italy, Spain and Sweden) between 1996 and 1999. Based on socio-biographical and life-history methods the study examined social risks in a comparative European context. The project developed the concept of "life-journeys" to characterize the typical experiences of subjects in six categories of risks related to exclusion, one of which was ethnic minorities and migrants (Chamberlayne & Rustin, 1999). The second study was carried out in 1999 in the context of a European-funded project carried out by the ECRE Task Force on Integration[1] with the aim of understanding refugee perspectives on integration in the EU—considered to be among the accepted durable solutions for refugees. A representative set of voices from refugees living in the 15 (at that time) European Member States was thought to be essential in understanding the impact of policy and services on integration (Mestheneos & Ioannidi, 1999a).

Researchers concluded that migration is a turning point in the "life journey" of an individual (Mestheneos & Ioannidi, 1999b), that migration is not a condition but a process that implies a new definition of identity for the individual, and that individual strategies exist for coping with migration (Spano, 1999). All people cannot overcome, in the same way, the barriers created by local communities. Some individuals are more able than others to deal with uncertainty, new cultures and situations, or the traumas of the past whereas others need more help and support and are even "paralyzed" by their obstacles and remain trapped in the margins of social life (Mestheneos & Ioannidi, 2002).

*"According to me to become a part of a society it is not just to live in it but to be a part of the system, you have to be accepted by the majority of the system as a part of it. If you are not, you will always be an outsider . . . To live on surviving it is not considered a life. Unfortunately we don't have this opportunity . . . ."*

(A male Kurdish refugee living 7 years in the Netherlands)

Feelings of superiority expressed by locals deprives many members of migrant and refugee communities from individual options and opportunities and even leads them to poverty as a result of the unavailability of educational opportunity and work. As migrants and refugees repeatedly state, the obligation to work in order to survive restricts them from any available opportunities to pursue formal education.

---

[1] The ECRE Task Force on Integration was a consortium of seven non-governmental organizations working under the auspices of ECRE - (European Council on Refugees and Exiles) which is also responsible for policy development. The partners in the Task Force and their areas of responsibility are as follows: the British Refugee Council - Employment, the World University Service - Education, the Italian Refugee Council - Health, the Dutch Refugee Council - Housing, the Greek Council for refugees - Community and Cultural Integration, France Terre d'Asile Vocational Training, the Flemish Refugee Council - Coordinating Secretariat.

Institutionalized racism is one of the most insidious and overwhelming obstacles to societal integration. Thus in all areas of employment, housing, training, education, and health, the assumption that migrants and refugees must be inferior, creates barriers to any kind of integration. Experiences of migrants' and refugees reveal how their 'otherness' is perceived by the local population and how this impacts efforts to earn a living in a different cultural setting.

*"People from Third World countries are looked down on as third or fourth class citizens, and that shouldn't be like that as we all live on Planet Earth"*
(A male Peruvian migrant living in Spain)

One of the greatest challenges of migrants and refugees involves obtaining a decent job in the local labor market. The perception shared by many African refugee men living in European countries is that they are denied the opportunity to demonstrate their abilities despite their qualifications and credentials. They feel exploited when they are offered menial jobs in the labor market and give examples of doctors and teachers from their countries who work as cleaners and street sweepers. Unskilled migrants often engage in dirty and dangerous jobs and are thus exposed to serious occupational health problems and prone to fatal accidents (Piper, 2005).

In Southern Europe the lack of social security drives undocumented migrants and refugees into all forms of insecure, temporary, and non-registered jobs regardless of their qualifications and leaves them vulnerable due to the lack of access to health services. Lack of health insurance has a dramatic effect on the receipt of care, as dire economic situations obviously do not provide access to health care. Furthermore, migrants and refugees often avoid public hospitals due to their legal status and seek help from Non Governmental Organizations (NGOs) only when the problem is so urgent that emergency medical help is required.

Migrants' reduced access to health care and resulting consequences for their health have been documented by various reports. Primary barriers include language, cultural differences in concepts of health and disease, correct description of symptoms, recognition of the need to seek treatment, and racism experienced when treatment is sought (Bollini & Siem, 1995).

Migrants and refugees recall countless experiences with the health sector and more often than not report feeling and being treated as "different." Dragan, a refugee from Bosnia living in Sweden described a disturbing experience with a Swedish physician and nurse. As a new arrival from a distant country, he underwent a thorough examination as *"a potential carrier of Mediterranean diseases."* Dragan felt compelled to voice and declare his dignity to avoid being categorized as a lower status of human being simply because of his refugee status (Peterson, 1999).

Issues raised mainly by migrant and refugee women in the context of health concerns involve cultural factors that cause them to be hesitant in seeking health care. In their remarks they stated feeling uncomfortable with the organization of health services and over the fact of having to go to a male doctor.

*"Once I went to the radiologist for an examination. He asked me to take my blouse off. I was shocked. How could I take my blouse off in the presence of a strange man? For me it was not logical but for him it was normal . . ."*

(A well educated female Sudanese Muslim refugee living in Austria)

Another Sudanese woman in the UK described the situation in a more detailed way and recounted the barriers that women encounter when seeking health care. She explained that in their home countries they go to female doctors but in the host country they do not have this choice and added the understandable difficulty of undergoing culturally embarrassing examinations and medical tests such as the PAP smear and commented on the lack of continuity in the primary health care clinics since one meets a different doctor in each appointment. As a qualified health worker herself, this woman raised another important cultural issue relating to perceptions of the doctor-patient relationship:

*"We are used to a doctor who touches us, listens to our chest, but here it's just conversation. And because we are foreigners and they are not touching us we think that maybe they are afraid to get infectious diseases like AIDS. We have all these things in our minds."*

(A female Sudanese refugee living in UK)

It is evident that problems arise primarily from difficulties in adapting to a new climate, cultural differences when confronting health problems, and dealing with health professionals. Apart from these difficulties, migrants' and refugees' experiences with treatment and hospitalization, as reported in the aforementioned studies, were good in nearly all of the EU member states, as many have had poor access to health services and treatment prior to their arrival in the host country.

Many migrants and refugees come from countries embroiled in civil war and conflict, or are controlled by totalitarian and repressive regimes. Factors that lead to the decision to migrate are also associated with specific health problems varying from malnutrition and torture to an increased vulnerability to the development of mental health problems (Mestheneos & Ioannidi, 1999a).

## Mental Health Problems for Migrants

The World Health Organization and the World Bank have highlighted that mental disorders represent five of the ten leading causes of disability worldwide, amounting to nearly one third of all health-related disabilities. Migrant and refugee populations are associated with increased vulnerability to mental health problems due to great pressures related to the decision to migrate or become a refugee (Minas, 2002). Migration has been known to affect mental health, in fact, in the United Kingdom, Irish, Caribbean and Pakistani men have higher rates of suicidal thoughts and inflict deliberate self-harm, while in Oslo, post-traumatic stress disorder affects 46.6% of refugees (Gavin, Kelly, O'Callaghan, & Lane, 2001). Migration does not necessarily cause migrants to display 'caseness' for depression or other psychological problems (McKay et al., 2003); however, they may find the experience of migration to be stressful and are likely to benefit from social support from both the already established migrant ethnic community and the host community.

Studies on refugee children (Rousseau, 1995; Westermeyer & Wahmanholm, 1996) have brought to light some consequences of their adaptation to a new society including depressive symptoms and other mental health problems. The need for further investigation on post-flight resettlement as well as on post-migration community environment was suggested (Mestheneos & Ioannidi, 2002). The need for further research is also stressed by Minas (2002) who states the necessity for systematic, coherent, and international collaborative research to understand the mental health needs of immigrants and refugees and how these needs can be met. Unfortunately, these issues are not on the list of priorities on national research funding bodies (Minas, 2002).

When discussing their experiences in the host country, many refugees refer to their psychological problems and the stresses they have been under. The need for sensitivity to mental health issues comes to light in the following quotes (Mestheneos & Ioannidi, 1999a):

*"I remember the first two months I could not sleep and the next day at work I was getting miserable and I had some hope that I should get over all this. Those strong continuous headaches . . . I had to go to the hospital and tried to explain everything in my broken language and the doctor could not do anything much, just prescribed some medicine which did not have any impact."*

(A male refugee living in Portugal referring to his health problems associated with his status)

The long wait for refugee status was mentioned as a critical factor in the depression experienced by many refugees. An educated Sudanese man in his 30s who lived in three different camps for asylum seekers, the last being in the north of Sweden, pointed out that waiting for the recognition of status (which lasted 15 months in his case and which often averages over 3 years for others) caused psychological problems including depression and frustration for some while leading some to suicide.

Minorities' mistrust of mental health services may deter them from seeking treatment. Sometimes clinicians are incompatible with the cultures of the clients they serve, which is interpreted by the ethnic minorities as a sign of insufficient care.

*"I doubt very much the effectiveness of this kind of treatment for people who are from traditional societies where custom, the wise and religion still have an important place in people's heads. Furthermore to go and display your life in front of a group of people with problems does not seem either healthy (sane?) nor the kind of thing that will*

*improve the situation . . . I think you can do a lot of harm when you distance people from their culture and in the end what is the result?"*

(A Rwandan refugee, expressing his skepticism about the psychotherapeutic treatment offered to his companion from the Antilles)

The influence of cultural factors on migrants and refugees' mental health is a complex one and reports present different aspects of this issue. Individuals who demonstrate cultural adaptation experience less stress than those confronting marginalization (Tabassum, Macaskill, & Ahmad, 2000). On the other hand some migrants are more commonly diagnosed with schizophrenia because of the lack of cultural awareness among clinicians or racism on the part of psychiatrists (Gavin, et al., 2001).

Some claim that few psychologists have the cultural knowledge that allows them to contribute to the study of individuals from non-mainstream cultures (Piper, 2005). Another problem area is that psychologists are less concerned about gender differences because their main interest focuses on adaptive processes and outcomes. Results from the few studies that exist on gender and psychological well being in the context of the United States, Canada and Europe suggest that women, mainly those with low socio-economic status facing particular risk factors, suffer from higher levels of stress than men (Piper, 2005). Additionally, ethnic/racial differences show Asian women in the U.S. and Canada suffering from higher levels of depression compared to women from other ethnic groups due to their experiences with greater social pressures and conflicting gender roles. Some mental problems are also related to sexual and reproductive health of women, which are evident in the case of victims of sexual and gender-based violence (Janssens et al., 2005).

## Health Disparities Among Female Migrants

Scholars in the past decades have brought female migration into focus as women represent about 50% of the estimated 175 million migrants worldwide (IOM, 2003) and migration is now viewed as a gendered phenomenon. Migrant women are 'triply disadvantaged' by race/ethnicity, status as a non-national, and gender inequalities (Piper, 2005). Gender is defined as

*"the widely shared expectations and norms within a society about appropriate male and female behavior, characteristics and roles, which ascribe to men and women differential access to power, including productive resources and decision making"*

(UNAIDS, 1999 p., 5)

The health of migrant women is reported to be worse than that of men from the moment they arrive in the host country and continues to deteriorate while living there. Women and girls suffer disproportionately from the consequences of war, civil unrest, poor health care, and violence. Protection of women is often defined in terms of male ideologies and interests without taking into consideration women's needs (WHO, 1998). Migrant women encounter higher health risks—in fact, a number of studies have highlighted specific health areas where groups of migrant women are affected, including reproductive health, HIV/AIDS and domestic violence (Ackerhams, 2003). Research findings indicate that women suffer higher maternal morbidity and mortality, experience poorer pregnancy outcomes, have less access to family planning services and counseling, show higher prevalence of unwanted pregnancy and induced abortion and are at a higher risk of STIs, including HIV/AIDS (Janssens et al., 2005).

Migrant and refugee women's health problems become more evident when attention is focused on their sexual and reproductive health, as this is one area where gender is the critical factor in health status. Because of traditional and cultural roles, migrant women are more dependent upon men for their daily survival and in many cultures they are viewed as property of and subordinate to men. This makes them vulnerable to sexual abuse and rape, which in many Third World countries is not even reported due to the social status of women. Sexual abuse puts women at greater risk for STIs and globally the most striking development is the recognition of the role that gender plays in the spread of the AIDS epidemic. As individual risk for HIV infection is influenced by cognitive, attitudinal and behavioral factors, women find themselves in an unequal position since gender norms and roles restrict their potential for taking control of their lives. Sexual practices occur in a context of unequal power relations as female sexuality in many cultures today is restricted and controlled by societal expectations and norms and the sexual position of women is subordinated to that of men. According to dominant ideologies of femininity, women are expected to be ignorant and innocent in sexual matters, to defer to men's sexual needs, not to take the initiative in sexual encounters and not to negotiate safe sex (Garcia-Sanchez & Rivadeneyra, 2003). Further, women are less able to refuse sexual relations, are frequently victims of different forms of violence, including sexual violence and depend economically or emotionally on partners who often maintain additional sexual contacts (Frasca, 2003).

In addition to women's vulnerability, marginalized sexual cultures are also central to the growth of the HIV pandemic (Dowsett, 2003). In cultures where women learn to please men, they engage in high-risk sexual behavior in order to satisfy their male partner. For example, in parts of west, central and southern Africa, women insert herbs and roots into their vagina to tighten their vaginal passage even though these agents cause inflammation and abrasions that increase the efficiency of HIV transmission. In cultures where virginity is highly valued, women practice alternative sexual behaviors such as anal sex, which increases their risk for infection (UNAIDS, 1999).

Migration itself places women at greater risk for infection because women traveling alone may have little choice but to sell sex for survival or to establish partnerships in transit or at destination countries simply for protection. Research conducted in Africa and Asia has shown that migration disrupts family life and creates a demand for prostitution, which in turn contributes to the spread of HIV/AIDS (Piper, 2005). In many cases, female heads of households often engage in sexual relationships in exchange for money or goods for their economic survival. In the Democratic Republic of Congo, women who migrate from rural to urban areas seek occasional sexual partners known as "spare tyres" in order to cover their immediate economic needs (UNAIDS, 1999).

The highest increase in HIV infections is seen among trafficked girls and women because the threat of violence forces them to perform sex acts that put them at greater risk than other sex workers. Trafficked girls and women have reported rape, forced unprotected sex and other violent sexual practices, which further increase their vulnerability and exposure to HIV/AIDS (Long, 2001).

## STI/HIV Prevention for Migrant Women

In the framework of the European project for the prevention of HIV/AIDS and other STIs named PHASE (prevention of HIV/AIDS and STIs among women in Europe) a number of target groups were defined for intervention activities. Among the 10 participating countries (Austria, Germany, Greece, Ireland, Italy, The Netherlands, Portugal, Spain, Sweden, and United Kingdom) a variety of groups emerged due to the different socio-economic and cultural contexts in which women live in different parts of Europe. However, there was a consensus among all countries for the development of specific actions to reach out to migrant women as an urgent priority.

It was clearly stated that in Europe's multi-cultural societies, migrant women lack access to information. In addition to language barriers, migrant women face cultural barriers that may prevent them from accessing information. Cultural differences emerge as one of the greatest obstacles to access to HIV/AIDS information for migrant groups (Ackerhams, 2003). Cultural diversities also determine differences in views on sexuality, gender relations and women's rights to make their own choices.

Since gender inequalities affect women's risk of infection, the health sector must work toward realizing gender equity through an empowerment process. In doing so, health care workers should take into account diverse needs and develop appropriate methods. In the case of migrant women, it is important to know that many of them have cultural backgrounds with a strong tradition of sharing their life-experiences exclusively with other women. It was suggested that in these cases educational material, prevention strategies, and empowerment processes should be provided through women or peer groups (van Mens, de Schutter, Garcia-Sanchez, & Pinzon-Pulido, 2002).

## Concluding Remarks

Migration can leave people vulnerable due to their precarious legal status, abusive working conditions, exposure to health risks due to lack of information, and lack of access to health care due to legal issues or insufficient funds to seek medical advice. It is evident that migrants' health risks are compounded by discrimination and restricted access to health information, health promotion, and health insurance. A different culture, language barriers and the insecure position in the host country do not permit migrants to adequately address specific health needs and further, make it difficult to access appropriate health information and services. Conversely, health practitioners may lack awareness about the complex needs of migrant populations. A recent study conducted in the Netherlands reveals that miscommunication should not be explained only by language barriers but that it often stems from not understanding each other, communicating from different perspectives, or differences in expectations from health care (Janssens et al., 2005).

In recent years attention has been placed on the increased disparities in access to care on the basis of racial and ethnic characteristics. The American Institute of Medicine, in a large scale analysis of racial and ethnic disparities concluded that bias, prejudice and stereotyping on the part of health care providers may contribute to discrepancies in care (Henry Kaiser Family Foundation, 2004). It appears that the primary manifestation of a society's value and attitudes towards 'otherness' are the ways in which they deliver health and social care to migrants and migrant communities. Some argue that if one of the chief responsibilities of public health is fostering policies to promote health, then countering racism should be considered a public health issue (McKenzie, 2003).

Increasing global flows and settlement of migrants and refugees with diverse socio-economic and socio-cultural backgrounds have helped to focus attention on migrant health. In the promotion of migrant and refugee health, it is a challenge for different societies to deal with multiple cultures, the concept of 'otherness,' and the interface of this with racism and xenophobia. Social exclusion, poverty and health are interrelated issues. As it was stated by the European Commission's communication of October 26, 1999:

*"Investment in health is widely accepted as a cornerstone of poverty reduction strategies . . . Poor health is seen as both a consequence and cause of poverty and inequality in opportunity or gender"*

(Janssens et al., 2005, p.85)

Better health for migrant populations can be achieved through the promotion of social integration and cohesion. In this case, there is a need to examine what is necessary to enhance cultural competency and to develop effective strategies in order to integrate the new communities and provide services for them so they can effectively integrate into the host society. Health professionals, policy makers, educators, and researchers in the provision of heath care and nursing have a crucial role to play in promoting the integration of migrants, but in order to accomplish this task successfully they need to possess the necessary transcultural competencies.

## References

Ackerhams, M. (2003). Health issues of ethnic minority and migrant women: Sexual and reproductive health in a multicultural Europe. *Entre Nous, The European Magazine for Sexual and Reproductive Health,* 55, 9-11.

Agrafiotis, D. (2003). *Health, Illness, Society.* Athens, Greece: Dardanos.

Ahmad, W. (Ed.) (1995). *Race and Health in Contemporary Britain.* Buckingham, UK: Open University press.

Annandale, A. (1999). *The Sociology of Health & Medicine: A Critical Introduction,* 2nd Ed. Cambridge: Polity press.

Arber, S. (1990). Opening the black box: Inequalities in women's health. In (P. Abbott & G. Payne, Eds.) *New Directions in the Sociology of Health,* Basingstoke, UK: Falmer Press.

Baker, D.W., Parker, R.M., Williams, M.V., Clark, W.S., & Nurss, J. (1997). The relationship of patient' reading ability to self-reported health and use of health services. *American Journal of Public Health,* 87, 1027-1030.

Bollini, P. & Siem, H. (1995). No real progress towards equity: Health of migrants and ethnic minorities on the eve of the year 2000. *Social Science Medicine,* 30(6), 819-828.

Bröring, G., Canter, C., Schinaia, N., & Teixeira, B. (2003). *Access to Care: Privilege or Right? Migration and HIV Vulnerability in Europe.* The Netherlands: NIGZ, European Project AIDS & Mobility.

Brown, P. (1996). *Perspectives in Medical Sociology,* 2nd Ed. Chicago, IL: Waveland press.

Bunton, R., Nettleton, S., & Burrows, R. (1995). *The Sociology of Health Promotion. Critical Analyses of Consumption, Lifestyle and Risk.* London, UK: Routledge.

Bury, M. (1997). *Health and Illness in a changing society.* London, UK: Routledge.

Chamberlayne, P. & Rustin, M. (1999). From biography to social policy. *Final Report* of the SOSTRIS (Social Strategies in Risk Societies) project. Center for Biography in Social Policy, Sociology Department, University of East London.

Cohen, R. & Kennedy, P. (2000). *Global Sociology.* New York, NY: Palgrave.

Cruikshank, K. & Beeves, D. (Eds.) (1989). *Ethnic Factors in Health and Disease.* London, UK: Wright.

Davis, T.C., Meldrum, H., Tippy, P.K.P., Weiss, B.D., & Williams, M.V. (1996). How literacy leads to poor health care. *Patient Care,* 30, 94-127.

Dowsett, G. (2003). Some considerations on sexuality and gender in the context of AIDS. *Reproductive Health matters,* 11(22), 21-29.

Fox, A.J. & Coldblatt, P.O. (1982). *Longitudinal Study: Socio-demographic Mortality Differentials 1971-1975 in England and Wales.* London, UK: HMSO.

Frasca, T. (2003). Men and women-still far apart on HIV/AIDS. *Reproductive Health matters,* 12(23), 12-20.

Freeman, H.P. (1993). Poverty, race, racism and survival. *Annual Epidemiology,* 3, 145-149.

Garcia-Sanchez, I. & Rivadeneyra, A. (2003). Best practices for the prevention of HIV/STIs in women in the general population in Europe. In (I. Garcia-Sanchez, L. van Mens, A. Rivadeneyra, & M. de Schutter, Eds.), *Best Practices in HIV/AIDS and STI prevention for women in Western Europe* (pp 7-14). Women's network PHASE. Utrecht: Plantijn Casparie.

Gavin, B.E., Kelly, B.D., O'Callaghan, E., & Lane, A. (2001). The mental health of migrants. *Irish Medical Journal,* 94(8), editorial.

Giddens, A. (1997). *Sociology,* 3rd Ed. UK: Polity Press.

Haour-Knipe, M. (2001). HIV/AIDS and migration: Myths and realities. In (M. Martini, Ed.) *HIV/AIDS. Prevention and Care among Mobile Groups in the Balkans* (pp. 143-149). Rome: IOM, International Organization for Migration.

Henry Kaiser Family Foundation (2004), Racial and Ethnic Disparities in Women's Health Coverage and Access to Care. Findings from the 2001 Kaiser Women's Health Survey. http://www.kff.org/women'shealth (accessed 9/7/2004).

Illsley, R. (1986). Occupational class, selection, the production of inequalities in Health. *Quarterly Journal of Social Affairs,* 2(2), 151-165.

Ioannidi, E. & Mestheneos, E. (2003). L'alterite comme obstacle a l'integration des refugies dans les pays de l'Union Europeenne. Colloque International de Sociologie: Alterite et societe. Athens, May 7-10. Insitut Francais d'Athenes.

IOM (2000). Migration and Health. *Newsletter 2,* Switzerland: International Organization for Migration.

IOM (2003). World Migration 2003. Geneva: International Organization for Migration.

Janssens K., Bosmans M., & Temmerman M. (2005) *Sexual and Reproductive Health and Rights of Refugee Women in Europe. Rights, Policies, Status and Needs. Literature Review.* Ghent: Academia Press, University of Ghent.

Le Grand, J. (1986). *Class and Health. Research and Longitudinal Data.* Cambridge: Tavistock.

Long, L. (2001). HIV/AIDS. A Gender Issue. In (M. Martini, Ed.) *HIV/AIDS. Prevention and Care among Mobile Groups in the Balkans* (pp. 175-182). Rome: International Organization for Migration.

McKay, L., Macintyre, S., & Ellaway, A. (2003). *Migration and Health: A Review of the International Literature. Medical Research Council, Social and Public Health Sciences Unit.* Occasional Paper No 12. Glasgow: University of Glasgow.

Mestheneos, E. & Ioannidi, E. (1999a). *Bridges and Fences: Refugee Perceptions of Integration in the European Union.* Final Report. ECRE Task Force on Integration. Brussels: OCIV.

Mestheneos, E. & Ioannidi, E. (1999b). Autochthonous and new minorities in Greece. In: Ethnic Minorities and Migrants. *SOSTRIS Working Paper 4.* Center for Biography in Social Policy. Sociology Dept., University East London, pp. 56-66.

Mestheneos, E. & Ioannidi, E. (2002). Obstacles to refugee integration in the European Union member states. *Journal of Refugee Studies,* 15(3), 304-320.

Minas, H. (2002). Migration and mental health. *Migration and Health,* Newsletter 1, Switzerland: International Organization for Migration.

Nettleton, S. (1995). *The Sociology of Health and Illness.* Cambridge: Polity press.

Pakulski, J. & Waters, M. (1996). *The Death of Class.* London, UK: Sage.

Peterson, M. (1999). Migration experience in an ambivalent society. In: Case Study Materials: Ethnic Minorities and Migrants. *SOSTRIS Working Paper 4.* Center for Biography in Social Policy. Sociology Department, University of East London, pp. 104-119.

Piper, N. (2005). Gender and Migration. Paper for the Policy analysis and Research Programme of the GCIM. National University of Singapore: Global Commission on International Migration.

Smaje, C. (1995). *Health, "Race" and Ethnicity.* London, UK: King's Fund Institute.

Spano, A. (1999). Migration as a process: journeys in time, space and identity. In: Case Study Materials: Ethnic Minorities and Migrants. *SOSTRIS Working Paper 4*. Center for Biography in Social Policy. Sociology Department, University of East London, pp.11-29.

Stern, J. (1983). Social mobility and the interpretation of social class mortality differentials. *Journal of Social Policy*, 12(1), 27-49.

Tabassum, R., Macaskill, A., & Ahmad, I. (2000). Attitudes towards mental health in an urban Pakistani community in the United Kingdom. *International Journal of Social Psychiatry*, 46(3), 170-181.

Tejero, E. & Torrabadella, L. (1999). Migration and emancipation: the tension between globalization and identity. In: Case Study Materials: Ethnic Minorities and Migrants. *SOSTRIS Working Paper 4*. Center for Biography in Social Policy. Sociology Department, University of East London, pp. 67-86.

Townsend, P. & Davidson, N. (1982). *Inequalities in Health, the Black Report.* London, UK: Pelikan books.

UNAIDS (1999). *Gender and HIV/AIDS: Taking stock of research and programs.* Best practice collection, Geneva: UNAIDS/99.16E.

UNAIDS (2001a). *Report on the HIV/AIDS Risk for Migrant Populations (Migrants and Refugees Have Greater Risk than Stable Populations)*, UNAIDS /13 March.

UNAIDS (2001b). *Migrants Right to Health.* UNAIDS, IOM. UNAIDS /16 E March.

UNAIDS (2004). http://www.unaids.org (accessed 9/1/2004).

UNDP (2004). *Human Development Report. Cultural liberty in today's diverse world.* UNDP.

Van Mens, L., de Schutter, M., Garcia-Sanchez, I., & Pinzon-Pulido, S. (2002). Current priorities and challenges to HIV/AIDS and STI prevention among women of the general population. In (L. Van Mens, M. de Schutter, I. Garcia-Sanchez, & S. Pinzon-Pulido, Eds.) *Prevention of HIV and STI's among women in Europe.* (pp. 133-135). Women's network PHASE. Utrecht: Plantijn Casparie.

Westermeyer, J. & Wahmanholm, K. (1996). Refugee children. In (R.J. Apfel & B. Simon, Eds.). *Mine Fields in Their Hearts: The Mental Health of Children in War and Communal Violence* (pp. 75-103). New Haven, CT: Yale University Press.

WHO (1998). *Health Issues of Minority Women Living in Western Europe.* WHO Meeting (November 21-25, 1997) Report, Copenhagen: World Health Organization.

# Chapter 4

# Social Networks, Social Capital, and HIV Risks Among Migrants

VARDA SOSKOLNE, PH.D.

## Introduction

Migration has become a global phenomenon, encompassing massive numbers of people in different parts of the world and has become one of the most important determinants of global health and social development (Carballo, Divino, & Zerci, 1998). The majority of migrations within or between countries involves people moving from less to more economically developed countries or regions. These types of migration are highly selective from a health point of view, termed the 'healthy migrant' selection: unhealthy persons are less likely to move, while the immigrants are healthy, and are even generally healthier than native populations in the new country, showing lower rates of chronic diseases and disabilities (Chen, Ng, & Wilkins, 1996). Despite this apparent advantage, immigrants are vulnerable to other health problems that often arise from social conditions created after immigration, particularly communicable diseases, such as tuberculosis (TB), sexually transmitted infections (STIs) and HIV/AIDS (Carballo et al., 1998). Mobility and migration have thus become an important factor in the global spread of HIV (Haour-Knipe & Rector, 1996). It is one of the structural factors within an ecological perspective that views the risk for disease in general, and to HIV in particular, as arising not only from individual factors but from a combination of factors that determine social vulnerability to disease (Parker, 1996). The social environment is, therefore, crucial to an immigrant's adjustment and integration and in determining outcomes in terms of health status.

Within the social environment, the nuclear family and larger kin and non-kin networks comprise the core systems in which an individual adopts a value orientation and the belief systems that shape the patterns of behavior towards life issues, one of which is health. Among immigrants, these values, beliefs and health behaviors can break down or become inadequate. One of the approaches in international migration theories views migration as an ongoing social process spanning space and time. Networks are developed between places of origin and destination as the microstructures at its core (Massey, Arango, Hugo, Kouaouci, Pellegrino, & Taylor, 1993). These networks provide pre- and post-migration information, support and assistance at the country of destination in many life domains. It is, therefore, reasonable to conclude that in all types of migration, whether voluntary or involuntary, legal or illegal, permanent or temporary, within or between countries, social networks shape the behaviors, including HIV risk behaviors, of migrants.

This chapter reviews several theoretical and empirical domains in order to understand the role of social networks and support to HIV/AIDS within the context of migration. The review includes the theoretical concepts of social networks, social support and social capital and research findings of these factors among migrant populations – their social relationships and health in general, and the role of social and sexual networks in HIV risk. A conceptual framework of the pathways that link social networks to health and HIV within the context of migration is presented. Focusing on voluntary temporary migration (e.g., migrant workers) or permanent immigration, the presentation will expand on these societal and interpersonal factors among migrants, their contribution to migrants' HIV vulnerability and other STIs, and the relevant implications for practice.

# Dimensions of Social Relationships

## Social Networks, Social Support and Social Capital

Social support has been conceptualized in *structural* terms as social networks, the objective existence of and interconnections between social ties, referring to the number and sources of support and the frequency of contact, and in *functional* terms, as the perceptions of the availability or adequacy of support (House, Landis, & Umberson, 1988). While networks and support measure the degree of integration in a social system at the individual level the concept of social capital is a dimension of the whole community. It is a feature of collective relationships that act as resources for individuals and facilitate collective action (Kawachi & Berkman, 2000).

Social Networks

Social networks are studied using network analysis methods that focus on the characteristics of *the patterns of ties* between actors in a social system. The information is gathered from the standpoint of a sample of focal persons in terms of network composition (e.g., age or gender), structure (e.g., which of the network members directly tied to a focal individual are also tied directly to each other), and content (e.g., the flow of specific resources between the network members) (Hall & Wellman, 1985). Such information provides data on the dyadic ties as well as on the overall networks in which these ties are embedded. Accordingly, measures of ties describe interaction that occur within the network and include, for example, strength (the quantity of resources), frequency, duration, multiplexity (the number of different resources exchanged), or reciprocity. Measures of the network include, for example, size, intensity (extent to which social relationships offer emotional closeness), density (the extent to which network members know and interact with each other), or homogeneity (the number of network members who have similar personal attributes, e.g., gender, mobility), as well as geographic dispersion, (Hall & Wellman, 1985; Heaney & Israel, 2002).

Another network conceptualization refers to "strong" and "weak" ties. Strong ties are formed between those who share similar characteristics and lifestyles, promote group solidarity and are socially valuable. Weak ties, however, which involve contacts with extended, non-intimate network ties, are not always less socially valuable as they may link individuals to other social networks for attainment of information or other benefits (Granovetter, 1973). In the last decade, the rapid increase in the use of the Internet worldwide has become an important factor in shaping the formation of social networks and the relevance of weak ties in many life domains. Face-to-face contacts are no longer the only way by which networks are formed and maintained.

Network analysis, employed for studying information networks and sexual networks, is particularly relevant for the understanding of transmission of health beliefs, knowledge and behaviors. The spatial extent of information networks may follow social and kinship activities as well as migration patterns (Cravey, Washburn, Gesler, Arcury, & Skelly, 2001), and are shaped by the geographic location and its infrastructure and technologies. Using simple techniques such as mapping social networks and sites in which people share their knowledge and beliefs can identify the socio-spatial knowledge network nodes for sharing information, whether in physical or in virtual space.

Sexual Networks

Social networks are the core for forming sexual networks; every sexual situation is a social transaction. Sexual networks consist of persons who are sexually connected directly or indirectly to one another. Social network analysis provides both the methods and analytical techniques to describe and illustrate the effects of sexual networks on STI transmission. The term "networks" is used in sexual network analysis in two different senses: on the one level, it is considered as a collection of individuals (dots or nodes) and sexual relationships (lines) that link persons within the network, using network analysis of the type of the individual's ties (e.g., steady and casual partnerships) and network characteristics (e.g., number of sexual encounters, density of sexual relationships). On the other level, that of mathematical modeling of sexual networks, subgroups of the population are viewed as the nodes of the network. Two nodes are connected if there is mixing between them (Krezschmar, Reinking, Brouwers, van Zessen, & Jager, 1994). Network analysis has also been applied to the study of networks among drug users (Lovell, 2002).

## Social Support

Social support is defined in more qualitative terms, usually divided into four broad types of supportive behaviors. *Emotional support*—expression of empathy, love, trust, and affection; *Instrumental support*—tangible aid and service; *Appraisal support*—help in decision-making, information that is useful for self-evaluation; *Informational support*—advice, suggestion, or information in the service of particular need (House et al., 1988). Others made the additional distinctions between the cognitive aspects of support-perception of available social support, and behavioral aspects—social support that is actually received within a specific context (Dunkel-Schetter & Bennet, 1990). It is important to add that not all networks are supportive; some ties can also be a source of conflict (Rook, 1984).

## Social Capital

Moving beyond individual level factors, social capital is a measure of social relationships at the collective level (neighborhood, community, society). Although the social capital concept has been defined differently by various authors (Kawachi & Berkman, 2000), the core concepts of social capital consist of civic engagement (i.e., the extent to which citizens involve themselves in their communities), and levels of mutual trust, norms of reciprocity and solidarity among community members (Putnam, 2000). Social capital thus refers to available resources (capital) that can accrue to people by virtue of their mutual acquaintance and recognition (social) and that can be used for a variety of productive activities (capital) (Macinko & Starfield, 2001).

In recent years, social capital has been viewed as a property of spatially-defined communities ranging from regions to states, demonstrating that in those that possess high levels of social capital, a number of beneficial outcomes are obtained. For example, lower levels of social problems (e.g. neighborhood violence and crime), better health and lower levels of mortality (Kawachi & Berkman, 2000). Yet, others argue that not all forms of social capital are positive. Cohesive communities might sometimes be characterized by distrust, fear, and exclusion of outsiders; as such, they may not be healthy for those who are outsiders or disagree with the majority (Baum, 1999).

# Social Relationships and Health

Since the late 1970s, when the first large-scale epidemiological studies showed that social ties are linked to mortality, numerous studies added compelling evidence that having larger social networks and greater support is associated with better psychological and physical health conditions (Heaney & Israel, 2002; House et al., 1988). Social relationships operate through multiple social and biological pathways, and have a general effect of decreasing vulnerability to disease (Berkman & Glass, 2000). They can have a direct effect on health by meeting the basic human needs for affection, contact and security, and by reducing interpersonal conflict and tension, thereby reducing stress. The second mechanism by which social relationships operate is by having a buffering (modifying) effect on the association between stress and health. Mobilizing social ties in the presence of stressors protects the individual from the detrimental effects of stress and provides access to goods and services that influence health behavior and health status (Berkman & Glass, 2000).

Social networks, the core of social relationships, can inspire health behaviors. They may act as the sources of new information by means of the norms and values they transmit to their members, or they can actively advocate on behalf of their members, (e.g., by seeking care services and other resources), or by providing the needed services themselves (Hall & Wellman, 1985). However, social networks may also have the potential to be detrimental to health, such as during breakdown of traditional values regarding health behaviors, and adoption of deleterious behaviors within a network. At the community level, higher levels of social capital *per se,* measured by norms of reciprocity and trust in social networks were associated with better self-assessed health and lower mortality rates (Kawachi & Berkman, 2000), as well as with STIs and AIDS (Holtgrave & Crosby, 2003).

Based on previous theories and models that posit that there are multiple factors that influence one another, and ultimately, the health of the individual, several ecological models have been proposed. These models conceptualized the role of social networks in the transactions between the individual and the environment, incorporating biological pathways in a social context. Berkman and Glass (2000) proposed a cascading causal process from the macro-social structural conditions (e.g., socio-economic, cultural, social change) through social networks at the mezzo-level, and psychosocial micro-level mechanisms (e.g., social support, person-to-person contact, access to resources) that impact health via psychological, behavioral, and physiologic pathways. Others outlined reciprocal relationships of social networks and social support to health via stressors, individual and community resources, and health behaviors (Heaney & Israel, 2002).

## Migration, Social Relations, and HIV

While the complex interconnections of social networks with health are not unique to a specific population, they are particularly relevant to migrant populations. Migration is a major social structural factor, often the result of social, economic or political changes that are linked to additional macro-level factors, such as poverty and inequality. Immigrants are "at risk for risks" (Link & Phelan, 1995); individuals who are poor, less educated, or socially isolated are more likely to engage in a wide range of health risk-behaviors, and to have limited resources to cope with disease. Such vulnerability is particularly relevant for understanding the risk of migrants to HIV infections. Higher infection rates have been reported among various immigrants to other countries or internal migrants (e.g., Gras, Weide, Langendam, Coutinho, & van den Hoek, 1999; Kaplan, Kedem, & Pollack, 1998; Thawatwiboonpol-Entz, Prachuabmoh-Ruffolo, Chinveschakitvanich, Soskolne, & van Griensven, 2000). Moreover, higher HIV rates in regions with high out-migration indicate that migration increases vulnerability to HIV, both for those who migrate and for their partners back home (Lurie, Williams, Zuma, Mkaya-Mwamburi, Garnett, Sweat, Gittelsohn, & Karim, 2003). With the recognition that HIV/AIDS has become a disease of the poor and the socially disadvantaged, including migrants (Gillies, Tolley, & Wolstenholme, 1996), the understanding of risk for HIV shifted from the earlier conceptualization as an individual risk to social vulnerability (Parker, 1996), and to combined ecological models (Sumartojo, 2000).

A conceptual model to explain the social vulnerability of migrants or immigrants to HIV infections was previously outlined (Soskolne & Shtarkshall, 2002). Nevertheless, the role of social networks has not been fully explored, despite the salience of social network analysis to the understanding of the spread of STI and HIV infections. The fundamental network hypothesis posits that the probability of *acquiring* and of *transmitting* such an infection is a function of partner choice and sexual practices, behaviors that take place within a social context—within a network of persons, that influences the risk of transmission and the propagation of disease (Rothenberg, 2001). Studies about social and sexual network analyses among other populations vulnerable to HIV infections (e.g., drug users, low-income women, and gay men), clearly demonstrated the importance of studying the role of social networks among immigrants.

## A Conceptual Framework of Pathways Linking Migration, Social Networks and HIV

An expanded conceptual framework is presented in Figure 4.1. It views social networks as a central link between migration and other structural and community factors, individual level factors and HIV infection. At the macro level, the vulnerability of migrants to HIV is influenced by the interconnectedness of migration with other social structural factors that facilitate HIV transmission, such as lower socio-economic status, limited power, and discrimination in the new society (Gillies et al., 1996; Parker, Easton, & Klein, 2000). Migration may thus lead to HIV risk via proximal, intermediate-level factors of social capital and community resources, and via shaping the structure and types of social networks at the individual level. The networks may be directly linked to sexual and other HIV-related risk behaviors, or are dynamically linked to these behaviors due to limited social support or other depleted psychological factors (e.g., self-esteem, coping, inadequate health

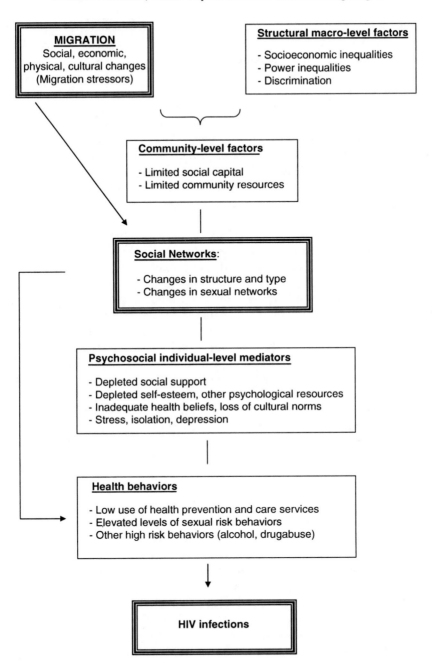

FIGURE 4.1. Framework of the associations between migration, social networks and HIV

beliefs), and higher levels of stress and psychological reactions (depression and isolation). The combination of these factors is thus associated with higher levels of HIV infection among migrants.

This framework is anchored in epidemiological models that view emerging infectious diseases, such as HIV/AIDS, as resulting from changes in the equilibrium between the agent (HIV), the host (the individual) and the environment. The proposed framework outlines how migration as an environmental factor is associated with infection via changes in the host (the social and sexual networks, sexual behavior), as well as via the spread of various strains of HIV. Migration can affect all the parameters (agent and host related) that determine the spread of HIV infections, as outlined in Anderson and May's (1991) model. Epidemic spread of HIV or other STIs requires a high reproductive rate (number of secondary cases generated by one primary case), which is determined by transmissibility of the virus, the duration of infectiousness, and the rate of change of sexual partners.

It is important to note that the proposed conceptual framework does not claim to encompass all the potential complex associations of HIV infections within the context of migration, but to outline the plausible connections between key variables. Furthermore, some of the associations are potentially bidirectional. In some countries, social networks have shaped migration patterns, so that out-migration has become a "culture of migration", such as in Jews from the former Soviet Union (Gitelman, 1997), or in Mexican communities (Kandel & Massey, 2002). In other populations, there may be out-migration of ill or HIV-infected persons to areas of lower infection rates in search for better care. Even so, the model presents the direction of the associations as related to health and risk for HIV post migration.

The following sections detail the available data among migrants regarding the pathways in the conceptual framework.

## Social Capital

Many authors have argued (see the review by Szreter & Woolcock, 2004) that social capital provides a missing causal link between social inequality and health. Migrants wishing to claim resources by virtue of being members of a particular social organization (having social capital), may find that these resources have become depleted. The migrants experience disruption of their old social and family systems, and have feelings of alienation, distrust and less solidarity. In addition, they suffer from a limited capacity to access social organizations and inability to create social capital in their new society (McMichael & Manderson, 2004). Although in some immigrant populations, where the motivation to migrate is transmitted across generations and among people through social networks (Kandel & Massey, 2002), social capital within their own community is high, it is often restricted, and without access into the larger society. Limited social capital and feelings of social alienation are often coupled with discrimination, stigmatization, and racism (O'Brien & Khan, 1996), which also characterize the HIV epidemic. Additionally, the sources of social capital are also important; not all are beneficial in terms of lower HIV-related risk. For example, social capital measured as organizational membership among internal migrants had positive benefits in terms of financial empowerment and social support, yet it had a negative effect on sexual health and HIV infections in certain age and gender groups, as it was associated with alcohol consumption and casual sex (Campbell, Williams, & Gilgen, 2002).

Social Networks of Migrants and Immigrants

Despite the high diversity of immigrant populations in various countries, the type and structure of their social networks are generally similar. Those are primarily composed of other immigrants—close and extended family members when they migrate to join their relatives, or other immigrant peers and friends when migrating alone. Often, the immigrants have fewer contacts in the larger society, as shown among immigrants from the former Soviet Union in Israel (Litwin, 1995; Soskolne, 2001), mainland Chinese immigrants in Hong Kong (Wong, 2002), Somalis in Australia (McMichael & Manderson, 2004), and Vietnamese in the United States (Gellis, 2003). Those who immigrate without their families often form fictive kin, defined as family-type relationships, based on close friendship ties that constitutes a type of social capital, and facilitates their incorporation into the host society (Ebaugh & Curry, 2000). The diverse social networks types that characterize different migrant populations may all reduce the short-term costs of settlement, providing social capital to assist the migrants in the initial stage of settlement, as well as additional organizational support from ethnic associations over time (Massey et al., 1993).

Using network analysis methods shows that these homogeneous and dense networks have both positive and negative consequences for the immigrants. New immigrants draw mainly on their informal networks of family members, relatives and close friends for different types of instrumental and emotional support (Sanders, Nee, & Sernau, 2002; Wong, 2001), and as sources for dissemination of health education messages (Levy-Storms & Wallace, 2003). However, the weakness of these strong ties may restrict the immigrants in accessing resources, such as locating only lower prestige jobs (Sanders et al., 2002), as well as in accessing health care services, in general, and HIV education programs in the larger society, in particular. This may be mainly salient among immigrant populations who rarely rely on formal networks for support except for information support (Wong, 2001), or among those who experience greater loss because of changes in traditional values and lack of social support. Thus, they may experience higher migration stress, increasing their vulnerability to infections.

## Sexual Networks and HIV-Related Risk Behaviors

The type of migration (with family or as individuals), and the ensuing characteristics of the social networks, are important in shaping sexual networks. Those who migrate by themselves tend to form multiple and concurrent (or simultaneous) sexual partnerships, that are mixed over places and type of partners. For example, male labor migrants have a higher prevalence of casual partners and of commercial sex work (CSW) partners than permanent residents in the same region, and have sex with their wives or non-CSW partners on their (rare) visits home (Campbell & Williams, 1999), comprising what was termed as "bridge populations" (Morris, Podhisita, Wawer, & Handcock, 1996). Those who migrated with the family usually behave differently. The availability of a regular partner is, probably, a protective factor. Yet, this is not true for all, since risky patterns also exist among migrant couples. For example, among married or cohabiting monogamous women, the sexual networks of their (unfaithful) partners, combined with a low use of condoms, put them at high risk (Salabarria-Pena, Lee, Montgomery, Hopp, & Muralles, 2003). Such concurrent (or simultaneous) sexual partnerships—not only the rate of partner acquisitions—contribute to propagation of HIV infection in a population, more than in serial monogamy pattern (Morris & Kretzschmar, 1997). A more in-depth examination of migrant risk behaviors reveals the significance of the type of social networks in creating sexual networks. Those who were members of stokvels (rotating credit associations) were found to have higher rates of risk behaviors and HIV infections than members of sports clubs, youth clubs, burial societies and churches (Campbell et al., 2002).

Studies among other populations vulnerable to HIV infections have demonstrated how network risk factors contribute to HIV transmission. Among drug users, networks composed of substance users and fewer kin (Lovell, 2002) or location in the densest part of a network (Nyamathi, Leake, Keenan, & Gelberg, 2000) were associated with risky behaviors, including exchanging sex for money or drugs. Similarly, network size and network density were associated with sexual risk behaviors among men who have sex with men (MSM) (e.g., Smith, Grierson, Wain, Pitts, & Pattison, 2004). Yet, even networking in virtual space may increase risk. Seeking sexual intercourse on the Internet, often followed by meeting in public restrooms was a risk factor for HIV infection among MSM (Rhodes, DiClemente, Cecil, Hergenrather, & Yee, 2002). The Internet makes it easier for people to find new partners, but information on sexual history is required only by some sites among those targeted at MSM (Wohlfeiler & Potterat, 2005). When no such information is provided, the potential for mixing of high and low-risk networks is elevated.

Network structure may be protective when it does not foster active propagation, thus contributing to low prevalence of HIV despite continued presence of sexual and drug-using risky behaviors (Rothenberg, Potterat, Woodhouse, Muth, Darrow, & Klovdahl, 1998). A hybrid pattern of dendritic risk networks (characterized by linear chains of connections with additional partners connected to each node, but not to each other usually associated with stable epidemic) and cyclic networks (which contain significant numbers of small groups of interconnected people and is associated with accelerating transmission) was associated with moderate HIV transmission (Potterat, Muth, Rothenberg, Zimmerman-Rogers, Green, Taylor, Bonney, & White, 2002). Identification of these patterns among immigrants is crucial for understanding how they contribute to elevated risk for HIV infections. Among populations who emigrate in family groups or among those who are less acculturated, sexual networking occurs predominately within the migrant population, most probably in a more cyclic network pattern. Some anecdotal evidence for such "sexual segregation" is known for the Ethiopian immigrants in Israel and may have contributed to increases in HIV prevalence rates (Kaplan et al., 1998). Among migrant workers, frequent visits to CSWs, often in the same locations, may represent another form of cyclic networks related to HIV infection (Thawatwiboonpol-Entz et al., 2000). While the current available data on sexual mixing patterns among migrants may suggest that cyclic sexual networks are more prevalent than dendritic networks, additional studies should examine them in more detail. These studies should further examine the use of the Internet for sexual networking among migrants. Those who have access to the Web may also take advantage of the anonymity it offers and expose themselves to higher risk for HIV.

### Social Support, Stress, Psychosocial Resource, Cultural Norms and Risk Behaviors

From a stress theory perspective (Lazarus & Folkman, 1984), life events leading to migration and the daily migration-related hassles of having to deal with continuous changes, depleted social capital and problematic cross-cultural interactions in a foreign environment, are stressful. The risk of HIV is just one of many stressors, often perceived as less important than others. Moreover, economic as well as psychosocial resources, such as social support, self-esteem, and control might be limited or inappropriate to the new social context. The role of social networks is, therefore, central.

The structure of networks can affect the extent to which migrants have direct or indirect access to supportive resources. Densely knit networks are structurally efficient for conserving existing, more sparsely knit resources; loosely bound networks are more efficient for accessing new and more varied resources (Hall & Wellman, 1985). Immigrants, particularly the less acculturated ones, are more likely to have densely knit networks that do not provide resources into the larger society, or are limited in the social support they can provide. This may limit immigrants' access to existing HIV prevention services in the new society, increasing the risk of exposure to HIV and their capacity to cope with it effectively. The evidence for this is still limited and not straightforward. Diverse social networks may provide greater access to support resources on the one hand, but on the other hand, such networks increase the likelihood of risky sexual networks among immigrants. For example, a study among young Latino gay men showed that lower social support in sexual matters and lower ethnic community attachments were associated with higher likelihood of engaging in unprotected anal intercourse (O'Donnell, Agronick, San Doval, Duran, Myint, & Stueve, 2002). Hence, the pathway from social networks to personal risk may involve limited personal resources that further impact on access to preventive health care programs and are insufficient to buffer the impact of migration stressors. These may be expressed in subsequent risky sexual behaviour, as well as in comprised biological host resistance in stressed immigrants, increasing their vulnerability to infections.

Culturally specific attitudes, norms, or values of the social networks of the immigrants may further explain HIV vulnerability. Norms of HIV risk and protective behaviors in countries of origin may differ considerably from norms in the new country. Many cultures frown upon open discussion of HIV and AIDS, as was found among Asian immigrants in the USA (Yoshikawa, Wilson, Hsueh, Rosman, Chin, & Kim, 2003) or Ethiopian immigrants in Israel (Soskolne & Shtarkshall, 2002). This may be because of strong taboos against discussion of the primary HIV risk behaviors—sexual intercourse (particularly among men), and injection drug use. On the other hand, other cultural values, such as the importance of familial interdependence, determine the support from family members regarding health issues, including HIV protective behaviors among Asian gay men (Choi, Kumekawa, Dang, Kegeles, Hays, & Stall, 2000). For immigrant women, the opinion of their social networks of female friends and family members were a major determinant of norms towards condom use, and subsequently their intention to use condoms (Salabarria-Pena et al., 2003). Immigrants may exhibit differential acculturation to a variety of communities as represented by members of social and sexual networks with which immigrants have contact. So far, findings regarding the relation of acculturation to risk behaviors are inconclusive. For example, among Latino immigrants, lower acculturation was related to a lower use of condoms among MSM (O'Donnell et al., 2002) and women (Salabarria-Pena et al., 2003), but also to a lower number of partners. These findings suggest that membership in a social network is not sufficient to explain HIV-related risk behavior. The network norms concerning condom use or drug use are the significant determinants of HIV risk behavior and subsequent levels of HIV seroprevalence in the immigrant community.

## Social Networks and Support Among Immigrants Living with HIV

While the conceptual model presented here relates to risk for HIV infection, social networks have a major role in coping, adjustment and sexual behavior of people living with HIV. Data on the role of networks among HIV-positive immigrants is scarce. Evidence from diverse populations of HIV-infected persons have shown that social support moderates risk behaviors (Kimberly & Serovich, 1999), and enhances adherence to highly active antiretroviral therapy (HAART) (Murphy, Marelich, Hoffman, & Steers, 2004), while poor or unsupportive contacts are linked to higher depressive symptoms (Schrimshaw, 2003) and to a more rapid progression to AIDS (Leserman, Petitto, Golden, Gaynes, Gu, Perkins, Silva, Folds, & Evans, 2000). Support cannot be provided unless the networks are informed about HIV status, a very difficult task for most people living with HIV, particularly those from stigmatized groups. Studies among gay men show that the majority disclose their HIV status to friends or main partners more than to their parents, and similar findings were found in a sample of HIV-positive Latino gay men, the majority of whom (90%) were immigrants (Zea, Reisen, Poppen, Echeverry, & Bianchi, 2004). Moreover, this study showed that acculturation to the U.S. was associated only with disclosure to parents but not related to disclosure to closest friends. These findings suggest that under the shadow of a double stigmatization—of HIV and homosexuality — the men less acculturated into U.S. society may adhere to norms limiting conversation about these topics within the family. Their main source of support shifts from the strong family ties attributed to Latinos to the network of friends.

## Conclusions and Implications

The prevalence of HIV and other STIs in a population is shaped by interactions between the pathogen, the behaviors of individuals in the population, and the prevention efforts that are developed to limit its impact. These interactions within the context of migration were the focus of this chapter. The ecological model presented here, with its social networks at its center, illustrates that associating migration with HIV is a dynamic and complex phenomenon that requires understanding of the underlying circumstances and mechanisms that affect HIV-related behaviors and HIV infections among migrants. The salience of social networks as a major link in these pathways is evident, as every sexual risk situation is a social transaction. Social and sexual core networks are important in the spread of HIV infections as well as in their prevention. Migrant networks might be more likely to include persons with undiagnosed HIV infection. Thus, understanding the structures of networks at the population and individual levels is required in order to characterize each immigrant population, to understand disease transmission, to identify risk factors and individual risks and to target prevention strategies as effectively as possible. HIV risk reduction efforts need to address the particular social (and sexual) network context of a migrant population. This may enable the development of interventions that work at the multiple levels of the factors in the proposed model.

The contribution of social networks, social support and social capital concepts is central to understanding of the social diffusion of health-related knowledge, attitudes, beliefs, and adoption of health behaviors. This implies that HIV health promoting interventions should be based on social models of change, in addition to individualistic models of interventions that are only partially sufficient to change risk behavior (Friedman, Des Jarlais, & Ward, 1994). Among migrants, this means that peer group and community subcultures need to be changed and social structural barriers removed in order to decrease risk for HIV. Several social theories, mainly diffusion models, leadership-focused approaches, social movements and social environment change (Friedman et al., 1994) have already been used as the basis for HIV prevention interventions, including immigrants. Based on the first two models several channels of communication have to be employed for the diffusion of cultural change within a social system, from mass media channels that are more effective in increasing knowledge of HIV, to interpersonal channels that are more effective in changing attitudes and behavior. The diffusion must rest on the use of "opinion leaders" of varying statuses within immigrant communities as the agents of change and role models for HIV-related behavior. It may be more difficult to identify leaders in migrant communities because they are often not cohesive, or where their traditional leaders have lost their status in the new country. Thus, the potential for changing risky practices of its members by the promotion of rapid diffusion of HIV information and support of safe sex norms is further limited.

Social network analysis may be employed to identify other "opinion leaders" among migrants. The contribution of these leaders as peer educators or cultural mediators was substantial in the development and implementation of HIV prevention programs among Ethiopian immigrants in Israel (Soskolne & Shtarkshall, 2002) and among Asian/Pacific Islander populations in the U.S. (Yoshikawa et al., 2003). Moreover, peer educators are central to the identification of the type and structure of social or sexual networks that should be the focus of interventions, where and how to intervene, and whether individual, group or even Internet-based HIV health promotions are recommended. Network interventions have been successful in disseminating HIV education messages in social and sexual venues and via the Internet for MSM, and in fragmenting sexual networks online, in order to pull low-risk men away from high-risk men (Wohlfeiler & Potterat, 2005). Enlisting persons who are HIV positive or at high HIV risk to recruit network associates in their social, sexual, and drug using networks was successful in identifying more HIV positive persons than those identified by conventional approaches (Centers for Disease Control, 2005). Similar network-based HIV risk reduction interventions among immigrants at risk for HIV should be encouraged.

Even so, such interventions are not sufficient. Additional changes in the social environment are required to remove structural barriers. There is a need for an environmental and geographical approach to reduction of sexual risk since many immigrant populations live in high-risk environments, with some variation in levels of risk between groups in those environments. It is therefore, the role and responsibility of a local authority or government to ameliorate disparities, and adopt broad-based strategies. It is essential to support outreach programs that are culturally targeted for the migrant populations to provide general HIV education to all sectors of the community, along with interventions in specific subgroups. In addition, decreasing structural barriers, for example by free distribution of condoms via peer-educators or even through informal social networks rather than via health facilities, may be encouraged. It is most important, however, that governments combine open moral commitment to aid HIV prevention programs among the migrants, with the necessary financial support to initiate changes and avoid unjustified stigmatization and discrimination.

## References

Anderson, R.M. & May, R.M. (1991). *Infectious Diseases of Humans: Dynamics and Control.* New York, NY: Oxford University Press.

Baum, F. (1999). [Editorial] Social capital: is it good for your health? Issues for public health agenda. *Journal of Epidemiology and Community Health,* 53, 195-196.

Berkman, L.F. & Glass, T. (2000). Social integration, social networks, social support, and health. In (L.F. Berkman & I. Kawachi, Eds.), *Social epidemiology* (pp. 137-173). New York, NY: Oxford University Press.

Campbell, C. & Williams, B. (1999). Beyond the biomedical and behavioural: towards an integrated approach to HIV prevention in the Southern African mining industry. *Social Science & Medicine,* 48, 1625-1639.

Campbell, C., Williams, B., & Gilgen, D. (2002). Is social capital a useful tool for exploring community level influence on HIV infection? An exploratory case study from South Africa. *AIDS Care,* 14, 42-54.

Carballo, M., Divino, J.J., & Zerci, D. (1998). Migration and health in the European Union. *Tropical Medicine and International Health, 3,* 936-944.

CDC (2005). Use of social networks to identify persons with undiagnosed HIV infection—seven US cities, October 2003-September 2004. *Morbidity and Mortality Weekly Report,* 54, 601-605.

Chen, J., Ng, E., & Wilkins, R. (1996). The health of Canada's immigrants. *Health Reports,* 7, 33-50.

Choi, K., Kumekawa, E., Dang, Q., Kegeles, S.M., Hays, R.B., & Stall, R. (2000). Risk and protective factors affecting sexual behavior among young Asian and Pacific Islander men who have sex with men. *Journal of Sex Education and Therapy,* 24, 47-55.

Cravey, A.J., Washburn, S.A., Gesler, W.M., Arcury, T.A., & Skelly, A.H. (2001). Developing socio-spatial knowledge networks: a qualitative methodology for chronic disease prevention. *Social Science & Medicine,* 52, 1763-1775.

Dunkel-Schetter, C. & Bennet, T.L. (1990). Differentiating the cognitive and behavioral aspects of social support. In (B.R. Sarason, I.G. Sarason, & G.R. Pierce, Eds.), *Social support: An interactional view* (pp. 267-296). New York, NY: Wiley.

Ebaugh, H.R. & Curry, M. (2000). Fictive kin as social capital in new immigrant communities. *Sociological Perspective,* 43, 189-209.

Friedman, S.R., Des Jarlais, D.C., & Ward, T.P. (1994). Social models for changing health-relevant behavior. In (R.J. DiClemente & J.L. Peterson, Eds.), *Preventing AIDS. Theories and methods of behavioral interventions* (pp. 95-116). New York, NY: Plenum Press.

Gellis, Z.D. (2003). Kin and nonkin social supports in a community sample of Vietnamese immigrants. *Social Work,* 48, 248-258.

Gillies, P., Tolley, K., & Wolstenholme, J. (1996). Is AIDS a disease of poverty? *AIDS Care,* 8, 351-365.

Gitelman, Z. (1997). 'From a northern country:' Russian and Soviet Jewish immigration to America and Israel in historical perspective. In (N. Lewin-Epstein, Y. Ro'i, & P. Ritterband, Eds.), *Russian Jews on Three Continents: Migration and Resettlemen.* (pp. 21-41). London, UK: Frank Cass.

Granovetter, M. (1973). The strength of weak ties. *American Journal of Sociology,* 78, 1360-1380.

Gras, M.J., Weide, J.F., Langendam, M.W., Coutinho, R.A., & van den Hoek, A. (1999). HIV prevalence, sexual risk behavior and sexual mixing patterns among migrants in Amsterdam, the Netherlands. *AIDS,* 13, 1953-1962.

Hall, A. & Wellman, B. (1985). Social networks and social support. In (S. Cohen & S.L. Syme, Eds.), *Social support and health* (pp. 23-41). Orlando, FL: Academic Press, Inc.

Haour-Knipe, M. & Rector, R. (1996). Introduction, In (M. Haour-Knipe & R. Rector, Eds.), *Crossing borders: Migration, ethnicity and AIDS* (pp. 1-14). London, UK: Taylor & Francis.

Heaney, C.A. & Israel, B.A. (2002). Social networks and social support. In (K. Glanz, B.K. Rimer, & F.M. Lewis, Eds.), *Health behavior and health education.* (pp. 185-209). San Francisco, CA: Jossey Bass.

Holtgrave, D.H. & Crosby, R.A. (2003). Social capital, poverty, and income inequality as predictors of gonorrhoea, syphilis, chlamydia and AIDS case rates in the United States. *Sexually Transmitted Infections,* 79, 62-64.

House, J.S., Landis, K.R., & Umberson, D. (1988). Social relationships and health. *Science,* 241, 540-545.

Kandel, W. & Massey, D.S. (2002). The culture of Mexican migration: A theoretical and empirical analysis. *Social Forces,* 80, 981-1004.

Kaplan, E.H., Kedem, E., & Pollack, S. (1998). HIV incidence in Ethiopian immigrants to Israel. *Journal of AIDS Human Retroviruses,* 17, 465-469.

Kawachi, I. & Berkman, L.F. (2000). Social cohesion, social capital, and health. In (L.F. Berkman & I. Kawachi, Eds.), *Social epidemiology* (pp. 174-190). New York, NY: Oxford University Press.

Kimberly, J.A. & Serovich, J.M. (1999). The role of family and friend social support in reducing risk behaviors among HIV-positive gay men. *AIDS Education and Prevention,* 11, 465-475.

Krezschmar, M., Reinking, D., Brouwers, H., van Zessen, G., & Jager, J.C. (1994). Network models: From paradigm to mathematical tool. In (E.H. Kaplan & M.K. Brandeau, Eds.), *Modeling the AIDS Epidemic: Planning, Policy and Prediction* (pp. 561-583). New York, NY: Raven Press, Ltd.

Lazarus, R.S. & Folkman, S. (1984). *Stress, Appraisal and Coping.* New York, NY: Springer Publishing Company.

Leserman, J., Petitto, J.M., Golden, R.N., Gaynes, B.N., Gu, H., Perkins, D.O., Silva, S.G., Folds, J.D., & Evans, D.L. (2000). Impact of stressful life events, depression, social support, coping, and cortisol on progression to AIDS. *American Journal of Psychiatry,* 157, 1221-1228.

Levy-Storms, L. & Wallace, S.P. (2003). Use of mammography screening among older Samoan women in Los Angeles county: A diffusion network approach. *Social Science & Medicine,* 57, 987-1000.

Link, B.G. & Phelan, J. (1995). Social conditions as fundamental causes of disease. *Journal of Health and Social Behavior, Special Issue*, 80-94.

Litwin, H. (1995). The social networks of elderly immigrants—an analytic typology. *Journal of Aging Studies*, 9, 155-174.

Lovell, A.M. (2002). Risking risk: The influence of types of capital and social networks on injection practices of drug users. *Social Science & Medicine*, 55, 803-821.

Lurie, M.N., Williams, B.G., Zuma, K., Mkaya-Mwamburi, D., Garnett, G.P., Sweat, M.D., Gittelsohn, J., & Karim, S.S. (2003). Who infects whom? HIV-1 concordance and discordance among migrant and non-migrant couples in South Africa. *AIDS*, 17, 2245-2252.

Macinko, J. & Starfield, J. (2001). The utility of social capital in research on health determinants. *Milbank Quarterly*, 79, 387-427.

Massey, D.S., Arango, J., Hugo, G., Kouaouci. A., Pellegrino, A., & Taylor J.E. (1993). Theories of international migration: A review and appraisal. *Population Development Reviews*, 19, 431-466.

McMichael, C. & Manderson, L. (2004). Somali women and well-being: Social networks and social capital among immigrant women in Australia. *Human Organization*, 63, 88-99.

Morris, M. & Kretzschmar, M. (1997). Concurrent partnerships and the spread of HIV. *AIDS*, 11, 641-648.

Morris, M., Podhisita C., Wawer M.J., & Handcock M.S. (1996). Bridge populations in the spread of HIV/AIDS in Thailand. *AIDS*, 10, 1265-1271.

Murphy, D.A., Marelich, W.D., Hoffman, D., & Steers, W.N. (2004). Predictors of antiretroviral adherence. *AIDS Care*, 16, 471-484.

Nyamathi, A., Leake, B., Keenan, C., & Gelberg, L. (2000). Type of social support among homeless women: Its impact on psychosocial resources, health and health behaviors, and use of health services. *Nursing Research*, 49, 318-326.

O'Brien, O. & Khan, S. (1996). Stigma and racism as they affect minority ethnic communities. In (M. Haour-Knipe & R. Rector, Eds.), *Crossing borders: Migration, ethnicity and AIDS* (pp. 102-117). London, UK: Taylor & Francis.

O'Donnell, L., Agronick, G., San Doval, A., Duran, R., Myint, U.A., & Stueve, A. (2002). Ethnic and gay community attachments and sexual risk behaviors among urban Latino young men who have sex with men. *AIDS Education and Prevention*, 14, 457-471.

Parker, R.G. (1996). Empowerment, community mobilization and social change in the face of HIV/AIDS. *AIDS, 10 (Suppl. 3)*, S27-S31.

Parker, R.G., Easton, D., & Klein, C.H. (2000). Structural barriers and facilitators in HIV prevention: a review of international research. *AIDS, 14 (Suppl. 1)*, S22-S32.

Potterat, J.J., Muth, S.Q., Rothenberg, R.B., Zimmerman-Rogers, H., Green, D.L., Taylor, J.E., Bonney, M.S., & White, H.A. (2002). Sexual network structure as an indicator of epidemic phase. *Sexually Transmitted Infections*, 78, *(Suppl. 1)*, i152-i158.

Putnam, R. (2000). *Bowling Alone: The Collapse and Revival of American Community*. New York, NY: Simon and Schuster.

Rhodes, S.D., DiClemente, R.J., Cecil, H., Hergenrather, K., & Yee, L.J. (2002). Risk among men who have sex with men in the United States: A comparison of Internet sample and a conventional outreach sample. *AIDS Education and Prevention*, 14, 41-50.

Rook, K.S. (1984). The negative side of social interaction. *Journal of Personality and Social Psychology*, 46, 1097-1108.

Rothenberg, R. (2001). How a net works: Implications of network structure for the persistence and control of sexually transmitted diseases and HIV. *Sexually Transmitted Diseases, 28,* 63-68.

Rothenberg, R.B., Potterat, J.J., Woodhouse, D.E., Muth, S.Q., Darrow, W.W., & Klovdahl, A.S. (1998). Social network dynamics and HIV transmission. *AIDS, 20,* 1529-1536.

Salabarria-Pena, Y., Lee, J.W., Montgomery, S.B., Hopp, H.W., & Muralles, A.A. (2003). Determinants of female and male condom use among immigrant women of Central American descent. *AIDS and Behavior, 7,* 163-174.

Sanders, J., Nee, V., & Sernau, S. (2002). Asian immigrants' reliance on social ties in a multi-ethnic labor market. *Social Forces, 81,* 281-314.

Schrimshaw, E.W. (2003). Relationship-specific unsupportive social interactions and depressive symptoms among women living with HIV/AIDS: Direct and moderating effects. *Journal of Behavioral Medicine, 26,* 297-308.

Smith, A.M.A., Grierson, J., Wain, D., Pitts, M., & Pattison, P. (2004). Associations between the sexual behaviour of men who have sex with men and the structure and composition of their social networks. *Sexually Transmitted Infections, 80,* 455-458.

Soskolne, V. (2001). Single parenthood, occupational drift and psychological distress among immigrant women from the former Soviet Union in Israel. *Women and Health, 33,* 67-84.

Soskolne, V. & Shtarkshall, R.A. (2002). Migration and HIV prevention programs: Linking structural factors, culture, and individual behaviour—an Israeli experience. *Social Science & Medicine, 55,* 1299-1309.

Szreter, S. & Woolcock, M. (2004). Health by association? Social capital, social theory and the political economy of public health. *International Journal of Epidemiology, 33,* 650–667.

Sumartojo, E. (2000). Structural factors in HIV prevention: Concepts, examples, and implications for research. *AIDS, 14 (Suppl. 1),* S3-S10.

Thawatwiboonpol-Entz, A., Prachuabmoh-Ruffolo, V., Chinveschakitvanich, V., Soskolne, V., & van Griensven, G.J.P. (2000). HIV prevalence, HIV subtypes, and risk factors among fishermen in the Gulf of Thailand and the Andaman Sea. *AIDS, 14,* 1027-1034.

Wohlfeiler, D. & Potterat, J.J. (2005). Using gay men's sexual networks to reduce sexually transmitted disease (STD)/human immunedeficiency virus (HIV) transmission. *Sexually Transmitted Diseases, 32, October Supplement,* S48-S52.

Wong, D.F.K. (2001). Differential functions and sources of social support of mainland Chinese immigrants during resettlement in Hong Kong. *Journal of Social Work Research and Evaluation, 2,* 319-332.

Yoshikawa H., Wilson, P.A., Hsueh, J., Rosman, E.A., Chin, J., & Kim, J.H. (2003). What front-line CBO staff can tell us about culturally anchored theories of behavior change in HIV prevention for Asian/Pacific Islanders. *American Journal of Community Psychology 32,* 143-156.

Zea, M.C., Reisen, C.A., Poppen, P.J., Echeverry, J.J., & Bianchi, F.T. (2004). Disclosure of HIV-positive status to Latino gay men's social networks. *American Journal of Community Psychology, 33,* 107-116.

# Part II
## Labor Induced Migration and Disease Diffusion

# Chapter 5

# Economic Migrants and Health Vulnerability

Mark N. Lurie, Ph.D.

## Introduction

In the midst of an increasingly global economy, a rising number of people are migrating to work, drawing increasing attention to the health impacts of labor migration. The connections between migration and health are complex, multi-faceted, and often difficult to unravel. How has labor migration shaped current global health crises, and how will it define the trajectories of these crises in the future?

The spread of disease in societies is shaped in large part by the political, social and economic environment in which people live. Migrant labor, a paramount and growing force, creates economic inequalities and influences policies, social institutions, familial structures, sexual networks, and individual behaviors in ways that threaten both the health of migrants and that of their communities.

In this chapter we begin by briefly exploring the extent of global labor migration and its economic impact. Thereafter we discuss the links between labor migration and disease, particularly focusing on southern Africa, and examine the different levels at which labor migration can cause health vulnerability. We then present two case studies that further explore the complex association between migrant labor and health vulnerability: the relationship between migration and tuberculosis (TB) in Norway, and the role of labor migration in the explosive spread of HIV/AIDS throughout South Africa. We conclude by making recommendations for effective interventions on the local, national, and regional scales.

## The Extent of Global Labor Migration

Migrant labor is a vast and growing global force. The United Nations estimates that the number of migrants worldwide has been increasing by 4-8% annually (SARDI & UNDP, 2004). In 2000, an estimated 175 million people, 2.9% of the world's population, were migrants predominantly motivated by economic need; by 2005, that figure was projected to be between 185 and

192 million (Omelaniuk, 2005). The International Labor Office (ILO) (2004) estimated that of the 175 million global migrants, immigrants, and refugees in 2000, approximately 86 million were economically active.

Estimates of the prevalence of migration should be cautiously interpreted. Illegal and undocumented migration, which is reported to be increasing in many parts of the world, is notoriously difficult to quantify. Many migrants find employment in the informal sector, and are unlikely to be counted in some official statistics. In many countries, the extent of internal migration may be far greater than international migration, and even more difficult to measure. In China alone it is estimated that there are more than 121 million internal migrants (National Statistic Bureau of China, 2001).

Migrant laborers are a central social and economic force both where they work and in the communities that they leave behind. The ILO estimates that 96 million people living outside their country of origin send US $73 billion back to their homes each year. For example, annually US $13.3 billion in remittances is sent to India and US $9.9 billion to Mexico from migrants in the United States (SARDI & UNDP, 2004).

Economically motivated migration follows the fault lines of economic inequality within and between countries. Mexicans motivated by economic need account for most of the northward migration of Latin Americans to the U.S.: the number of legal Mexican born immigrants in the U.S. rose from 750,000 in 1970 to 10 million in 2000 (United Nations Secretariat, 2005). The recent, rapid transition of several countries in Southeast Asia to a market economy has created disparities in standards of living, leading to increased migration within and between these countries (UNAIDS & IOM, 1998). In many regions, better economic and educational opportunities in cities lure rural workers to urban environments (Montgomery, Stren, Cohen & Reed, 2003).

A potent example of how economic disparity drives migration is the flux of health care workers—doctors, pharmacists, and nurses—out of resource poor settings. A recent study found that alarming proportions of health care workers in African countries intend to migrate: 49.3% in Cameroon, 61.6% in Ghana, 37.9% in Senegal, 58.3% in South Africa, 26.1% in Uganda, and 68% in Zimbabwe (Awases, Gbary, Nyoni & Chatora, 2004). Prior to Lithuania's entry into the EU, the Lithuanian Department of Health found that 61% of doctors in training and 27% of current doctors planned to work abroad once Lithuania joined the EU; among those, 15% of doctors in training and 5% of practicing doctors firmly intend not to return (Krosnar, 2004). Factors driving this migration include better training opportunities, higher income and efforts by countries in the developed world to fill vacant positions in their own health care systems (Bala, 2005; Chaguturu & Vallabhaneni, 2005; Krosnar, 2004). The loss of health care workers leaves crippling gaps in health care systems of developing countries already struggling to combat mounting health crises, such as TB and AIDS (Schubert, 2003).

# Labor Migration and Health: Levels of Causation

Historically, population movement has played a significant role in the spread of disease. Notably syphilis, carried across the Atlantic by colonialists, played a key role in decimating the Native American population (Brandt, 1985; Patterson & Runge, 2002). Colonial forces, in turn, faced high mortality rates from new exposure to diseases in India, the South Pacific, Africa, and the Americas (Curtin, 1989).

Today, given the interconnection of the global economy, the association between mobile populations and the spread of disease is just as strong, if not more so, than during the colonial era (Denduangboripant, Wacharapluesadee, Lumlertdacha, Ruankaew, Hoonsuwan, Puanghat, & Hemachudha, 2005; Dougan, Payne, Brown, Fenton, Logan, Evans, & Gill, 2004; Fagbo, 2002; Lurie, 2000; Poudel, Okumura, Sherchand, Jimba, Murakami, & Wakai, 2003; Reyburn, Rowland, Mohsen, Khan, & Davies, 2003; White, 2003). For example, the incidence of Mucocutaneous leishmaniasis in the Cuzco region of Peru increased after a gold rush beginning in 1975 drew scores of migrant laborers into the leishmaniasis-endemic region of Madre de Dios (Guthmann, Calmet, Rosales, Cruz, Chang, & Dedet, 1997; Triteeraprapab & Songtrus, 1999). During the 2003 SARS outbreak, the Chinese government was particularly concerned about the potential role of migrants spreading SARS to new areas (Biao, 2004). More recently, the highly pathogenic H5N1 avian flu virus has sparked renewed concern about the potential for the rapid spread of a highly infectious disease (Aldhous & Tomlin, 2005; Fouchier, Kuiken, Rimmelzwaan, & Osterhaus, 2005; Meltzer, 2004; Stohr & Esveld, 2004).

Labor migration unfolds in a vast diversity of patterns and conditions in different industries and different regions. Amidst various forms of migrant labor, certain common conditions and structures link migrant labor and disease vulnerability. Here, we examine three different levels of disease causation operating in migrant settings: superstructural, structural, and environmental (Sweat & Denison, 1995).

## *Superstructural Factors: Poverty and Social Marginalization*

Superstructural forces are macro social, economic, and political forces that shape the distribution of resources and opportunities. Labor migration emerges from and creates systems of economic inequality, political oppression, marginalization, and social fragmentation, all of which can render migrants at greater risk of sexual coercion, unhealthy working and living conditions, and exploitation and violence. Women, in particular, are at risk, and in many countries appear to comprise the majority of informal, trans-border traders. Although migration provides opportunities for women's economic empowerment, it can also render them socially and economically vulnerable, and consequently at risk for contracting STIs (Ybanez, 1999a). Some female traders, such as those crossing the border between Haiti and the Dominican Republic, may be coerced into sex to obtain passage from customs officials at border crossings (Inter-American Commission on Human Rights, 1999; Severino & de Moya, 1999; Wilson, 2001). Female migrant farm laborers often cannot report sexual abuse, sexual coercion, and rape on commercial farms for fear of losing their jobs (Crush, Mather, Mathebula, Lincoln, Maririke, & Ulicki, 2000).

## Structural Factors: Laws, Policies, and Regulations

Structural factors—laws, policies and regulations—enforce and perpetuate the systems of inequality and oppression that place migrants at risk. Few governments have instituted policies protecting the legal rights of migrants and providing them with health education and services (Duckett, 2001). For example, rarely do domestic workers have any kind of written contract, paid leave, benefits or medical aid, and they are frequently subject to poor living and working conditions, harassment, and abuse (Beresford, 1998; Hubbard & Girvan, 1996). Sometimes, in countries such as the U.S., Costa Rica, and Singapore, even the valid legal status of a domestic worker does not necessarily ensure that they are covered by all national labor laws (Piper, 2005).

In places where government policies do formally protect the health rights of migrants, these policies are often inadequate or may not be properly implemented. A study of two counties in South Florida found that commercial farms did not adequately implement state and federal laws regarding pesticide exposure, and failed to report cases of farm workers suffering symptoms of pesticide poisoning (Murphy-Greene, 2002). Even if offered health services by host countries, migrants often bear the brunt of the treatment costs (Piper, 2005).

Without legal rights, migrants may feel reluctant to seek out formal health services (Duckett, 2001). Some employers of migrant laborers use illness as grounds for dismissal, driving migrant workers to self-medicate and avoid formal health services (Ybanez, 1999b). For example, in the South African gold mines, there are examples of workers who became too sick to work having been "retrenched" absolving mining companies of the expense of their treatment.

## Environmental Factors: Conditions of Living, Working, and Moving

The environment in which migrant laborers move, work, and live is largely shaped by systems of social and economic inequality, as poverty, discrimination, and lack of legal protection precipitate unhealthy living and working conditions. Migrants are subject to poor working conditions, and are also vulnerable to sexual exploitation, coercion and violence from employers, host communities, and other migrants. Moreover, while the link between migrant labor and high-risk sexual behavior requires further exploration, migrants' frequent and lengthy absences from home is likely to "disrupt their familial and stable sexual relationships" (Decosas et al., 1995). The mobility of migrant laborers creates vast and complex social and sexual networks that link disparate communities. These disparate communities often have significantly different health and disease profiles—for instance, higher prevalence of TB and HIV in urban areas—exposing migrants, and subsequently their home communities, to increased risk of disease transmission.

Direct health risks arise from the paucity of regulations governing migrant working conditions. Two hundred migrant workers from several villages in the Henan Province of China acquired severe pneumoconiosis in quartz factories in Jiangsu Province because of the lack of protective measures in the mine. A 1996 study reported that as many as 70,000 female workers at the shoemaking factories in China's Fujian Province had suffered from benzene poisoning (Biao, 2004). South African gold miners face a 1-in-3 chance of being seriously injured and a 1-in-40 chance of being killed by underground rock fall. Migrant farm workers can face exposure to dangerous levels of pesticides; in California, for example, pesticide-related illness is an important cause of acute morbidity in migrant farm workers (Das, Steege, Baron, Beckman, & Harrison, 2001; Reidy, Bowler, Rauch, & Pedroza, 1992).

The living conditions of domestic workers, their separation from their partners and families, their vulnerability to sexual exploitation, and their lack of access to medical care likely has a serious impact on their reproductive health and risk of STI infection. A 2001 South African study found that 36% of domestic workers live in the house where they work, while only 25% said they live in their own house (Peberdy & Dinat, 2004). Employers often place restrictions on domestic workers having male and other visitors, and prevent husbands, partners and children from living with or visiting them. Filipino domestic workers in Hong Kong report sexual advances by their employers, lack of medical attention, inadequate eating arrangements, and poor sleeping accommodations, sometimes on the floor or near the bathroom (Ybanez, 1999c).

In a variety of other migrant industries, workers must also leave their spouses, families, and communities for extended periods of time. In South Africa, more than 90% of mine workers live in single-sex hostels (Crush, 1995), often in close proximity to commercial sex workers (Campbell, 2000). Foreign workers on the mines are generally able to return home less frequently than their South African counterparts, and their partners are less likely to be able to visit them on the mines (Lurie, Williams, Zuma, Mkaya-Mwamburi, Garnett, Sturm, Sweat, Gittelsohn, & Karim, 2003a). Formal migrant labor systems that are dominated by men frequently create a market for commercial sex (Campbell, 2000; Quinn 1994). The prominence of commercial sex and alcohol-related business create conditions that render both migrant and non-migrant members in surrounding communities vulnerable to HIV (Williams, Taljaard, Campbell, Gouws, Ndhlovu, van Dam, Caraël, & Auvert, 2003) and other STIs (Kark, 1949).

Several studies have linked the early spread of HIV in Southern Africa to migrant laborers working on construction projects, highlighting the health risks faced by another sector of migrant laborers. For example, a 1992 study on the Katse Dam Project in Lesotho reported that 5.3% of construction workers were infected with HIV, compared with 0.8% prevalence in mountain villages of the region. A 2001 report found approximately 160 sex workers, daily, around a more recent dam construction site in Mohale (Wilson, 2001). In Malawi, too, road construction projects have been associated with the spread of HIV (IOM, 2003). Commercial fishermen can also work for extended periods away from their communities, families, and regular partners. These workers often frequent and support alcohol and commercial sex industries in fishing ports, rendering them susceptible to STI contraction (Samnang, Leng, Kim, Canchola, Moss, Mandel, & Page-Shafer, 2004). For example, fishermen in Sihanouk Ville, a port and fishing area in Cambodia, have an overall HIV prevalence of 16.1%, more than twice that of the general Khmer population (Samnang et al., 2004). In Uganda, the first cases of AIDS were identified in 1985 in fishing villages along the shores of Lake Victoria. Sexual networking was investigated in one Ugandan fishing village in order to better understand HIV infection dynamic (Pickering, Okongo, Bwanika, Nnalusiba, & Whitworth, 1997). Pickering and associates found that casual, paying partners accounted for 42% of sexual contacts among married women and 80-100% of sexual contacts among single women. Finally, the conditions of migrant labor can affect the health of children of migrant laborers. While remittances from migrant workers can increase familial resources and improve children's access to education, better living conditions, and health services, the familial fragmentation caused by absent parents may have detrimental affects on child health, especially in situations where extended families cannot mitigate the impact of absent parents (Collinson, Lurie, Kahn, Wolff, Johnson, & Tollman, forthcoming; Kanaiaupuni & Donato, 1999).

# Case Studies

## Migration and Tuberculosis Transmission in Western Europe

The case of TB control and migration policy in Western Europe provides a revealing example of the role of migrant labor in the spread of infectious diseases. In 2004, 10 countries from Eastern and Central Europe joined the European Union and Romania and Bulgaria joined in early 2007. Western Europe, with its better employment opportunities and higher average income, will face rising rates of immigration. As many as 3 to 4 million migrants, about half of them economically motivated, are projected to arrive in Western European countries from new member states in the 25 years following expansion (Anon, 2004).

The number of TB cases and deaths in Western Europe and other industrialized countries decreased steadily during the 20th century. However, in the past two decades these rates have stopped decreasing or are increasing in many countries, and some attribute this change to increasing migration from countries with elevated TB prevalence (Heldal, Dahle, Sandven, Caugant, Brattaas, Waaler, Enarson, Tverdal, & Kongerud, 2003). Rising rates of multi-drug resistant (MDR) TB in Eastern Europe have raised concerns that increasing migration between EU countries will result in the spread of multi-drug resistant TB throughout the continent (Dahle, 2005).

In Norway, immigration in the 1990s was almost double that of the 1980s—50,000 new immigrants arrived in the 1990s, primarily from Yugoslavia, Iraq, and Somalia. TB incidence rose significantly in Norway from 4.7/100,000 in 1997 to 6.6/100,000 in 2001. Genetic studies have allowed researchers to track the course of TB incidence and transmission. One such study found that foreign-borne patients account for an increasing proportion of new TB cases in Norway: more than 70% of TB patients between 1999 and 2001 were found to be of foreign origin, compared to 53% of cases between 1994 and 1998. Most of these cases were reactivations of latent infections that occurred before arriving in Norway (Dahle, Sandven, Heldal, & Caugant, 2003). A similar DNA fingerprinting study in Denmark found that Somalian immigrants accounted for a high percentage of TB cases between 1992 and 1999, and that 74.9% of these cases were most likely infected before their arrival. This research indicates that migrants with latent TB infections account for an increasing proportion of TB cases in both Denmark and Norway, and a similar trend might be expected in other Western European countries, too, as migration from high-prevalence countries continues to increase.

Further data from both Denmark and Norway, however, indicate the complexity of TB transmission. In Norway, native-born Norwegians were *more likely* to transmit TB to immigrants than vice versa: six out of nine outbreaks that included both foreign-born and native-born Norwegians were of Norwegian origin. Further, most outbreaks of TB within Norway were found to be of Norwegian origin, from strains that had been in Norway for many years (Dahle et al., 2003). Similarly, in Denmark, although a large percentage of TB patients were Somali, only .9% of Danish TB patients were probably infected by Somalis (Lillebaek, Andersen, Bauer, Dirksen, Glismann, de Haas, & Kok-Jensen, 2001). Thus, transmission from migrants to native-born individuals appeared to be uncommon in both countries, perhaps in part because of the patterns of mixing.

These findings have significant implications for policies aimed at addressing connections between migration and TB. Given that transmission of TB from migrants to native Norwegians accounts for such a small proportion of new cases, regulations that limit migration and the rights of migrants would hardly provide greater protection. On the contrary, such policies could further marginalize migrants and make it more difficult for them to access the care they need, thus increasing the probability that those with latent infections will develop active and infectious TB. Even if migrants were more likely to transmit TB, ensuring that entering migrants received high quality health care and TB treatment would most effectively prevent further disease transmission. While the role of migrant movement in introducing infectious diseases to new areas has been extensively documented, this case illustrates that the trajectory of transmission facilitated by migration is not necessarily straightforward, and may depend on numerous complex factors. Why did increasing numbers of TB-positive migrant workers entering Norway not lead to TB outbreaks there? Why does labor migration fuel infectious disease epidemics and other health crises in other contexts? To answer these questions, we must look deeply at the structures of migrant labor systems, and the conditions in which migrant laborers work, live, and move between communities.

## Dynamic Structures and Patterns of Migrant Labor and Disease: The Case of HIV in Southern Africa

Imperfect estimates of the prevalence of migration in Southern Africa are that there are more than 2.5 million legal, and many more illegal migrants, drawn to work in South Africa's mines, factories and farms from rural areas within South Africa and from neighboring countries (Zwi & Bachmayer, 1990). Large-scale migration to industries in South Africa is a regional issue with far-reaching consequences. Migration patterns in South Africa were an integral part of the way in which government, with the support of industry (in particular the mining industry), structured South African society from early in the 20th century. This "social engineering" culminated in the system of apartheid, which was formalized in 1948. During the early decades of the 20th century, the movement of labor was strictly controlled so as to ensure a continuing supply of cheap black workers for agriculture, industry and commerce (Wilson, 1972) while simultaneously protecting the relative privilege of white workers (Lurie, 1992). The demise of apartheid and the rise of democracy has already changed the pressures and demands for labor, and it is still not clear precisely what form and patterns labor migration will take in the new South Africa.

The dynamic nature of migration in South Africa can best be understood by examining the way in which sources of rural livelihoods changed over the course of the last century. In the mid 1930s, 40-50% of rural subsistence food requirements were still met by rural production (May, 1990). Over the next 40 years, however, remittances from family members working in urban areas increased in importance. By 1970, agricultural production in these rural areas had declined to the point where only 10% of the total income for most rural households came from agriculture, with the remainder coming from remittances by family members employed as migrant laborers. In KwaZulu/Natal, for example, by the late 1980s, remittances from migrant workers made up over three-quarters of rural household income (May, 1990).

The patterns of migration in South Africa have changed considerably over the last century. In the early decades of the last century, migrant workers tended to work in the mines or other sectors of the economy for a few years after which time they would return permanently to their rural homes. In 1936, for example, the chance that by the time a migrant was 45 years old, he would have ceased to engage in migrant labor was greater than 75% (Natrass, 1976). Today, migrant labor tends to be a more long-term phenomenon, with more frequent trips home. Several factors have combined in recent years to encourage easier and more rapid movement of people in South Africa. These include the lifting of apartheid laws that restricted the movement of the majority of the population, the development of a significant transportation infrastructure, and the negotiation of more flexible work contracts resulting from strengthened trade unions. All of these events have made it easier for people to become migrants, and for migrants to return home more frequently than they could in the past.

In several parts of the world, geographic mobility, migration and widespread population displacement have been identified as significant risk factors in the transmission of HIV (Decosas et al., 1995). A number of studies have shown that migrants are at greater risk of infection with HIV and other STDs than are non-migrants, both in South Africa (Jochelson, Mothibeli, & Leger, 1991; Lurie et al., 2003a; Lurie, Williams, Zuma, Mkaya-Mwamburi, Garnett, Sweat, Gittelsohn, & Abdool Karim, 2003b) and elsewhere (Decosas et al., 1995; Hunt, 1989; Lurie, Hintzen, & Lowe, 1995; Nunn, Wagner, Kamali, Kengeya-Kayondo, & Mulder, 1995; Quinn, 1994). In an early study of HIV seroprevalence in a rural KwaZulu/Natal community, people who had recently changed their place of residence were three times as likely to be HIV infected compared to those who had not (Abdool Karim & Abdool Karim, 1992).

Studies in South Africa conducted by Lurie and associates (2003a, 2003b) provide insight into the link between migration and HIV. HIV prevalence among migrant men was found to be 25.9% compared to 12.7% among non-migrant men, so that migrant men were 2.4 times more likely to be HIV-infected than non-migrant men. In multivariate analysis, the main risk factors for being HIV-infected among men were being a migrant, ever having used a condom, and having lived in four or more places during the course of a lifetime. The study also found very high rates of HIV among women; overall 17.5% of women were HIV-infected (Lurie et al., 2003a). The study further examined patterns of HIV concordance and discordance among migrant and non-migrant couples, offering a mirror into the dynamics of HIV transmission during a mature epidemic. Migrant couples were 2.28 times more likely than non-migrant couples to have one or both partners infected (35% versus 19%) and over twice as likely to be HIV-1 discordant (27% versus 15%) (Lurie et al., 2003b).

It has long been assumed that in the context of southern African migration, HIV transmission largely occurs uni-directionally from returning migrant men—who themselves became infected while away—to their rural partners when they return home. But if this were the case, it would be the man who was the infected partner in all migrant HIV discordant couples. However, among HIV discordant couples in this study, the female was the infected partner in 29% of the cases; this did not differ by migration status of the couple (Lurie et al., 2003b). Clearly a woman who is HIV-infected—and whose primary partner is not HIV-infected—could not have been infected by her partner. Additionally, women whose partners were migrants were as likely to be HIV-infected compared to women whose partners were not migrants, suggesting that rural transmission is playing a large role in the spread of HIV as well (Lurie et al., 2003a). The study raises questions about the sexual networks of rural women, and challenges the common assumption of uni-directionality of HIV transmission in the context of large-scale population mobility. This finding highlights the importance of understanding the rural, as well as the urban, dynamics of the epidemic, and implies that successful prevention efforts should concentrate not only on the urban 'receiving' areas but on the rural 'sending' areas as well.

These finding are particularly pertinent given the mature stage of the South African epidemic. It is likely that early in the epidemic, the role of migration was critical in disseminating of the virus from urban to rural areas, and that this role was relatively more important compared to that during the more mature stage of the epidemic (Coffee, Garnett, & Lurie, 2000). Nevertheless, migration still appears to be an independent risk factor for men at a mature stage in the epidemic, even against the background of extremely high HIV prevalence. This highlights the importance of migration as one explanation for the size and rapidity of spread of the southern African AIDS epidemic, during all of its stages.

## Recommendations for Interventions

The two case studies provide evidence for the complexity of the relationship between migration and the spread of disease in diverse settings. The South African case study highlights the impact of migration on the health of not only those travelling, but on all communities involved in the migration process. Assessing the health impact of migration in other industries and other regions is critically important; the impact of migration on disease risk and transmission is likely to be different under different migratory, social, cultural, economic and political conditions. Understanding the mechanisms behind the spread of disease through migration is an essential step toward addressing and preventing these adverse health consequences. While small-scale interventions can confront local health concerns, their effectiveness is limited, given the national and regional nature of migration.

Small-scale interventions target high-risk groups in key locations. Interventions in South African mining towns have provided STI treatment and education specifically to female sex workers, while other interventions have used peer educators as a means of stimulating discussion and debate at the workplace (Williams et al, 2003). Workplace interventions are likely to grow in importance, particularly in Southern Africa where mining companies are taking the lead in delivering effective antiretroviral therapy to HIV-infected workers. Indeed, in some work settings, industry's need for a healthy workforce has stimulated the growth of company-run health clinics, which are often better staffed and equipped than clinics in the public sector. Unfortunately, well-designed evaluations aimed at measuring the impact of such workplace programs have been few and far between.

Also on a local scale, organizing grassroots efforts has proven to be an effective means of empowering both migrants and their communities to proactively address and transform the health vulnerabilities they face. In the Cuzco region of Peru, when the government did not effectively respond to a leishmaniasis outbreak in 1975, affected migrants organized patients' associations, which provided a mutual support structure for learning about, advocating for, accessing, and taking treatment together. Within this context, these associations played a crucial role in encouraging sick, marginalized migrant laborers to seek out the medical care they needed (Guthmann et al., 1997). Some migrant workers in China are actively organizing grassroots activities through which migrant workers are taking ownership over their own health care and building alternative structures to fill the gaps in government health care services (Biao 2004).

On a national scale, policy changes can play a crucial role in improving the general living conditions of migrants, which in turn would positively impact their health. Such policies might include regulating safe working conditions for migrant laborers, ensuring that they have secure legal rights, and protect-ing them from discrimination and sexual violence. Additionally, the estab-lishment of humane monitoring systems to diagnose and treat migrants as they enter a country is crucial to protecting the health of both migrants and the communities they move between.

In recognizing the potential of infectious disease to spread along migration routes, it is important not to indict migrant workers as the agents of disease spread whose movements must be contained. If not carefully designed to promote the health of migrants and the health of the communities they move between, migration policies can have detrimental health effects by marginalizing migrants from the health and social support services they need (Duckett, 2001). A potent example of this is the U.S. internment of HIV-positive Haitian refugees in Guantanamo Bay. Following a violent 1991 coup in Haiti, 34,000 Haitian refugees were denied asylum in the U.S., most of whom were interned at Guantanomo Bay and subjected to mandatory HIV testing (Farmer, 2005). Two-hundred and sixty-eight HIV-positive Haitians were put in an "HIV detention camp," where detainees reported that they were confined to cramped barbed wire enclosures, forced to eat food with maggots, and beaten when they demonstrated to demand better living conditions. Judge Sterling Johnson, who ruled on the case in 1993, called the conditions of HIV-positive detainees "cruel and unusual punishment" (Farmer, 2005).

While interventions targeting high-risk migrant groups, such as those mentioned above, may have an impact on HIV prevention, they frequently do not address the deeper conditions that put individuals and entire communities at risk. If the chain of disease transmission is to be broken, interventions must be aimed at people both in the areas sending and receiving labor. A successful case of a small-scale intervention that addresses the problematic social structures associated with disease transmission is that of the Lonmin Platinum mine in Rustenburg, South Africa. This mine has started to replace single-sex hostels with more family-friendly housing, a move that could greatly reduce risk-related behaviors caused by the separation of migrants from their families. Mathematical models show that eliminating single-sex mine hostels would be cost-effective and could have a substantial impact on HIV transmission (Gebrekristos, Resch, Zuma, & Lurie, 2005). Today, more than 90% of mine workers still live in single-sex hostels.

Highly effective interventions will change the broader social and economic structures that make migrant labor dangerous, i.e. the roots of the connection between migration and disease. For example, facilitating local development and economic empowerment in rural and urban resource-poor areas would eliminate the need for workers to migrate in the first place, allowing them to remain with their families, communities, and social support structures. These deeper socio-economic transformations will require considerable resources, time, and political will to affect, and their greatest results will be long-term (Sweat & Denison, 1995). As labor migration plays an increasingly prominent role in shaping social and economic structures and determining health vulnerability, these more comprehensive interventions aimed at structural factors that help facilitate HIV transmission are urgently needed.

*Acknowledgements.* The author would like to thank Ari Johnson for the significant contribution he made to this chapter, and Emily de Moor for editorial assistance.

## References

Abdool Karim, Q. & Abdool Karim, S.S. (1992). Seroprevalence of HIV Infection in Rural South Africa. *AIDS*, 6, 1535-1539.

Aldhous, P. & Tomlin, S. (2005). Avian flu special: Avian flu: Are we ready? *Nature*, 435, 399.

Anon (2004). The coming hordes: fears of migration from east to west. *The Economist* (January 15).

Awases, M., Gbary, A., Nyoni, J., & Chatora, R. (2004). *Migration of Health Professionals in Six Countries: A Synthesis Report.* South Africa: World Health Organization Regional Office for Africa. http://www.afro.who.int/dsd/migration6countriesfinal.pdf (accessed 11/22/2005).

Bala, M.M. (2005). Poland is losing its doctors. *British Medical Journal,* 331, 235.

Beresford, B. (1998). Domestic Workers and the Law. (October 16). *Mail & Guardian.*

Biao, X. (2004). Migration and health in China: Problems, obstacles, and solutions. *Asian Metacentre Research Paper Series,* No. 17. http://www.populationasia.org/Publications/Research_Papers.htm (accessed 11/21/2005).

Brandt, AM. (1985). *No Magic Bullet: A Social History of Venereal Disease in the United States since 1880.* Oxford: Oxford University Press.

Campbell, C. (2000). Selling sex in the time of AIDS: The psycho-social context of condom use by sex workers on a Southern African mine. *Social Science and Medicine,* 50(4), 479-494.

Chaguturu, S. & Vallabhaneni, S. (2005). Aiding and abetting – nursing crises at home and abroad. *New England Journal of Medicine,* 353(17), 1761-1763.

Coffee, M., Garnett, G., & Lurie, M. (2000). Modelling the impact of circular migration on the rate of spread and the eventual scale of the HIV epidemic in South Africa. Poster presented at the *XIII International AIDS Conference,* Durban, South Africa.

Collinson, M., Lurie, M., Kahn, K., Wolff, B., Johnson, A., & Tollman, S. (forthcoming). Health Consequences of Migration: Evidence from South Africa's Rural North-East (Agincourt). In (M. Tienda, S.E. Findley, S. Tollman, & E. Preston-Whyte, Eds.). *African Migration and Urbanization in Comparative Perspective.* Princeton: Princeton University and Wits University Press.

Crush, J. (1995). Mine migrancy in the contemporary era. In (J. Crush & W. James, Eds.), *Crossing Boundaries: Mine Migrancy in a Democratic South Africa.* Cape Town: IDASA/IDRC.

Crush, J., Mather, C., Mathebula, F., Lincoln, D., Maririke, C., & Ulicki, T. (Eds.), (2000). *Borderline Farming: Foreign Migrants in South African Commercial Agriculture,* South African Migration Project, Migration Policy Series No.16. http://www.queensu.ca/samp/samppresources/samppublications/policyseries/policy16.htm (accessed 11/22/2005).

Curtin, P.D. (1989). *Death by Migration: Europe's Encounter with the Tropical World in the Nineteenth Century.* Cambridge: Cambridge University Press.

Dahle, U.R. (2005). TB in immigrants is not public health risk, but uncontrolled epidemics are. *British Medical Journal,* 331, 237.

Dahle, U.R., Sandven, P., Heldal, E., & Caugant, D.A. (2003). Continued low rates of transmission of *Mycobacterium tuberculosis. Journal of Clinical Microbiology,* 41(7), 2968-2973.

Das, R., Steege, A., Baron, S., Beckman, J., & Harrison, R. (2001). Pesticide-related illness among migrant farm workers in the United States. *International Journal of Occupational and Environmental Health,* 7(4), 303-312.

Decosas, J., Kane, F., Anarfi, J.K., Sodji, K.D., & Wagner, H.U. (1995). Migration and AIDS. *Lancet,* 346(8978), 826-828.

Denduangboripant, J., Wacharapluesadee, S., Lumlertdacha, B., Ruankaew, N., Hoonsuwan, W., Puanghat, A., & Hemachudha, T. (2005). Transmission dynamics of rabies virus in Thailand: Implications for disease control. *BMC Infectious Diseases,* 5, 52.

Dougan, S., Payne, L.J., Brown, A.E., Fenton, K.A., Logan, L., Evans, B.G., & Gill, O.N. (2004). Black Caribbean adults with HIV in England, Wales, and Northern Ireland: An emerging epidemic? *Sexually Transmitted Infections,* 80(1), 18-23.

Duckett, M. (2001). *Migrants' Right to Health.* Joint United Nations Programme on HIV/AIDS and the International Organization for Migration. Geneva: The Joint United Nations Programme on HIV/AIDS (UNAIDS).

Fagbo, S.F. (2002). The evolving transmission pattern of Rift Valley fever in the Arabian Peninsula. *Annals of the New York Academy of Sciences,* 969(1), 201-204.

Farmer, P. (2005). *Pathologies of Power.* Berkeley: University of California Press.

Fouchier, R. Kuiken, T., Rimmelzwaan, G., & Osterhaus, A. (2005). Global task force for influenza. *Nature,* 435, 419-420.

Gebrekristos, H.T., Resch, S.C., Zuma, K., & Lurie., M.N. (2005). Estimating the impact of established family housing on the annual risk of HIV infection in South African mining communities. *Sexually Transmitted Diseases,* 32(6), 333-340.

Guthmann, J.P., Calmet, J., Rosales, E., Cruz, M., Chang, J., & Dedet, J.P. (1997). Patients' associations and the control of leishmaniasis in Peru. *Bulletin of the World Health Organization,* 75(1), 39-44.

Heldal, E., Dahle, U.R., Sandven, P., Caugant, D.A., Brattaas, N., Waaler, H.T., Enarson, D.A., Tverdal, A., & Kongerud, J. (2003). Risk factors for transmission of Mycobacterium tuberculosis. *The European Respiratory Journal,* 22(4), 637-642.

Hubbard, D. & Girvan, L. (1996). *The Living and Working Conditions of Domestic Workers in Namibia.* Namibia: Gender Research and Advocacy Project with the Legal Assistance Centre. http://www.lac.org.na/grap/grapDW.htm (accessed 11/22/2005).

Hunt, C., (1989). Migrant Labor and Sexually Transmitted Disease: AIDS In Africa. *Journal of Health and Social Behavior,* 30, 353-373.

Inter-American Commission on Human Rights. (1999). *Report on the Situation of Human Rights in the Dominican Republic.* http://www.cidh.oas.org/countryrep/DominicanRep99/Table.htm (accessed 11/22/2005).

ILO (2004). Towards a fair deal for migrant workers in the global economy. *International Labor Conference, 92nd Session.*

IOM (2003). *Mobile Populations and HIV/AIDS in the Southern African Region: Recommendations for Action.* Pretoria: Southern African Regional Poverty Network/International Organization for Migration. http://www.sarpn.org.za/documents/d0000365/index.php (accessed 11/22/2005).

Jochelson, K., Mothibeli, M., & Leger, J. (1991). Human immunodeficiency virus and migrant labor in South Africa. *International Journal of Health Services,* 21(1), 157-173.

Kanaiaupuni, S.M. & Donato, K.M. (1999). Migradollars and mortality: The effects of migration on infant survival in Mexico. *Demography,* 36(3), 339-353.

Kark, S. (1949). The social pathology of syphilis in Africans. *South African Medical Journal,* 23, 77-84.

Krosnar, K. (2004). Could joining EU club spell disaster for the new members? *British Medical Journal,* 328, 310.

Lillebaek, T., Andersen, A.B., Bauer, J., Dirksen, A., Glismann, S., de Haas, P., & Kok-Jensen, A. (2001). Risk of Mycobacterium tuberculosis transmission in a low-incidence country due to immigration from high-incidence areas. *Journal of Clinical Microbiology,* 39(3), 855-861.

Lurie, M. (1992). *Preserving White Privilege: Industrial Unrest on the Witwatersrand, 1913.* University of Florida: Master's Thesis.

Lurie, M. (2000). Migration and AIDS in Southern Africa: A review. *Southern African Journal of Science.* 96(6), 343-347.

Lurie, M., Williams, B., Zuma, K., Mkaya-Mwamburi, D., Garnett, G., Sturm, A.W., Sweat, M.D., Gittelsohn, J., & Abdool Karim, S.S. (2003a). The impact of migration on HIV-1 transmission: A study of migrant and non-migrant men, and their partners. *Sexually Transmitted Diseases,* 40(2), 149-156.

Lurie, M., Williams, B., Zuma, K., Mkaya-Mwamburi, D., Garnett, G.P., Sweat, M.D., Gittelsohn J, & Abdool Karim S.S. (2003b). Who infects whom? HIV concordance and discordance among migrant and non-migrant couples in South Africa. *AIDS*, 17, 2245-2252.

Lurie, P., Hintzen, P., & Lowe, R. (1995). Socioeconomic Obstacles to HIV Prevention and Treatment in Developing Countries. *AIDS*, 9, 539-546.

May, J. (1990). The Migrant Labour System: Changing Dynamics in Rural Survival. In *The Political Economy of South Africa*. Cape Town: Oxford University Press.

Meltzer, M.I. (2004). Presentation at WHO consultation on priority public health interventions before and during an influenza pandemic. Geneva: World Health Organization Meeting, March 16-18 (www.who.int/csr/disease/avian_influenza/consultation/en/).

Montgomery, M.R., Stren, R., Cohen, B., & Reed, H.E. (Eds.) (2003). *Cities Transformed: Demographic Change and its Implications in the Developing World*. London, UK: Earthscan.

Murphy-Greene, M.C. (2002). The occupational safety and health of Florida farm workers: environmental justice in the fields. *Journal of Health and Human Services Administration*, 25(3), 281-314.

National Statistic Bureau of China (2001). 2000 nian zhongguo nongcun liudong renkou xin tezheng' (New characteristics of rural floating population in China in 2000). *Zhongguo Guoxing Guoli (Chinese National Situation and National Power)*, 9.

Natrass J. (1976). *The Migrant Labour System and South Africa's Economic Development, 1936-1970*. University of Natal: Unpublished Doctoral Dissertation.

Nunn, A., Wagner, H., Kamali, A., Kengeya-Kayondo, J.F., & Mulder, D.W. (1995). Migration and HIV-1 seroprevalence in a rural ugandan population. *AIDS*, 9, 503-506.

Omelaniuk, I. (Ed.). (2005). *World Migration 2005: Costs and Benefits of International Migration*. France: Clerc SAS/International Organization for Migration.

Patterson, K.B. & Runge T. (2002). Smallpox and the Native American. *American Journal of the Medical Sciences*, 323(4), 216-222.

Peberdy, S. & Dinat, N. (2004). *Domestic workers in Johannesburg: Worlds of Work and Health*. Paper presented at the "HIV and the Workplace" symposium (June). Johannesburg, South Africa: University of the Witwatersrand.

Pickering, H., Okongo, M., Bwanika, K., Nnalusiba, B., & Whitworth, J. (1997). Sexual behaviour in a fishing community on Lake Victoria, Uganda. *Health Transition Review*, 7(1), 13-20.

Piper, N. (2005). *Gender and Migration*. Geneva: Global Commission on International Migration. http://test.gcim.org/attachements/TP10.pdf (accessed 3/30/2006).

Poudel, K.C., Okumura, J., Sherchand, J.B., Jimba, M., Murakami, I., & Wakai, S. (2003). Mumbai disease in far western Nepal: HIV infection and syphilis among male migrant-returnees and non-migrants. *Tropical Medicine and International Health*, 8(10), 933-939.

Quinn, T. (1994). Population Migration and the Spread of Types 1 and 2 Human Immunodeficiency Virus. *Proceedings of the National Academy of Sciences*, 91, 2407-2414.

Reidy, T.J., Bowler, R.M., Rauch, S.S., & Pedroza, G.I. (1992). Pesticide exposure and neuropsychological impairment in migrant farm workers. *Archives of Clinical Neuropsychology*, 7(1), 85-95.

Reyburn, H., Rowland, M., Mohsen, M., Khan, B., & Davies, C. (2003). The prolonged epidemic of anthroponotic cutaneous leishmaniasis in Kabul, Afghanistan: "bringing down the neighbourhood." *Transactions of the Royal Society of Tropical Medicine and Hygiene*, 97(2), 170-176.

Samnang, P., Leng, H.B., Kim, A., Canchola, A., Moss, A., Mandel, J.S., & Page-Shafer, K. (2004). HIV Prevalence and risk factors amoung fishermen in Sihanouk Ville, Cambodia. *International Journal of STD & AIDS*, 15(7), 479-483.

Schubert, C. (2003). Nurses disappearing from developing nations. *Nature Medicine* 9, 979.

Severino, I.L. & de Moya, E.A. (1999). *Migratory Routes from Haiti to Dominican Republic: Implications for HIV/AIDS and Human Rights of Infected People.* Santo Domingo, Dominican Republic: Patronato de Lucha Contra el SIDA (PLUS), Inc

SARDI & UNDP (2004). *Situational Assessment on Migration and HIV/AIDS: A Generic Tool.* South Asian Research and Development Initiative & UNDP. http://www.mobilityandhiv.org/docs/saardi.pdf (accessed 11/22/2005).

Stohr, K. & Esveld, M. (2004). Will vaccines be available for the next influenza pandemic? *Science*, 306(5705), 2195-2196.

Sweat, M.D. & Denison, J.A. (1995). Reducing HIV incidence in developing countries with structural and environmental interventions. *AIDS*, 9 (suppl A), S251-257.

UNAIDS & IOM (1998). Migration and AIDS. *International Migration*, 36(4), 445-468.

Triteeraprapab, S. & Songtrus, J. (1999). High prevalence of bancroftian filariasis in Myanmar-migrant workers: a study in Mae Sot district, Tak province, Thailand. *Journal of the Medical Association of Thailand*, 82(7), 735-739.

United Nations Secretariat, Population Division of the Department of Economic and Social Affairs. (2005). In International Organization for Migration, *World Migration Report 2005.* http://www.iom.int/iomwebsite/Publication/Servlet SearchPublication?event=detail&id=4171 (accessed 11/22/2005).

White, R. (2003). What can we make of an association between human immunodeficiency virus and population mobility? *International Journal of Epidemiology*, 32(5), 753-754.

Williams, B.G., Taljaard, D., Campbell, C.M., Gouws, E., Ndhlovu, L., van Dam, J., Caraël, M., & Auvert, B. (2003). Changing Patterns of knowledge, reported behaviour and sexually transmitted infections in a South African gold mining community. *AIDS*, 17, 2099-2107.

Wilson, D. (2001). *Lesotho and Swaziland HIV/AIDS Risk Assessments at Cross-Border and Migrant Sites in Southern Africa.* Arlington: Family Health International IMPACT Project.

Wilson, F. (1972). *Labour in the South African Gold Mines 1911-1969.* Cambridge: The University Press.

Ybanez, R.F.C. (1999a, 6 May). Addressing the needs of families of migrant workers in the Philippines. *CARAM News*. http://caramasia.gn.apc.org/page.php?page=publications/c_issue6philippinefam&title=CARAMASIA.ORG%20::%20 Publications%20: :%20Newsletter (accessed 3/30/2006).

Ybanez, R.F.C. (1999b). *Breaking Borders: Bridging the Gap between Migration and HIV/AIDS.* Manila, Philippines: Kalayaan, Inc. and CARAM-Asia.

Ybanez, R.F.C. (1999c, 23-27 October). *Conditions in Labor Migration that Contribute to the HIV Vulnerability of Migrant Workers: A Case Study of Filipino Domestic Workers in Hong Kong.* Paper presented at the Fifth International

Congress on AIDS in Asia and the Pacific (ICAAP). Kuala Lumpur: Kalayaan, Inc. and CARAM-Asia. http://caramasia.gn.apc.org/page.php?page=publications/ Ritchie_HK_conditions&title=CARMASIA.ORG%20::%20Publications% 20::%20Papers for further information, see http://caramasia.gn.apc.org/reports/ Labor%20 Migration%20&%20HIV-AIDS.pdf (accessed 11/22/2005).

Zwi, A. & Bachmayer, D. (1990). HIV and AIDS in South Africa: What is an appropriate public health response? *Health Policy and Planning*, 5(4), 316-326.

# Chapter 6

## Military Personnel: On the Move and Vulnerable to HIV/AIDS and Other STIs

Stuart J. Kingma, M.D. and Rodger D. Yeager, Ph.D.

## Introduction

> *"Disease is woven intricately into the fabric of war. The story of one cannot be told without the other and yet, each succeeding generation of history, soldier and scholar alike, seems destined to repeat the errors of history and fail to perceive the impact of disease."*
>
> (Ognibene, 1987)

Throughout time, military populations have formed one of the largest and most mobile sectors of society. At present, the world's armed forces comprise more than 20 million men and women in active service. In an ever more contentious post-Cold War era, national militaries perform an increasingly prominent, mobile and visible role. In the late 1990s, 36 countries were actively engaged in armed struggles, eight confronted emergent international conflicts, and 13 were embroiled in internal civil disorders.

To a greater extent than in the past, national military personnel are also employed in multinational interventions in response to domestic and international conflicts. By June 2004, 16 United Nations peacekeeping operations were underway in Africa, Asia, the Caribbean, Europe, and the Middle East, involving a total of over 56,000 troops and police drawn from 97 countries. These figures may well expand, both in missions and in personnel involved, since five additional missions were, at that time, in preparation or under consideration (Côte d'Ivoire, Burundi, Haiti, Iraq, and Sudan). Figures from 2002 indicate that, in addition to UN peacekeeping operations, another 30 non-UN peacekeeping, observer, and enforcement missions were deployed in these regions.

### The Hidden Enemy for the Military: Disease and Infection

Just as militaries have always figured centrally in human affairs, disease has presented a perennial problem for military populations and for civilians with whom they come in contact. Troops may find themselves far from home in biological environments that are hostile to their immune systems, in adverse

93

physical conditions of weather, climate, and human nutrition, and in disrupted social settings that serve as ideal breeding grounds for infectious bacteria, viruses, and parasitic organisms.

During the 12th Century Crusades, bubonic plague and famine reduced one Christian army from 100,000 to 5,000 troops. In 1741, the Austrian army surrendered Prague to the French because 30,000 defenders had fallen to typhus. During the Napoleonic wars, four French soldiers died of disease to every one killed in action. In the first month of the Russian campaign alone, dysentery and typhus stripped Napoleon's Grand Armée of an estimated 80,000 men. Between 1853 and 1856, some 2,000 Crimean War combatants succumbed to wounds but more than 50,000 died of typhoid, typhus, dysentery, and cholera.

Similarly, one-half of all U.S. soldiers who died in World War I, about 43,000, were victims of the 1918-1919 influenza pandemic. During World War II, the case rate of dysentery in the U.S. armed forces rose from about 20,000 to over 500,000, of dengue fever from fewer than 700 to more than 84,000, and of malaria from about 8,000 to nearly 461,000.

More recently, malaria and dengue attacked American troops in Somalia, and UN peacekeepers were on high alert for malaria and typhus in post-war Bosnia. U.S. Air Force personnel serving in Guam have been diagnosed with leptospirosis (Worth, 2004).

Multinational forces in Kuwait were beset by sand-fly fever (leishmaniasis) during Operation Desert Storm and, by early March 2004, more than 500 cases of leishmaniasis had been diagnosed in U.S. soldiers serving in Iraq. It is the largest outbreak in the history of the American military since World War II. With large-scale military operations still underway in that country, the number of those who may become infected could reach 750 to 1,250 or more (Turner, 2004).

As products of wartime, with its political, social and economic disintegration, large refugee and internally displaced populations often share the same space and vulnerability to disease with combatants and peacekeepers. By the beginning of 2004, such conditions had produced some 17 million asylum seekers, refugees, and others of 'concern to the UN High Commissioner for Refugees (2004).

The last two decades have seen an alarming resurgence of tuberculosis (TB) throughout the world – in the industrialized West, but even more dramatically in Africa and South-East Asia. TB kills more young people and adults than any other infectious disease; someone dies of TB every 10 seconds (Aït-Khaled & Enarson, 2003). TB is also a challenging infection among military populations, many of whom live together in close quarters. TB is the sixth leading cause of death in the Philippines, and it was recently reported that the high rate of TB infection in the Philippine army is causing real concern, particularly as soldiers often move around the country and could spread the disease (BBC News, 2004). Part of the concern about the resurgence of TB is the increasing prevalence of multidrug-resistant TB (MDR-TB).

Since World War II, advances in medicine have rendered many infectious diseases less dangerous. Particularly in industrialized societies, reduced threat of epidemics has turned public health concerns more toward curative medicine than toward disease prevention. The trend is also seen with regard to a group of diseases that have always been part of military life, and especially on deployment—the sexually transmitted infection (STI).

## Sexually-transmitted Infections

The World Health Organization (WHO) estimated that 340 million new cases of STIs occurred in adults worldwide in 1999. The largest number of new infections occurred in the region of South and Southeast Asia, followed by Sub-Saharan Africa and Latin America and the Caribbean. However, the highest rate of new cases per 1,000 population occurred in Sub-Saharan Africa. Of the incidence of new STIs in adults in 1999, WHO estimated that Chlamydia infections accounted for 92 million cases, gonorrhea for 62 million, syphilis for 12 million, and trichomoniasis for 173 million (WHO, 2001).

During World War I, STIs were second only to influenza as a cause of lost productivity in U.S. forces. Between 1929 and 1939, the average time lost from duty in recovery from a case of gonorrhea was 38 to 50 days. Monthly morbidity reports from the Army list venereal disease as the number-one diagnosis among common diseases reported from 1965 to the end of the Vietnam War (Emerson, 1997).

In the past three decades, however, one STI has emerged and proliferated to pandemic proportions for which medicine has, as yet, no cure. This is the Human Immunodeficiency Virus (HIV), which results in the Acquired Immunodeficiency Syndrome (AIDS). Today, in many parts of the world, HIV and AIDS together with other infectious diseases pose a far more serious threat to militaries than the inherently hazardous nature of their occupation.

## Policy Issues

### The Military Workplace

The armed forces recruit young men and women at a time of their greatest risk to HIV, in the 15 to 25 year age group where more than half of all new infections occurs. The military risk environment is further enhanced by the mobility and absences from home and community that military life demands. In the less-developed world at least, the military workplace imposes a heightened vulnerability to HIV infection and onward transmission, with the dynamic of transmission being similar to that seen in long-distance transport workers and migrants employed in the mining sector. Military installations also inevitably attract gatherings of sex workers.

The military risk environment is further enhanced during missions that military contingents are increasingly called upon to carry out, responding to internal and cross-border armed conflicts that are so often accompanied by massive displacements of civilian populations, circumstances that create complex humanitarian emergencies. During the late 1990s, 16 such wars raged in Africa (40% of the world total) and 14 in Asia (30%). As members of regional and international peacekeeping forces, soldiers operate in infectious disease-endemic areas to assist civilian relief workers in efforts to improve public health and to restore reasonably normal social and economic activities.

Always at the top of the list among wartime and post-wartime infectious diseases are STIs. HIV is now among those STIs, and HIV is five to 20 times more likely to be transmitted in the presence of other STIs. In peacetime, military STI rates are generally two to five times higher than in surrounding civilian populations (UNAIDS, 1998), and under wartime and immediate post-wartime conditions military infection rates may soar.

And yet, militaries are still significantly excluded from the targeted bilateral and multilateral assistance that is absolutely necessary to slow the spread of HIV and AIDS (although this is now changing). In the past, exclusion might have been justified by the argument that militaries, which receive their own support, were not proper recipients of humanitarian and development assistance. Now, these militaries are manifestly part of a global humanitarian and developmental crisis. At this point the critical issues are how to convince donors completely to eliminate this deadly bias in foreign assistance, and how to convince the commanders and political supervisors of militaries to receive foreign aid to place HIV/AIDS prevention and management at the top of their wish lists.

## Command and Control

Command and control structures, central features of all formal organizations, are especially visible and important in the armed forces, and incorporate both advantages and disadvantages for HIV/AIDS prevention and management. The military's well-developed span of control and chain of command hierarchies provide the means to induce change over a wide range of behaviors. And yet changes in sexual behavior, difficult to bring about in the best of circumstances, may be especially difficult to achieve for off-duty soldiers and sailors and for troops who are deployed in operational areas. In these circumstances, it is naïve simply to rely on written codes of conduct. More proactive approaches are needed to mobilize military discipline and behavioral regulation on behalf of HIV prevention.

Two factors have further weakened the capacity of military organizations to control the spread of HIV, especially in regions like Africa where the disease has reached epidemic proportions within civilian populations. First, military commanders and medical officers respond to somewhat different mandates, with commanders more interested in maintaining deployable force strength, while medical officers are more concerned with maintaining a healthy fighting force. The second factor operating here has blurred the obvious linkage between these goals.

Unlike other infectious diseases such as dysentery and malaria, HIV is not an immediate deterrent to combat. In adults, a long asymptomatic phase occurs after the infection is first acquired. There are no symptoms during the initial "window period," which may last for up to 12 weeks, even as the circulating viral load steeply climbs and HIV-specific antibodies begin to appear. At the end of the window period, serological testing will reveal the change to "HIV-positive." The asymptomatic phase continues even as immune function begins to decline and may last for up to 10 years of physical fitness before the onset of symptomatic AIDS.

Thus, HIV began as a "slow plague" (Gould, 1993), one that initially lulled force commanders and civilian leaders into a mistaken belief that their countries were not seriously endangered by the virus. This false sense of security and indeed public denial of the problem have since all but evaporated, not least because of heavy losses within the officer corps and the civilian leadership themselves. In spite of a growing understanding of the impact of the epidemic on the security sector, however, military command commitment to HIV control remains heavily oriented toward an illusory "quick-fix" through the use of pre-recruitment testing and screening.

Practical and effective responses are absolutely vital to military commanders and to the troops under their command. Together with the Civil-Military Alliance to Combat HIV and AIDS (CMA), the UN's Department of Peacekeeping Operations (DPKO) has emphasized the pressing need to sensitize senior officers to the top priority of HIV prevention in the conduct of peacekeeping operations (DPKO & CMA, 2000). In late October 2002, the AIDS Control Organization of the Indian Armed Forces released its own *Commander's Handbook, Fighting AIDS on a War Footing* (The Times of India News Service, 2000).

A greater effort is still required, of necessity externally funded and otherwise supported, to convey the same sense of urgency and capacity for change to the command structures of Asian, African, and other resource-deprived national militaries, for within these ranks can be found the primary troop contributors to UN peacekeeping missions.

## Training and Service

Compulsory pre-recruitment HIV testing and screening (and refusing recruitment to those with HIV-positive results) is being adopted by more and more by African militaries. It has been justified partly out of concern that they cannot afford the economic loss that AIDS brings, overwhelming their medical services and necessitating major personnel replacement and training costs. The real problem, in fact, is that such militaries lack the financial and technical resources to devise and implement recruitment policies that transform

HIV's long asymptomatic period from a loss into a gain. Policy reform in this area would significantly reduce the twin evils of social stigmatization and employment discrimination and would help to maximize the overall contributions of young adults seeking military service. Without the necessary means to accomplish this end, militaries must fall back on exclusionary recruitment policies that waste human potential even as they deny basic human rights.

Particularly in Africa, compulsory pre-recruitment HIV testing and screening have also been justified partly on the grounds of a largely intuitive notion that, in and of themselves, strenuous military training and service under harsh conditions weaken the human immune system and accelerate the progression of HIV infection to symptomatic AIDS.

One report from Malawi concluded that "a soldier loses about five kilograms of weight after training which makes him/her more susceptible to infections associated with HIV/AIDS" (*The Chronicle Newspaper*, 2001). A more careful but as yet un-replicated study in Zimbabwe compared the effects of training on HIV-positive and HIV-negative army recruits. It found that after only three weeks of strenuous activity, HIV-positive recruits had smaller abdominal, waist, thigh, and calf circumferences and more abnormal blood conditions, abdominal disorders, upper respiratory infections, and the like, compared to their HIV-negative counterparts (Mudambo, 1999). Aside from the rather brief time frame allocated to this examination, the study did not consider the stage of infection of each HIV-positive subject. Blood tests for viral load and CD4 cell count were not reported. In the absence of these diagnostic benchmarks, it remains difficult to determine the impact of military training and service on the progression of HIV in the armed forces recruitment pool in Africa.

In light of the assumptions that have been made in this regard, the CMA has urged for several years that the armed forces, particularly in Africa, study this issue that is clearly important and has policy implications. Interestingly, several studies, carried out on American, Canadian, and French military trainees, were reported in the period of 2000-2003 on changes in immune functions induced by rigorous training.

The U.S. Army Ranger Training Course is one of the most physically demanding military training courses. It lasts for 62 days and involves food restriction, sleep deprivation, geographical challenges (forest, mountain, swamp and desert exposures), and prolonged low-intensity physical work. Recruits participating in this course have demonstrated a leukocytosis, a decrease in the number of and percentage of T cells (helper, suppressor, and pan T cells), a suppression of lymphocyte proliferation, a decrease in release of the soluble interleukin-2 receptor to phytohemagglutinin, an impaired delayed-type hypersensitivity skin test, and an increase in the incidence of infection (mainly, cellulitis of the lower extremities and upper respiratory infections) (Shephard et al., 2001).

Food restriction makes a major contribution to the observed immunosuppression in these demanding exercises, with energy expenditure greatly exceeding energy input. Among environmental stressors, heat may compound the exercise-induced suppression of immune function (Shephard & Shek, 2000). Likewise, cold exposure can interact with heavy exercise to augment the depression of immune function (Shephard & Shek, 1998).

The French Armed Forces reported on research designed to determine whether the immune and hormonal systems were affected by a rigorous five-day military course that followed three weeks of combat training in a population of 26 male soldiers of the French Military Officer School, (mean age, 21 ± 2 years). The combination of continuous heavy physical activity and sleep deprivation led to energy deficiency. At the beginning of the training program and immediately after the combat course, saliva samples were assayed. Secretory immunoglobulin A was lower and circulating interleukin-6 was increased by the end of the course, which was attributed to sympathoadrenergic stimulation. Dehydroepiandrosterone sulphate, prolactin, and testosterone levels fell significantly (Gomez-Merino et al., 2003).

These results suggest that prolonged and repeated exercise such as that encountered in a rigorous military training program does indeed induce some measure of immune impairment. Related studies, however, seem to indicate that basic infantry training does not appear to affect immune function in the same way. One study examined 23 male subjects enrolled in an 18.5-week Canadian qualification-level, regular infantryman training course. They found an increase in cell function (natural killer cell activity and lymphocyte proliferation), no change in cell-mediated immunity, and a relatively stable incidence of infection during the course. The conclusion was that the pattern of basic infantry training examined in this study does not compromise the soldier's health (Brenner et al., 2000). The physical component of basic infantry training is likely to have been much less than that experienced in the more specialized courses in these other reports.

In summary, there are few data to indicate the impact of this type of intensive and stressful training, with its consequences on the immune system, in relation to either the susceptibility to or progression of HIV infection. At present there is only anecdotal evidence to support an adverse and accelerated impact of military training, or military life itself, on HIV-infected individuals, but further research in this area is clearly needed.

## Deployment and Combat

It seems reasonable to conclude that length of deployment in HIV-endemic areas is independently and directly associated with risk of HIV infection. Although little empirical evidence is presently available to confirm this hypothesis, at least one case study from Africa may be sufficient to make length of deployment an important policy issue for national military and peacekeeping commanders to resolve.

During the 1990s, Nigerian ground forces were deployed as the major component of the sub-regional Economic Community of West African States Ceasefire Monitoring Group (ECOMOG) in Liberia and Sierra Leone. An epidemiological study of troops engaged in this campaign was conducted by

Brigadier General A. Adefolalu, Commandant and Chief Consulting Surgeon at the Nigerian Army Medical Command School Headquarters in Lagos. Adefolalu concluded that HIV prevalence among Nigerian Army troops increased from less than 1% in 1989/90 to 5% in 1997, and by 1999 to 10%. The years 1998 and 1999 coincided with a return of troops from ECOMOG operational areas, and among them the HIV prevalence rate was 12%. The Adefolalu study also included a comparative analysis of HIV incidence and the lengths of soldiers' duty tours in the turbulent Operation Sandstorm area of Sierra Leone. Incidence rates among these troops increased from 7% after one year in the operational area to 10% after two years, and to more than 15% after three years of deployment, for a cumulative annual risk factor of about 2% (Adefolalu, 1999).

An effective response to the length-of-deployment issue depends on whether militaries can acquire the necessary tools to lower their soldiers' risk of infection while serving in war zones made additionally dangerous by HIV. This means shorter tours of duty in conflict and immediate post-conflict theaters of operation, together with constant reinforcement of HIV prevention education, including squad-level peer education, and proactive condom promotion and distribution extending into the post-deployment period. These are not technically complicated or even necessarily expensive, but at present they are well beyond the means of most militaries in developing countries.

## Complex Humanitarian Emergencies and Peacekeeping

Once HIV has become firmly established through heterosexual contact, it can spread rapidly in societies that are at peace and where free movement of people and trade is the norm. But HIV and many other infectious diseases thrive almost unchallenged in the complex humanitarian emergencies that are created and sustained by socio-economic and political disintegration, communal strife, and armed conflict. Combat places refugees and internally displaced persons (IDPs) in situations of vulnerability to the spread of infectious diseases.

In central Africa, for example, the migration of Hutu refugees from the civil war in Rwanda to camps in Zaire provoked eruptions of cholera, dysentery, and other highly communicable diseases. Unable to address the problem effectively, Zaire pushed for the repatriation of Hutu refugees, who were reluctant to return in the face of threats from Rwanda's new Tutsi rulers. While the political game played out, the squalor of the camps continued to breed disease (Moodie et al., 2000).

By the end of 2000, the UN High Commissioner for Refugees (UNHCR) had reported nearly 5.5 million refugees and IDPs in Africa and more than seven million in Asia (Population Data Unit, PGDS/DOS, UNHCR, 2002). What had become a culture of violence partly because of HIV and AIDS also helped to extend the chances of acquiring the virus. This reflects the structural nature of the HIV risk environment for populations trapped in complex humanitarian emergencies, a risk environment that persists long after the fighting has ended.

HIV risks are extremely important factors to consider when peacekeeping forces are sent in to sustain the peace between contending parties and to help restore public order. Countries that both contribute and host peacekeepers have recognized that HIV transmission is a two-way street. Troops can bring the virus home with them and they can transmit it to comrades-in-arms and civilians in the field.

The UN Security Council confirmed these realities at its opening session on January 10, 2000. For the first time in UN history, the Council recognized a public-health problem, HIV/AIDS in Africa, as a threat to international peace and security (UN Security Council press release, 2000). Following similar alarms raised in the General Assembly, attempts were made to strengthen HIV prevention activities in the DPKO at pre-deployment training sites and for peacekeepers already in the field. Actual commitment has, however, been slow to match up to this rhetoric. HIV/AIDS prevention remains under-funded in the DPKO, which is forced to rely on troop-contributing states to provide the necessary levels of prevention education, testing and counseling, condom promotion and monitoring of use, and STI treatment. This obligation is impossible for most contributing militaries to fulfill without substantial external assistance. Bilateral cooperation to relieve the problem is specifically called for in Security Council Resolution 1308 of July 2000 (UN Security Council, 2000), but affluent UN members have been slow to respond.

In April 2000, the U.S. National Intelligence Council (NIC) released a declassified version of the Central Intelligence Agency's (CIA's) own first-ever intelligence estimate related to public health, concerning the global impact of infectious diseases. This report described the HIV/AIDS pandemic as a direct threat to U.S. national security (CIA, 2000). In late 2002, a further report issued by the NIC/CIA and a paper prepared for the independent Center for Strategic and International Studies (CSIS) focused immediate security attention on the next wave of the HIV/AIDS pandemic in the populous regional giants of China, Ethiopia, India, Nigeria, and Russia (DCI Strategic Warning Committee, 2002). Further justification should not be necessary for a substantial commitment of bilateral and multilateral assistance toward the creation and maintenance of an HIV-free international peacekeeping force. In Africa, a failure to move in this direction will result in a catastrophic loss of regional force strength, "effectively shifting the burden of peacekeeping operations . . . to non-African countries (including the United States)" (Price-Smith, 2002).

## Demobilization

The Chinese and Russian armed forces have demobilized the world's largest number of troops in recent years but, from the standpoint of HIV/AIDS prevention and management, the human stakes of demobilization are still highest in Sub-Saharan Africa. Following decades of relentless poverty and economic downturn, socio-political instability and warfare, Africa now faces the challenging issue of how to retire thousands of soldiers from duty and to reintroduce them into civilian society. The problem is further complicated by the fact that HIV incidence and prevalence rates may be higher in military than in civilian populations, and African civilian as well as military populations are already inundated by HIV/AIDS. Nevertheless, "if demobilisation programmes do not include prevention and peer counselling, the reintegration of HIV-positive soldiers into new communities and the return of combatants to their original villages may result in a major proliferation of the virus" (Mendelson-Forman & Carballo, 2002, p. 79).

In a way similar to military service itself, demobilization presents not only a problem for HIV/AIDS prevention and control but also an advantage. Regular troops and even guerilla forces are readily identifiable and subject to cantonment (temporary or semi-permanent military quarters), where HIV prevention education and counseling can be administered and where voluntary testing, care, and transitional support can be provided before they are sent home. It may also be possible to convert former combatants into fighters in the war against HIV and AIDS. According to Mendelson-Forman & Carballo (2002):

*In Sub-Saharan Africa, where the resources for HIV prevention are limited at best and non-existent at worst, the structured and externally financed demobilisation of military personnel presents a number of opportunities for innovative and creative solutions. Many of the region's armies are capable of delivering healthcare and providing community education and logistical support to villages. With sound training and follow-up supervision, some demobilised military personnel could work with active duty forces to become 'agents of change', specifically in regard to HIV prevention. They could be trained in the organisation of discussion groups, the provision of counselling and the marketing and distribution of condoms, and they could assist in carrying out urgently needed community-based surveillance of changing attitudes and behaviour regarding HIV/AIDS.*

These new functions would help to change local attitudes toward returning war veterans from perceptions of foreboding to expressions of support. They would likewise improve African governments' standing with bilateral and multilateral aid partners that more-or-less formally mandate military downsizing as a condition of development assistance, but are also concerned about the spread of HIV/AIDS that can result. The quandary is that considerable foreign aid is needed to activate this linkage between demobilization, public health and development, and here the record to date is spotty.

One of Africa's largest demobilization and reinsertion exercises has occurred in Nigeria. Although the U.S. Agency for International Development (USAID) and the British Department for International Development (DFID) provided assistance in this effort, little if any funding was assigned to HIV prevention and control (Yeager & Kingma, 2000). On the other hand, USAID and the U.S. Department of Defense are now including HIV activities in their demobilization support for African defense ministries and health-care agencies. Similar initiatives are being planned and implemented by other official development agencies (Mendelson-Forman & Carballo, 2002).

It would also be highly beneficial if the mandate of the multilateral Global Fund to Fight AIDS, Tuberculosis, and Malaria could be expanded specifically to address pressing demobilization issues in Africa and elsewhere. Item 1.10 of the Fund's official scope of action may provide an avenue for this commitment: "For areas in conflict or distress, the Fund will develop special criteria to support technically sound proposals designed to address critical HIV/AIDS, TB, and malaria problems" (Global Fund, 2003). But unless the levels of such assistance are significantly raised and applied in an informed manner, what has been invested thus far may become a wasteful example of too little and too late.

## Operational Issues

### *Prevention Education*

"With no vaccine, and no cure, education is all we have" (Gould, 1993). Written more than a decade ago by a scholar of HIV and its global diffusion, this statement remains largely valid today. When the ultimate goal is to transform behavior in highly sensitive areas of human life, simple information transfer is not the same as education. Motivational learning does not result from episodic didactic lectures and briefings, but rather from on-going interactive relationships linking teachers and students at all levels, with peer education among both groups providing constant reinforcement. Unfortunately, this is the most difficult and expensive form of learning to offer on a mass scale.

In 2000, the CMA published the results of a global survey of military HIV/AIDS policies and practices (Yeager, Hendrix, and Kingma, 2000). The survey found that, while most reporting militaries carried out STI/HIV prevention education, the majority relied on infrequent (yearly or less often) large-group briefings and on the passive distribution of written materials. Virtually no militaries reported using peer-educational techniques. The study also revealed that while 90% of militaries provided pre-deployment STI/HIV briefings to their troops, only half matched these sessions with post-deployment briefings despite long-standing evidence that the post-deployment period carries special risk of STI transmission (Yeager et al., 2000).

Notwithstanding improvements in some countries, there is little evidence that STI/HIV prevention education has broadly advanced since that survey, and for good reason. One major problem for low-income, high-incidence countries lies in finding sufficient financial resources to mount comprehensive STI/HIV and sexuality education for children and adolescents during their school years. The same resource constraint faces the defense sector which often lacks the resources to pursue full-scale, interactive and repeated STI/HIV prevention education during recruit and officer training, including before and after deployment and at military discharge. This implies that sufficient funding will have to be found to train large numbers of civilian and military STI/HIV prevention instructors and peer educators, using curricula and teaching methods that are already available and tested for effectiveness or are now being developed (Ruscavage & Purnell, 1999; Ruscavage & Yeager, 2002).

## Condom Promotion and Provision

*"In a world with an HIV pandemic, the latex condom emerges as the only practical and responsible strategy"*

(Gould, 1993)

Ensuring the maximum consistent employment of latex condoms through their widespread promotion, practical usage instruction, and ready availability is absolutely essential to breaking the pattern of STI/HIV infection through sexual intercourse. Moreover, the value of this particular weapon in the war against AIDS has been greatly enhanced by the recent development of an efficient and effective female condom. Embodying highly organized command and control structures, militaries are relatively well placed to promote and distribute these crucial barrier devices.

In the earlier CMA survey, two shortcomings that appeared then remain today. First, condom promotion methods were similar to those for STI/HIV prevention education, with most respondents mentioning only group briefings and written materials (Yeager et al., 2000). Second, there are simply not enough funds available to facilitate active condom promotion, to distribute condoms free of charge and in sufficient numbers, and to monitor consistent condom use in the armed forces.

Beyond these operational issues are questions of religious and cultural beliefs and practices that prohibit or ridicule condom use, encourage multiple sex partners, and foster invasive and usually non-sterile procedures such as female circumcision and ritual scarification. Vulnerability to HIV transmission, by civilians and soldiers alike, is enhanced by the risk-taking propensities of young men and women and the resolve-weakening effects of alcohol and drug use. Only after these particulars are understood can informed action be taken. Such has been the case in Thailand, which suffered a very high HIV incidence and prevalence rates until the early 1990s when a culturally sensitive safe-sex campaign was mounted and the use of condoms became common practice.

The theme cannot be repeated often enough: PREVENTION WORKS and the best tool that we have to pursue prevention interventions at this time is a barrier to the sexual transmission of HIV—the condom.

## Testing and Counseling

When the global CMA survey was completed in the late 1990s, experience in HIV antibody testing by African militaries was in its infancy as compared with militaries in Asia and other world regions. African militaries ranked lowest in actually having formal testing policies, in offering voluntary testing, and in requiring testing at any point in uniformed service from recruitment to discharge (Yeager et al., 2000).

Since then compulsory military testing and screening have increased dramatically in Africa. This new interest is spurred by the burgeoning costs of AIDS care, as well as the financial burden of retraining to fill the positions of people lost to AIDS. Compulsory testing and screening have likewise gained importance by the attention recently given to the deployment of African forces in UN and other peacekeeping missions, and by an admittedly unenforceable UN recommendation that these troops should test negative for HIV. This is in spite of the UN's advice that, except under very special circumstances, mandatory testing practices fail to achieve the goals to which they are addressed. The UN likewise holds that, more often than not, mandatory testing practices are in violation of basic human rights to privacy and freedom from stigmatization and discrimination.

Non-voluntary testing and screening are increasingly used to exclude HIV-positive individuals from recruitment and career advancement, and thus to preserve force readiness and deployment capacity while easing the strain on military medical and training budgets. Universal testing is also defended as a deterrent to HIV infection in countries where military service offers an important employment option. It is a means of yielding surveillance data for future efforts at HIV prevention and vaccine development. Periodic mandatory testing is also viewed as the way to identify HIV-infected serving personnel, to adjust their in-service duty assignments until such time as medical discharge is indicated, and to identify personnel and their partners for counseling and care.

The CMA survey revealed that testing in the armed forces has been widely used for protecting blood supplies, for complying with deployment and training restrictions, for promotion in rank, and for screening assignment to duties requiring high performance standards (e.g., aircraft pilots, commandos, and tank commanders). The study added that "a majority of responding militaries fail to test their personnel periodically, which raises the question, for them, of whether any of these purposes can be adequately served through testing" (Yeager et al., 2000).

Indeed, most military and civilian organizations in resource-poor countries have neither the medical capacities nor the financial means effectively and humanely to satisfy the protocols of either mandatory or voluntary testing programs. Foremost among these is the need for confidential contact tracing and pre-test/post-test counseling of HIV-positive *and* HIV-negative personnel, including their partners and families. Periodic testing for viral load and antibody/CD4 cell count of HIV-infected individuals enables military and civilian health agencies to assess the progress of infection and preserve their occupational and natural lives for as long as possible. Testing combined with counseling aimed toward employment- and life-extending treatment and care further provides an effective strategy for stemming the onward flow of HIV infection (Valdiserri, 1997).

Whether testing and counseling are compulsory or voluntary, neither will create positive effects unless rules of confidentiality and informed consent are tightly defined and strictly followed. Cases abound of social ostracism, rejection from insurance and other services, denial of job entry, and dismissal from employment simply because of an HIV diagnosis—which may be inaccurate in the first place, especially if administered only once.

Some African militaries now face a drying up of their recruitment pools as a result of their sometimes thoughtless disclosure of test information and their dismissal of still-healthy recruits, trainees, and soldiers for no disclosed reason. The problem lies in a lack of funding and other assistance (a) to train examining personnel, counselors and commanders; (b) to provide counseling for all tested soldiers and their families; and (c) to offer meaningful in-service duty options. African militaries are not insensitive to these needs. What they lack are the means to fulfill them.

## Treatment, Care, and Support

In that AIDS is, or soon will be, a leading cause of death in the militaries and civil societies of developing countries, questions arise as to the competing values of national security versus equal treatment, care, and support for all patients suffering from AIDS-related and other infectious diseases. Defense ministries must also seek a viable balance between military readiness and public health for their own personnel and dependents.

Of real concern in the context of the global resurgence of tuberculosis is the deadly link between TB and HIV. Because of the special and particular ways in which these two infections affect the immune system, they are increasingly important as risk factors with mutual impact. HIV infection is the most powerful risk factor that increases the likelihood of development of TB in a person previously infected with *Mycobacterium tuberculosis*. The risk of developing TB is 10 times higher in an HIV-positive individual than in a sero-negative individual living in the same conditions. Tuberculosis is a common complication of HIV infection—one of the more important of the opportunistic infections found in AIDS patients. The case-fatality rate is higher for HIV-positive TB patients than for HIV-negative patients (Aït-Khaled & Enarson, 2003).

TB is a leading cause of death among people who are HIV-positive, accounting for about 13% of AIDS deaths worldwide. In Africa, over the past 10 years HIV has been the single most important factor determining the increased incidence of TB (WHO, 2004).

All across Eastern and Southern Africa, even in upper-middle income countries such as Botswana and South Africa, AIDS has overwhelmed rural and urban treatment, care, and support facilities (Yeager, 2002). In the civilian and military hospitals of these countries not even enough hospital beds are available to accommodate AIDS patients. Financial and technical assistance is urgently needed to enable the civilian and military sectors to find equitable solutions to several critical and controversial problems. Should military AIDS patients receive priority free care and ARV therapies? Under what conditions should long-term medical benefits be extended to discharged military AIDS patients and their dependents? Should military widows and orphans receive favored treatment in the provision of financial, legal, educational, and other protective benefits? Whatever their specifics, workable answers to these questions will have to involve close, capacity-building collaboration between civilian and military health services, made possible by external assistance to each.

## Civil-Military Collaboration

Success in the prevention and management of HIV and AIDS requires the establishment of close linkages between military organizations and civilian agencies, especially in less-developed countries. As the CMA survey concluded:

*Civil-military cooperation can make available to civilian practitioners relatively sophisticated military epidemiological data bases. It can also ease the financial burden placed on military resources and broaden the ability of militaries to offer long-term care through referral to civilian medical facilities. In all countries, the most effective overall goal may be the adoption of long-term, multi-sectoral approaches to the control of HIV/AIDS, which treat the disease not only as an immediate threat to public health but also as a challenge to social, economic, and political stability and thus to national security in the broadest possible sense*

(Yeager et al., 2000)

Throughout the world, realization is growing that militaries are central to the war against the HIV/AIDS pandemic. High-prevalence countries that pursue vigorous HIV prevention programs in the defense sector tend also to show results in restraining the pandemic across all segments of society. There is also growing evidence that when the military is actively represented on national AIDS councils, HIV prevention progresses more rapidly in both the armed services and civil society.

Nationally and/or locally, countries whose militaries and civilian agencies collaborate freely are likely to be those where incidence curves are flattening out and where prevalence rates may actually be declining. Countries such as Cambodia, Morocco, Senegal, Tanzania, Thailand, Uganda, and Zambia offer valuable insights into best practices and lessons learned for adaptation and application on a wider scale. Thailand and Senegal provide cases in point.

Thailand has endured one of the oldest HIV/AIDS epidemics in Asia, but has also been cited as one of the first countries to achieve stable and indeed declining surveillance curves. Thailand's first AIDS case was reported in 1984 and its first military case in 1987. Between 1985 and 1990, a comprehensive national prevention and care program was implemented with the Royal

Thai Army (RTA) taking the lead in several areas. The HIV/AIDS program launched by the RTA was designed around six main components:

- prevention of new HIV infections;
- supportive measures for already-infected personnel;
- treatment in military medical facilities;
- multi-sectoral coordination with civilian agencies;
- international cooperation with other militaries; and
- material support for medical research and development.

Preventive measures encompass HIV prevention education, HIV/AIDS awareness classes introduced into all military curricula, peer-group interventions targeted toward STI clinic attendees and other personnel at high risk, comprehensive anti-discrimination education, and extension of HIV/AIDS prevention and management efforts out into the communities from which it draws new recruits. Research and development include AIDS vaccine trials, in which the Thai Armed Forces Research Institute of Medical Sciences (AFRIMS) cooperates with international bodies such as the HIV Prevention Program of the U.S. Department of Defense.

Senegal retains low HIV/AIDS rates, largely because of its early and concerted response to the West African HIV2 epidemic. In spite of the fact that Senegalese rural and urban areas share the same risk factors with neighboring countries exhibiting higher rates of infection, here the surveillance curves remain flat with less than 1% prevalence. This success can be attributed to vigorous HIV/AIDS prevention and care programs in the military as well as in civilian society. Africa's premier HIV virology laboratory is located in Dakar, and its director is also a colonel in the Army of Senegal.

From the outset, the Senegalese government has presented a very open public approach to HIV prevention, complete with a campaign involving condom promotion, distribution, and education on proper use. Nowhere is this more evident than in the armed forces. HIV prevention is strongly reinforced each time an army contingent prepares for a peacekeeping mission, with overwhelmingly positive results.

## Inter-Military Cooperation

Sharing of data and lessons learned is essential to the prevention and management of HIV/AIDS in the armed services of less-developed countries, which are among the most vulnerable groups to infection worldwide. Between 1995 and 2003, this premise has guided the work of the CMA through 11 regional technical and policy workshops convened in Africa, Asia, the Caribbean, Eastern Europe, and Latin America (Leonard, 2001). One result of these workshops has been the establishment of three networks of technical cooperation among the militaries of Eastern and Southern Africa, Francophone Africa, and Anglophone West Africa (Yeager & Kingma, 2001). The purpose of this networking is to facilitate communication across national boundaries, aimed toward information sharing on HIV/AIDS prevention and management.

Individual countries have also undertaken such initiatives. Thailand, for example, is one of the most active states in Asia engaged in military-to-military cooperation. The RTA and the Thai Ministry of Health Public Health Service have been engaged by the United Nations Children's Fund (UNICEF) to carry out several missions in China to help local authorities in the development of plans for HIV/AIDS prevention and care. In 1995, officers of the RTA and AFRIMS participated in a UN Department of Peacekeeping Operations (DPKO) mission to Cambodia with subsequent follow-up visits. The goal was to help the Cambodian Ministry of National Defence to devise and implement an AIDS control plan.

Seasoned Senegalese military-medical staff members have regularly conducted technical-support missions to countries that had launched their military HIV/AIDS prevention and control programs somewhat later than Senegal.

## Conclusions

Many countries in the world's less-developed regions are haltingly emerging from decades of political instability and authoritarianism, socio-cultural ferment, economic stagnation and mass poverty, and international dependency. A new era of reform has begun and security-sector reform is very much a part of the process, but all of these nascent advances are threatened by the unrelenting crisis of HIV/AIDS and other infectious diseases such as TB and malaria. The good news is that at long last prevention and mitigation of these maladies have become priorities of both the defense and development communities. In the words, for example, of former World Bank President James Wolfensohn, spoken at the January 10, 2000 opening session of the UN Security Council, "we face a major development crisis, and more than that, a security crisis. For without economic and social hope we will not have peace, and AIDS surely undermines both. We need to break that vicious circle of AIDS, poverty, conflict, AIDS. For the truth is that not only does AIDS threaten stability, but when peace breaks down it fuels AIDS" (World Bank Group, 2000).

The less happy news is that, while the civil-military programmatic and policy requirements to break the burgeoning AIDS pandemic are well understood in Africa and elsewhere, the political and financial resolve to do so remains woefully inadequate.

Across the global human landscape, the only effective and cost-effective weapons to combat HIV are found in its prevention through changes in behaviors that are often grounded in deeply-held attitudes, values, and beliefs. The magnitude of the task at hand, compounded by the vaccine-eluding adaptability of the virus, means that traditional inter-sectoral distinctions mean little in the struggle to overcome this deadly enemy. The pandemic presents a clear and present danger not only to public health, socio-economic advancement and political stability, but also to basic human security no matter how it is defined and to the national security of even the least-affected affluent countries that control most of the world's wealth and power. This realization should prompt a well-founded sense of urgency in the war against HIV and AIDS.

## References

Adefolalu, A. (1999). *HIV/AIDS as an Occupational Hazard to Soldiers—ECOMOG Experience* (unpublished paper presented at the 3rd All Africa Congress of Armed Forces and Police Medical Services, Pretoria, South Africa, October 1999).

Aït-Khaled, N. & Enarson, D.A. (2003). *Tuberculosis: A Manual for Medical Students.* International Union Against Tuberculosis and Lung Disease / World Health Organization. World Health Organization Document WHO/CDS/TB/99.272.

BBC News (2004). *High Rate of TB Infection in Philippine Army.* (September 1, 2004).

Brenner, I.K.M., Severs, Y.D., Rhind, S.G., Shephard, R.J., & Shek, P.N. (2000). Immune function and incidence of infection during basic infantry training. *Military Medicine*, 165, 878-883.

Central Intelligence Agency (2000). *The Global Infectious Disease Threat and its Implications for the United States.* (National Intelligence Council, report NIE 99-17D, Washington).

Director of Central Intelligence Strategic Warning Committee (2002). *The Next Wave of HIV/AIDS: Nigeria, Ethiopia, Russia, India, and China.* (National Intelligence Council, report ICA 2002-04-D, Washington).

Emerson, L.A.C. (1997). Sexually transmitted disease control in the armed forces, past and present. *Military Medicine*, 162, 87-91.

Global Fund (2003). http://www.globalfundatm.org/overview.html

Gomez-Merino, D., Chennaoui, M., Burnat, P., Drogou, C., & Guezennec, C.Y. (2003). Immune and hormonal changes following intense military training. *Military Medicine*, 168, 1034-1038.

Gould, P. (1993). *The Slow Plague: A Geography of the AIDS Pandemic.* Cambridge, MA and Oxford, UK: Blackwell Publishers.

Leonard, L. (2001). *An External Evaluation of Activities, Accomplished Events, and Achievements of the Civil-Military Alliance to Combat HIV & AIDS (CMA),* January 1995-March 2001 (unpublished report to the Ford Foundation).

Mendelson-Forman, J. & Carballo, M. (2002). A policy critique of HIV/AIDS and demobilisation, *Conflict, Security and Development*, 73-92.

Moodie, M., Taylor, W.J., Baek, G., Ban, J., Fogelgren, C., Lloyd, S., Swann, J., & Chung, Y. (2000). *Contagion and Conflict: Health as a Global Security Challenge.* Washington, DC: The Center for Strategic & International Studies.

Mudambo, Dr. (1999). *The Effects of Strenuous Exercise on HIV Positive Individuals* (unpublished paper).

Ognibene, A.J. (1987). Medical and infectious diseases in the theater of operations. *Military Medicine*, 152(1), 14-18.

Population Data Unit, PGDS/DOS, UN High Commissioner for Refugees (2002). http://www.unhcr.ch/

Price-Smith, A.T. (2002). *Pretoria's shadow: The HIV/AIDS pandemic and national security in South Africa.* Washington, D.C.: Chemical and Biological Arms Control Institute.

Ruscavage, D. & Purnell, P. (1999). *HIV Prevention and Behavior Change in International Military Populations*. Rolle, Switzerland: Civil-Military Alliance to Combat HIV & AIDS.

Ruscavage, D. & Yeager, R. (2001). *HIV Prevention in Conflict and Crisis Settings*. Rolle, Switzerland: Civil-Military Alliance to Combat HIV and AIDS.

Shephard, R.J. & Shek, P.N. (1998). Cold exposure and immune function. *Canadian Journal of Physiological Pharmacology*, 76, 828-836.

Shephard, R.J. & Shek, P.N. (2000). Immune dysfunction as a factor in heat illness. *Critical Review of Immunology*, 19, 285-302.

Shephard, R.J., Brenner, I.K.M., Bateman, W.A., & Shek, P.N. (2001). Basic recruit training: health risks and opportunities. *Military Medicine*, 166, 714-720.

*The Chronicle Newspaper* (June 12, 2001). Lilongwe, Malawi.

The Times of India News Service (October 28, 2002). Cited in: Gupta, R. (2002). Communicable diseases, risky sex and alcohol and drug abuse in India: Implications for health, development and security. (Los Alamos Report No. ALUR-02-5305, Los Alamos National Laboratory, Los Alamos, New Mexico).

Turner, J. (2004). Army treating hundreds of leishmaniasis cases. http://www4.army.mil/ocpa/read.php?story_id_key=5726

UNAIDS (1998). *AIDS and the Military*. Geneva: UNAIDS Point of View.

UN High Commissioner for Refugees (2004). http://unhcr.ch/cgbin/texis/vtx/statistics.

UN Security Council (2000). Press release SC/6781, January 10, 2000, New York.

UN Security Council (2000). UN Security Council resolution 1308 (2000) on the responsibility of the Security Council in the maintenance of international peace-keeping and security: HIV/AIDS and international peacekeeping operations. http://www.un.org/docs/scinfo.htm.

Valdiserri, R.O. (1997). HIV counseling and testing is evolving its role in HIV prevention. *AIDS Education and Prevention* 9 (Supplement 2), 2-13.

WHO (2001). Global prevalence and incidence of selected curable sexually transmitted infections: Overview and estimates. Geneva: World Health Organization.

WHO (2004). Tuberculosis—WHO Fact Sheet N° 104. http://www.who.int/mediacentre/factsheets/fs104/en/.

World Bank Group (2000). News release 2000/172/S, January 10, 2000, Washington.

Worth, K. (2004). Leptospirosis cases traced to Sigua Falls. Pacific Daily News. (April 24, 2004).

Yeager, R. (Ed.) (1997). *Third African Regional Seminar on HIV/AIDS Prevention in Military Populations,* 2-7 March 1997, Windhoek, Namibia, proceedings. Rolle, Switzerland: Civil-Military Alliance to Combat HIV & AIDS.

Yeager, R. (2002). HIV/AIDS: *Implications for Development and Security in Sub-Saharan Africa* (unpublished paper). http://www.certi.org/cma.

Yeager, R. & Kingma, S. (2000). *A Civil-Military Response to the HIV/AIDS Epidemic in Nigeria* (unpublished report prepared for the U.S. Agency for International Development/Washington).

Yeager, R. & Kingma, S. (2001). HIV/AIDS: Destabilising national security and the multi-national response. *International Review of Armed Forces Medical Services*, 74, 3-12.

Yeager, R., Hendrix, C.W., & Kingma, S.J. (2000). International military human immunodeficiency virus/acquired immunodeficiency syndrome policies and programs: Strengths and limitations in current practice. *Military Medicine*, 165, 87-92.

# Chapter 7

## Selling Sex in the Era of AIDS: Mobile Sexworkers and STI/HIV Risks

NATALYA TIMOSHKINA, M.S.W., PH.D. CANDIDATE,
ANTHONY P. LOMBARDO, M.A., PH.D. CANDIDATE, AND
LYNN MCDONALD PH.D.

## Introduction

Women in the sex trade are commonly perceived to be at a higher risk for sexually transmitted infections (STI) and have been historically blamed for the spread of diseases. Public concerns and indignation against sex trade workers have increased dramatically in the past two decades in light of the HIV/AIDS epidemic. Activists for sexworkers' rights have long argued that, in industrialized countries, the majority of female sexworkers practice safe sex and are not a high risk group for STIs/HIV (e.g., McKeganey & Barnard, 1996; Morgan-Thomas, Brussa, Munk, & Jirešová, 2006). However, as will be discussed further in the text, reliable statistical data supporting this argument is limited and rather dated. Furthermore, situations vary in many parts of the developing world where STI/HIV prevalence among commercial sexworkers is significantly higher than among the general population (UNAIDS, 2004). Risks of contracting STIs/HIV are also higher for transgender/transsexual and male sexworkers (UNAIDS, 2004; UNAIDS & WHO, 2005) who may have sex with both men and women, thus representing a risk for both homosexual and heterosexual STI/HIV transmission (UNAIDS, 2002). Sexworkers who inject drugs are especially vulnerable to STI/HIV risks (UNAIDS, 2004; UNAIDS & WHO, 2005). In fact, the overlap between the commercial sex trade and intravenous (IV) drug use is considered by many experts to be the primary driving force behind the spread of the HIV epidemic (UNAIDS, 2004; UNAIDS & WHO, 2005).

Active internal (mostly from rural to urban areas) and transnational migration of both sexworkers and their clients exacerbate the problems identified above. A number of studies found that long distance truck-drivers, seasonal agricultural workers, migrants working in mines, and other temporary migrants who frequently used services of sexworkers had higher prevalence of STIs/HIV (Population Information Program, 1996; UNAIDS & WHO, 2004, 2005). In recent years, many countries around the world also have seen a dramatic increase in the number of foreign women entering the sex trade. Each year, thousands of females, who travel from poorer to richer countries in search of a better life and adequate sources of income for themselves and their families, end up in the sex industry. Many women are trafficked into the sex trade by criminal structures though the use of violence, abuse of authority, debt bondage, and deception; others enter the trade voluntarily, but are often unaware of the harsh working and social conditions that await them in the host countries, or the degree of control that would be exercised over them (Wijers & Lap-Chew, 1997).

The presence of migrant women in the sex trade has altered all aspects of the industry, and posed a serious challenge to immigration and law enforcement systems of host nations. The fact that thousands of women and children are trafficked from and within regions with rapidly growing HIV/AIDS epidemics (e.g., Sub-Saharan Africa and Eastern Europe) is a matter of serious international concern, especially considering that mobile sexworkers often function as "bridge population groups" linking high and low STI/HIV prevalence groups (Hamers & Downs, 2003) that pose potentially explosive health risks.

Migrant sexworkers remain largely outside of the legal, medical and social services structures. Undocumented status, poor language skills, absence of support networks, limited understanding of foreign laws and regulations, and subjection to xenophobia result in the extreme marginalization of migrants, putting them at a greater risk of abuse and exploitation. In addition, migrant sexworkers are more likely to be affected by the negative social dynamics of the sex trade, marked by discrimination on the basis of race, nationality, class, age, and specific place in the industry's hierarchy (Morgan-Thomas et al., 2006). All this makes migrants working in the sex industry particularly vulnerable to STI/HIV (Matteelli & El-Hamad, 1996; Morgan-Thomas et al., 2006; UNAIDS, 2005).

This chapter addresses mobile sexwork and the STI/HIV risks associated with it. The extent of trafficking and mobile sexwork are discussed from a global perspective and data on STI/HIV prevalence rates among sexworkers worldwide are highlighted in order to provide the context for STI/HIV and sexworkers. The chapter continues on to mobile sexwork and STI/HIV risks in particular, concluding with a discussion on responses to STI/HIV among sexworkers that have been undertaken thus far, and what other responses are required.

## The Extent of Trafficking and Mobile Sexwork

There are many configurations, views and definitions of trafficking. Some experts believe that only those forced into the sex trade under false pretences should be viewed as trafficked; others perceive coercion as irrelevant and place emphasis on the issue of sexual exploitation, thus considering all sexworkers to be trafficked to one extent or another (Andrees & van der Linden, 2005). On the other side of the debate are sexworkers' rights activists who argue that the term "trafficking" should be scrapped altogether because it carries negative connotation and portrays migrant sexworkers as passive objects of exploitation rather than active subjects who control their own destiny and have a human right to work in the sex industry (Doezema, 1999). The issue is further complicated by the fact that sexworkers' personal circumstances change and evolve over time. For example, at the initial stage of their involvement in the sex trade, some workers experience forceful trafficking, but later manage to escape their exploitive situations and remain in the trade on their own terms (Andrees & van der Linden, 2005). There are also disagreements among experts on whether the term "trafficked" should be used to refer only to those sexworkers who are transported across national borders, or should be applied to both international and internal migrants. In this context, the term "mobile sexworkers" seems to be most appropriate as it encompasses both international and internal migration, and both forceful and voluntary involvement in the trade. Due to the lack of consensus on the issue; however, the terms "trafficked," "migrant," and "mobile" sexworkers are often used in the literature interchangeably.

The United Nations (2000) estimates that as many as five to seven million people are being trafficked annually worldwide. Women and girls comprise about 80% of trafficking victims; up to 50% of these females are minors, and 70% are believed to be trafficked into the sex industry (USDOS 2004, 2005). Western Europe, North America, and Australia are among the main destination regions for trafficked women and children for the purposes of the sex trade.

Conservative calculations placed the number of trafficked children in 2000 at approximately 1.2 million (IPEC 2002). About 1.8 million children were in forced prostitution and pornography worldwide, especially in Latin America, the Caribbean, the Asian-Pacific region, and in developed economies (IPEC, 2002; UNICEF 2005). It has been suggested that the number of children in prostitution could be as high as 10 million (Willis & Levy, 2002).

In most states of the European Union (EU), the number of migrant sexworkers, representing at least 50 different nationalities, is already much greater than that of the local ones (Morgan-Thomas et al., 2006). In Spain, for example, 82% of all sexworkers are migrants: 54% of them come from Africa, 33% from Latin America, 9% from Central Europe, and the rest mainly from Asia (TAMPEP, 2004). In addition, foreign nationals represent half of female transsexual and 27% of male sexworkers in the country (Rodriguez-Arenas, 2002). In the Netherlands, migrants, who come primarily from Eastern Europe, account for 80% of those working in all types of the sex industry (TAMPEP, 2004). In Germany, migrants comprise about 60% of sexworkers (Morgan-Thomas et al., 2006). In France, in 2002, an estimated 57% of sexworkers were migrants: 43% of them were from Africa, 42% from Central and Eastern Europe, 14% from Latin America, and 1% from Asia (TAMPEP, 2004). In Italy, the majority of female sexworkers are trafficked from Africa (with almost 60% of all migrant sexworkers being from Nigeria) and Eastern Europe (TAMPEP, 2004). In Greece, in 1999, out of an estimated 10,000 non-registered sexworkers, 6,000 were believed to be migrants (EUROPAP, 2000).

Distribution of nationalities and patterns of mobility in the European sex trade are becoming increasingly complex, largely due to the expansion of the E.U. and frequent changes in immigration regulations and visa regimes. Until three years ago, for instance, Albanian sexworkers could be found almost exclusively in Italy and Greece, while today there are fewer of them in Italy and more in Belgium, France and Germany (Morgan-Thomas et al., 2006). Almost half of 100 migrant sexworkers (mainly from Eastern Europe and Latin America) interviewed in Frankfurt, Germany, and Antwerp, Belgium, reported that they had worked in as many as 13 different countries, both within and outside the EU (van der Helm, 2002).

From 14,500 to 17,500 persons, primarily women and children, are trafficked into the U.S. annually (USDOS, 2005). Most come from Southeast Asia, Latin America and the former Eastern Bloc countries, and end up in the commercial sex trade (O'Neill-Richard, 1999). At least 600 foreign women and girls are trafficked into the Canadian sex trade each year and up to 2,200 migrants are smuggled to the U.S. to toil in brothels, sweatshops, etc., yet these numbers may be only a fraction of the actual total (Canadian Press, 2004). Thailand, Cambodia, the Philippines, Russia and other Eastern European nations, Korea, and Malaysia serve as the principal source regions for trafficking in persons to Canada (Royal Canadian Mounted Police, 2004). Within the country, hundreds of Aboriginal women are trafficked from reserves to large urban centers, such as Vancouver.

Approximately 1,000 women are trafficked annually into prostitution in Australia (Australian Centre for the Study of Sexual Assault, 2005). These women originate mainly from Thailand, as well as China, Indonesia, Malaysia, Vietnam, Columbia, and the former Soviet Union; many women holding Thai passports are believed to have been previously trafficked to Thailand from Myanmar (Australian Centre for the Study of Sexual Assault, 2005).

Active migration of sexworkers—both forced and voluntary—also occurs within the developing world. In Asia, for example, thousands of female and male Nepalese sexworkers go to work in India (Simkhada, 2002); large numbers of women from Cambodia, Laos, Myanmar and Vietnam work in brothels in Thailand, while sexworkers from Thailand and the Philippines work in Japan and Singapore (Population Information Program, 1996). China has become a destination country for trafficking in women and girls from Burma, North Korea, Vietnam, and Russia (USDOS, 2005). A similar situation exists in Africa. For instance, many women from Côte d'Ivoire work in prostitution in Ghana (Population Information Program, 1996), while both female and male sexworkers from Ghana, as well as Burkina Faso, Mali, Liberia and Nigeria are involved in the trade in Côte d'Ivoire (Family Health International, 2005; Ghys, P.D., Diallo, M.O., Ettiegne-Traore, V., Kale, K., Tawil, O., Caraël, M., Traore, M., Mah-bi, G., De Cock, K.M., Wiktor, S.Z., Laga, M., & Greenberg, A.E., 2002), while sexworkers from Lesotho routinely cross the border to South Africa (Robinson & Rusinow, 2002). In Cotonou, capital of Benin, approximately 40% of commercial sexworkers are migrants from the surrounding countries of Nigeria, Togo, Ghana, and the Ivory Coast (African AIDS Awareness Campaign, 2005). Extremely high mobility of sexworkers has been recorded also within Latin America, particularly among Central American countries (Belize, Guatemala, El Salvador, Honduras, Nicaragua, Costa Rica, and Panama) and Mexico (Dreser, Caballero, Leyva, & Bronfman, 2002).

Since 1989, there has been a noticeable shift in the sources of supply to the global sex industry. With the collapse of the Socialist regimes and wars in the Balkans that produced substantial numbers of migrants and refugees, countries of the former Eastern Bloc became the primary sender states, supplementing and replacing previously significant sources of women from Asia and Latin America (Caldwell, Galster, & Steinzor, 1997; IOM, 1998). It has been suggested that two-thirds of the estimated number of women and children annually trafficked for prostitution worldwide come from Eastern and Central Europe (Hughes, 2000; McClelland, 2001). According to U.S. government sources, every year over 100,000 women are trafficked from the former Soviet Union, with an additional 75,000 from Eastern Europe (Miko, 2000). Some experts argue that the former Soviet republics—Moldova, Ukraine, and Russia in particular—have replaced Thailand and the Philippines as the epicenter of the global business in trafficking women (Baker, 2002; IOM, 2001; Miko, 2000).

## STI/HIV Prevalence Among Sexworkers

There are no available statistical data on health status of commercial sex trade workers. This could be explained by the clandestine nature of the sex trade that makes this population highly marginalized and hard to reach, especially when it comes to migrant sexworkers, most of whom work in the host countries illegally. Studies on STI/HIV prevalence among sexworkers are scant and usually based on small, non-representative samples in select cities. The numbers of infected sexworkers vary greatly, not only from country to country but from city to city, and the available studies generally do not differentiate between local and migrant sexworkers. Some highlights of STI/HIV prevalence rates among sexworkers around the world are noted below (a more comprehensive review of these data is beyond the scope of this chapter).

## Africa

In Africa, the lowest HIV prevalence among commercial sexworkers was recorded in the capital of Madagascar—0.1% in 2001 (UNAIDS & WHO, 2004), and was also low among sexworkers in Morocco (2.3 in 2003) and Sudan (4.4%) (Sudan National AIDS Control Program, 2004). In Mauritius, HIV infection levels among female sexworkers were estimated at 3-7% (UNAIDS, 2005). In Algeria, these levels ranged from 1.7% in the northern city of Oran to 9% in Tamanrasset, in the south, where they rose sharply from 2% in 2000 (UNAIDS & WHO, 2005). Infection levels of 21% were recorded in 2002 among female sexworkers in the capital of Burkina Faso, Ouagadougou, which was a steep decline from 59% in 1994 (Kintin et al, 2004 cited in UNAIDS & WHO, 2005). In 2000, HIV prevalence stood at 21.0% in the capital of Mali and at 25.5% in the capital of Kenya (UNAIDS, 2004).

In other areas, HIV prevalence among sexworkers is significantly higher. Prevalence in the range of 30-40% has been reported among sexworkers in Senegal (UNAIDS, 2004; Gomes do Espirito Santo & Etheredge, 2005), Guinea (UNAIDS, 2004), Angola and Niger (UNAIDS & WHO, 2004). Approximately half of the commercial sexworkers in South Africa are believed to be HIV-positive (UNAIDS, 2004). The prevalence rate is 60.5% for HIV in Porto-Novo, the capital city of Benin (UNAIDS, 2004); the 1999 data on female sexworkers in the city of Cotonou also showed prevalence rates of 40.6% for HIV, 20.5% for gonorrhea, 5.1% for Chlamydia, and 1.5% for syphilis (Alary et al., 2002).

The highest HIV prevalence on the African continent was found among sexworkers in Sierra Leone (71%) and urban sexworkers in Ethiopia (74%) (UNAIDS, 2004). In Ghana as well, surveys in 1999 found HIV prevalence rates of 74.2% among street-based and 27.2% among home-based sexworkers in Tema and Accra; a very high rate of 83% was reported among sexworkers in Kumasi (UN-OCHA Integrated Regional Information Networks, 2005).

## Asia

Arguably the most comprehensive data on STI/HIV prevalence among sexworkers come from Asia. In the capital of Laos, HIV prevalence among sexworkers was recorded as low as 1.1% in 2001 (UNAIDS, 2004). In China, in the capital city of Beijing, prevalence was also extremely low—0.2% in 2000 (UNAIDS, 2004). Yet, prevalence is higher in male sexworkers: according to a recent survey, 5% of male sexworkers in the southern city of Shenzhen were HIV-positive (UNAIDS & WHO, 2005). A study on female sexworkers conducted in Guangzhou in 1998-1999 also found high ST' prevalence: 32% for Chlamydia, 14% for syphilis, 12.5% for trichomoniasis, and 8% gonorrhea (van den Hoek et al., 2001).

In Bangladesh, HIV prevalence in urban female sexworkers has stayed between 0.2% and 1.5%, and prevalence of other STIs has declined to under 10% in 2002 (Ministry of Health and Family Welfare Bangladesh, 2004). In the capital city of Dhaka, however, HIV prevalence among sexworkers was 20% in 2004 (UNAIDS, 2004). In addition, as of 2001, about 43% of female sexworkers and 18.2% of male sexworkers in Central Bangladesh had syphilis (The World Bank Group, 2003).

In the Malaysian capital of Kuala Lumpur, HIV prevalence of 10% was recorded among sexworkers (an increase from 6.3% in 1996) (UNAIDS & WHO, 2004). In Thailand, the first country to implement the 100% Condom Use Prevention Program, HIV prevalence among brothel-based sexworkers declined from 43% in 1997 to just over 10% in 2003 (UNAIDS, 2004; UNAIDS & WHO, 2005), while in the capital it was as low as 2.6% in 2002 (UNAIDS, 2004). HIV prevalence of 16% was found in sexworkers in Vietnam, although levels of infection in the cities of Hai Phong, Ho Chi Minh City, Hanoi and Can Tho were higher (Ministry of Health Viet Nam, 2005). In Cambodia, HIV prevalence among brothel-based sexworkers dropped from 43% in 1998 to 21% in 2003 (Saphonn et al., 2005 cited in UNAIDS, 2005; National Center for HIV/AIDS, Dermatology and STIs, 2004).

In Indonesia, HIV infection levels among female sexworkers vary widely—from 0% in the capital of Jakarta to 8–24% in other parts of the country (UNAIDS, 2004). HIV prevalence among transgender sexworkers (*waria*) in Jakarta rose and was nearly 22% in 2002 (UNAIDS, 2004); among male sexworkers, it was approximately 4% (Pisani et al., 2004; Riono & Jazant, 2004). Studies conducted in 2003 also found that an average 42% of sexworkers in seven cities were infected with gonorrhoea and/or Chlamydia (Monitoring the AIDS Pandemic Network, 2004).

In Myanmar, HIV prevalence among sexworkers has remained steady around 25% since 1997; in 2004, 27% of sexworkers (one in four) were found to be HIV-positive (UNAIDS & WHO, 2005). In the capital of Nepal, HIV prevalence among sexworkers ranged from 17.0% to 36% in 2002, while in other urban areas it could be as high as 36% (UNAIDS, 2004; UNAIDS & WHO, 2005). In Pakistan's main trading city of Karachi, 36% of male sexworkers were found to be infected with syphilis (Ministry of Health Pakistan, Department for International Development, & Family Health International, 2005); HIV prevalence, however, was 0% (Baqi et al., 1999).

In various parts of India, HIV prevalence rates among sex trade workers vary considerably. For example, in Kolkata's Sonagachi red-light district (in West Bengal), HIV prevalence among commercial sexworkers was under 4% in 2004 (UNAIDS & WHO, 2005). In Mumbai, however, HIV infection rates among female sexworkers are extraordinary high—from 52% to 70% (AVERT, 2005; National AIDS Control Organization, 2004).

## Oceania

Statistics on STI/HIV prevalence among sexworkers in Oceania are scant. Commercial sex trade workers in Australia reportedly have the lowest rate of HIV/AIDS amongst sexworkers in the world, and virtually all cases of HIV infection are attributed to IV drug use. To date, no cases of HIV transmission from sexworkers to clients have been recorded in the country (Scarlet Alliance, 2005). A 1991-1998 study in Sydney found an HIV prevalence rate of 6.5% among 94 male sexworkers, a rate higher than that of female sexworkers (0.4%), but lower than homosexual men who were not sexworkers (23.9%) (Estcourt et al., 2000). In the capital of Papua New Guinea, HIV prevalence among sexworkers was estimated at 16.0% in 2000 (UNAIDS, 2004), while studies in East Timor in 2003 found that one quarter of commercial sexworkers in Dili had gonorrhea and/or Chlamydia, and 60% were infected with HSV2 (UNAIDS & WHO, 2005).

## Western Europe

There are very few recent statistics on STI/HIV prevalence among sexworkers in Western Europe as most data come from studies conducted between the 1980s and early 1990s. The available estimates suggest that HIV prevalence among female sexworkers in the region is low, yet the rates are generally higher among male, drug-injecting, and transgendered/transsexual sexworkers.

One survey of 896 female sexworkers in nine European nations found an average HIV prevalence of 5.3%-31.8% for IV drug users and 1.5% for non-drug users (European Working Group on HIV Infection in Female Prostitutes, 1993). In Greece, in the mid to late 1990s, an HIV prevalence of as low as 0.4% was recorded among registered sexworkers and 0.22% among non-registered workers (EUROPAP, 2000). In Vienna, Austria, only 0.8% of sexworkers were HIV positive in 1986, and all of the infected workers were either IV drug users or had drug-injecting sexual partners (Kopp & Dangl-Erlach, 1986 cited in Hawk, 1998).

Estimates from the Netherlands vary; a small study of 32 non-drug using female sexworkers in Amsterdam, found no cases of HIV; in contrast, 24% of a group of 25 transsexual/transvestite sexworkers were HIV-positive (Gras et al., 1997 cited in Hawk, 1998). A larger study carried out in Rotterdam in 2002-2003 found that 7% of sexworkers and almost 12% of those working the streets were HIV-positive (UNAIDS & WHO, 2004). In the U.K., HIV prevalence was very low even among drug-injecting sexworkers. Studies on IDU sexworkers in Glasgow, for instance, found prevalence of no more than 2.5% (Green & Goldberg, 1993; McKeganey et al., 1992). Among London-based male sexworkers, however, HIV prevalence was around 25% (Tomlinson, Hillman, Harris, & Taylor-Robinson, 1991).

Estimates on HIV infection in female sexworkers in Belgium range from 0.3% to 1.16%, and from 17.4% to 38.5% for male sexworkers (EUROPAP, 2000). A recent study in Antwerp, Belgium, found an HIV prevalence rate of 10.8% among 120 male sexworkers (Leuridan, Wouters, Stalpaert, & Van Damme, 2005). In Spain, estimates on HIV prevalence among female sexworkers vary between 1.2-12.6% for non-drug users and between 18.6-45% for IDUs (EUROPAP, 2000). A study of 418 male sexworkers from 19 Spanish cities, conducted between 2000 and 2002, found HIV prevalence rates of 12.2%; 67% of these male sexworkers were of foreign origin (Belza, 2005).

## Eastern Europe

Data on STI/HIV prevalence rates among sexworkers in Eastern European countries is largely unavailable. In the past several years, however, countries of the former Soviet Union have seen a dramatic increase in the number of people living with HIV, with the commercial sex trade and drug injection being the driving forces behind the spread of the epidemic.

Low rates of HIV prevalence have been reported among sexworkers in Lithuania (0.5%) (UNAIDS, 2004), and in Poland and the Czech Republic (under 1%) (EuroHIV, 2003). Studies on street-based sexworkers in Moldova found an HIV prevalence of 5% (WHO Regional Office for Europe, 2004).

In Russia, HIV prevalence of 14% and 15% was found among sexworkers in the cities of Moscow and Ekaterinburg respectively (WHO Regional Office for Europe, 2004; EuroHIV, 2003). For drug-injecting female workers; however, the figures are believed to be considerably higher (Smolskaya et al., 2004a cited in UNAIDS & WHO, 2004). In the Ukraine, HIV prevalence among non-injecting female sexworkers in the cities of Odessa and Donetsk is estimated at 17%, while 35%-67% of drug-injecting sexworkers in cities are believed to be HIV-positive (Ukrainian AIDS Center, 2005).

In the former Soviet republics of the Caucuses and Central Asia, HIV infection rates among sexworkers also vary: 4.6% in Kazakhstan (EuroHIV, 2005; UNAIDS & WHO, 2004); 6%-11% in Azerbaijan (WHO Regional Office for Europe, 2004); 7.5% in Armenia (UNAIDS, 2004); and 10-28% in Uzbekistan (Todd et al., 2005 cited in UNIADS & WHO, 2005).

The highest STI rates among sexworkers in Eastern European region were reported in Bulgaria: according to one study, 43% of female sexworkers showed evidence of one or more STI (Tchoudomirova, Domeika, & Mardh, 1997).

## Latin America and the Caribbean

HIV prevalence among sexworkers in Latin America and the Caribbean is generally low, although the commercial sex trade is believed to be the driving force behind the spread of the epidemic in the region (UNAIDS, 2004). HIV prevalence has been reported at only 0.3% in Mexico in 1999 (UNAIDS, 2004); 0.8% in Colombia in 2001-2003 (UNAIDS & WHO, 2005); 0.5-1% in Bolivia in 2002 (Carcamo, 2004 cited in UNAIDS & WHO, 2005); 1% in Nicaragua; and 2% in Panama (UNAIDS & WHO, 2005). In Ecuador, the 2002 prevalence was under 2% (UNAIDS & WHO, 2005), although in the capital city it was as high as 14% in 2002 (UNAIDS, 2004). In the Dominican Republic, HIV infection levels range from 3–4% among sexworkers in Santo

Domingo to 12.4% in the southern province of Bani (UNAIDS, 2004; UNAIDS & WHO, 2005).

In most Central American nations, street-based sexworkers are at least twice as likely to be infected with HIV as those working in brothels and out of hotels and bars (UNAIDS & WHO, 2004). In Guatemala, for example, HIV prevalence among street sexworkers was recorded at 15%, compared to 3.6% among sexworkers in brothels; in Honduras, these levels were measured at 14% and 4% respectively (UNAIDS & WHO, 2004). HIV prevalence among street sexworkers in San Salvador and Puerto de Acajutla, El Salvador, was 16% (UNAIDS & WHO, 2005). One of the highest HIV infection levels among female sexworkers in Latin American region was found in Suriname— 21% in 2005 (UNAIDS & WHO, 2005).

In Brazil, levels of HIV infection among female sexworkers are estimated at 6.1% (Chequer, 2005 cited in UNAIDS & WHO, 2005), with higher prevalence recorded in those working in the cities of San Paolo and Santos: overall, 7% of sexworkers there were HIV-positive, but among those living in slums and especially among illiterate women, HIV levels reached 18% and 23% respectively (Gravato, Morell, Areco, & Peres, 2004 cited in UNAIDS & WHO, 2004). Levels of HIV prevalence among transvestite sexworkers in Brazil have been reported between 60.7–63% (Inciardi & Surratt, 1997 and studies cited therein).

## North America

In Canada, there are currently no official estimates on STI/HIV prevalence among sexworkers, but there is also no existing epidemiological evidence to show regular transmission of HIV from sexworkers to their clients (Canadian HIV/AIDS Legal Network, 2005). The situation could be more complex in Vancouver's Downtown Eastside – an area that evidently has the highest HIV infection rate in North America, and is plagued by chronic poverty, crime and drug use (Duddy, 2004). It has been reported that female sexworkers in that area, almost 70% of whom are Aboriginal, have been disproportionately affected by the local AIDS epidemic (Duddy, 2004).

The available information on HIV prevalence among sexworkers in the U.S. is rather dated. One study conducted in the 1980s, tested 1,396 female sexworkers in six American cities and found HIV seroprevalence ranging from 0% to 47.5% depending on the particular city and level of IV drug use (CDC, 1987). Research on brothel-based sexworkers in Nevada showed that, as of 1993, out of 20,000 HIV tests, no woman tested positive (Albert et al., 1995). Studies on male sexworkers conducted in the late 1980s found seroprevalence from 11% to as high as 50% (Bastow, 1995; Elifson, Boles, & Sweat, 1993; Simon et al., 1994). A study of 53 transvestite sexworkers in Atlanta, Georgia, between 1990 and 1991, found highly elevated rates of HIV among the transvestite sexworkers versus non-transvestite sexworkers (68% vs. 27%, respectively) (Elifson, Boles, Posey et al., 1993).

## Mobile Sexwork and STI/HIV Risks

The presence of migrants in local sex trade industries of many nations is not a temporary or static phenomenon but a rapidly growing trend. Yet, in most countries, current legal and social policies in the areas of sexwork, immigration, and STI/HIV prevention do not reflect this. Basic human rights of migrant sexworkers are routinely violated. In most parts of the world, prostitution is an illegal and highly stigmatized activity, and there exist discriminatory, often repressive policies and attitudes towards persons with HIV/AIDS. Mandatory registration and medical check-ups of sexworkers in countries where prostitution is legalized (such as Greece and southern Germany) have proved to be oppressive and counterproductive, as they drive sexworkers further underground (EUROAP, 2000). Many countries also have strict laws against illegal migration, which put migrant sexworkers at high risk of arrest and deportation. Migrants are also subjected to xenophobia and discrimination. In the Netherlands, for instance, where prostitution is legalized and regulated, a new law was introduced in October 2000 that prohibits owners of brothels to employ women from non-EU countries and who have no permit to stay (van der Helm, 2002). As a result, migrant sexworkers are becoming increasingly dependent on international criminal structures/ traffickers, which directly affects their already unenviable working conditions. Moreover, it forces sexworkers to frequently move between various cities and countries to avoid being caught, thus contributing to the potential spread of infections.

Many experts consider migrant sexworkers to be particularly vulnerable to the risks of STI/HIV transmission (EUROPAP, 2000; Matteelli & El-Hamad, 1996; Morgan-Thomas et al., 2006; UNAIDS, 2005). Even when migrant sexworkers come from areas where STI/HIV prevalence is lower than in their host countries, they face an increased risk for infections for several reasons. First, many migrants are new to the sex trade and lack awareness of potential health risks and safe sex practices. Second, illegal and clandestine status of most foreign sexworkers prevents them from accessing health-care services and makes them more vulnerable to abuse from clients who refuse to wear condoms. Finally, due to their desperate economic situation, migrants are more likely to engage in unprotected sex if clients are willing to pay more (Matteelli & El-Hamad, 1996; Morgan-Thomas et al., 2006). Indeed, higher risks of STIs/HIV in migrant sexworkers "have been associated with the least favorable working conditions, the highest financial needs, the lowest levels of well-being and job satisfaction and greater experience of violence and victimization in the sex industry" (EUROPAP, 2000, p. 6).

A study by van Haastrecht and associates (1993) that tested 201 non-drug using female sexworkers in the Netherlands found that although HIV prevalence among them was very low (1.5%), all HIV-infected women were recent migrants from AIDS-endemic countries. In Madrid, Spain, the 1998-2003 data on immigrant male and female sexworkers, most of who came from

Sub-Saharan Africa, the region with the most serious HIV/AIDS epidemic in the world, showed that 5% of the workers were HIV-positive (UNAIDS & WHO, 2004). In addition, an increase in syphilis among sexworkers in some European countries, such as Portugal, has been linked to migration from the former Eastern Bloc where there are substantial epidemics (EUROPAP, 2001).

The fact that infected migrant sexworkers return or are deported to countries that do not have adequate STI/HIV treatment programs only adds to the problem. In Ghana, for instance, "many rural women who left for Côte d'Ivoire and became sexworkers brought HIV home with them to their villages, which now have a high prevalence of HIV" (Population Information Program, 1996, p. 11). Rates of HIV infection among Nepali sexworkers under the age of 18 working in Mumbai, India, have been recorded as high as 72% (UNAIDS, 2000), and now in many parts of Nepal returnees from Mumbai are automatically stigmatized as AIDS carriers (Simkhada, 2002).

The overlap between the mobile sex trade and IV drug use is a serious driving force behind the spread of the HIV epidemic. For example, in Rome, Italy, high rates of HIV prevalence—74% (Gattari et al., 1992 cited in Inciardi & Surratt, 1997)—among South American transsexual sexworkers were significantly associated with the use of injected drugs (Spizzichino, 1993 cited in Matteelli & El-Hamad, 1996). Further, studies conducted between 1997 and 1998 found an HIV prevalence rate of 20% among 40 transvestite sexworkers in Rome, 65% of who were from South America (Spizzichino et al., 2001; Verster et al., 2001).

## Conclusions

This chapter has provided an overview of the changing nature of trafficking and mobile sexwork, and how mobile sexworkers, in particular, are impacted by STIs/HIV. The intersection of increasing mobility patterns and STI/HIV prevalence rates puts mobile sexworkers in a particularly perilous position with respect to their health. Preventive interventions specifically aimed at mobile sexworkers are urgently needed to protect the sexworkers themselves as well as to help stem the transmission of STIs/HIV to their contacts.

There are already some examples of successful safe sex programs for sexworkers. For instance, 100% condom use programs implemented in a number of countries—such as Thailand, Bangladesh, and parts of India (e.g., the red-light district of Sonagachi in Kolkata)—helped to significantly reduce STI/HIV prevalence among sexworkers (UNAIDS, 2004). Another highly effective STI/HIV prevention initiative is the TAMPEP/EUROPAP project in Europe that specifically targets migrant sexworkers (Morgan-Thomas et al., 2006). Yet, much more needs to be done.

In most countries, services for migrant sexworkers are virtually non-existent. Even sexworkers' organizations, which are active in many parts of the world, have very little contact with migrants, who generally view their involvement in the industry as temporary and do not wish to associate themselves with sexworkers (Brussa, 1998; Pheterson, 1996). In addition, the relationships between local and foreign sexworkers are often quite negative, as local women tend to blame migrants for driving down prices and violating professional standards by engaging in unprotected sex (Chapkis, 1997; McDonald & Timoshkina, 2004). At the same time, it is virtually impossible for migrant sexworkers to form their own, independent organizations due to their illegal status and high mobility (Morgan-Thomas et al., 2006).

Programs are therefore urgently needed to address the unique needs of mobile sexworkers in STI/HIV prevention. Confidential, culturally sensitive, non-judgmental services should be made available to migrants regardless of their willingness to leave the sex trade and return to their home countries. Such services should include: anonymous STI/HIV testing; distribution of condoms and safe sex information materials in relevant languages; substance abuse treatment and harm-reduction programs for IV drug using workers; and general health services. Emphasis should be placed on regular and continuous outreach in all workplaces of migrant sexworkers.

Furthermore, services for migrants working in the sex trade should not be limited to health promotion. The only way to address the multitude of problems facing migrant sexworkers is to create services that are holistic. Drop-in centers and crisis/help lines for migrant sexworkers should be established to provide various types of counseling and referrals. Counseling should be combined with housing and legal protection services, language courses, vocational training, and educational programs. The services for migrants working in the sex trade should employ cultural mediators, cultural advocates and peer educators who possess knowledge of migrant sexworkers' needs and are able to develop trusting relationships with the workers (Morgan-Thomas et al., 2006). Migrant sexworkers should be actively involved and integrated into the service delivery system. It is essential to promote formation of migrant sexworker peer support and self-help groups that would allow them to build self-efficacy, and empower them to take control over their working and living conditions. As well, it is imperative to build bridges of understanding and cooperation between local and migrant sexworkers to eliminate xenophobic attitudes towards migrants and their discrimination within the sex industry.

Services for migrant sexworkers should function in collaboration with government and law enforcement officials, health-care professionals, and the general public who should be educated about the realities of the sex trade and the situation of migrants in it to de-stigmatize sexwork and, consequently, to increase accessibility and effectiveness of services and responses to STI/HIV. But services alone can provide only temporary solutions. The problems surrounding mobile sexwork call for the development of adequate policies, specifically those governing immigration and the commercial sex trade that will address the needs of migrant sexworkers within the framework of human rights and social justice. Non-governmental organizations should take a leadership role in the international migrant sexworkers' rights and advocacy initiatives, and should engage in comprehensive program evaluation and dissemination of best practices. These initiatives should be informed by rigorous, methodologically sound quantitative and qualitative research. The collection of routine statistical data on STI/HIV prevalence rates among sexworkers worldwide is particularly important.

## References

African AIDS Awareness Campaign. (2005). *Cotonou: Nights under a streetlamp.* http://overland.naomba.com/cotonou.html (accessed 12/26/2005).

Alary, M., Mukenge-Tshibaka, L., Bernier, F., Geraldo, N., Lowndes, C.M., Meda, H., Gnintoungbe, C.A., Anagonou, S., & Joly J.R. (2002). Decline in the prevalence of HIV and sexually transmitted diseases among female sexworkers in Cotonou, Benin, 1993-1999. *AIDS*, 16, 463-470.

Albert, A.E., Warner, D.L., Hatcher, R.A, Trussell, J., & Bennett, C. (1995). Condom use among female commercial sexworkers in Nevada's legal brothels. *American Journal of Public Health*, 85, 1514-1520.

Andrees, B. & van der Linden, M.N.J. (2005). Designing trafficking research from a labour market perspective: The ILO experience. In (F. Laczko & E. Gozdziak, Eds.), *Data and research on human trafficking: A global survey* (pp. 55-73). Geneva: International Organization for Migration.

Australian Centre for the Study of Sexual Assault (2005). *Trafficking in women for sexual exploitation (ACSSA Briefing no. 5, June).* Melbourne: ACSSA.

AVERT (2005). *HIV and AIDS in India.* http://www.avert.org/aidsindia.htm (accessed 12/26/2005).

Baker, P. (2002). In struggling Moldova, desperation drives decisions: Europe's poorest country is major source of human organ sellers and workers to sexual slavery. *Washington Post*, A14 (November 7).

Baqi, S., Shah, S.A., Baig, M.A., Mujeeb, S.A., & Memon, A. (1999). Seroprevalence of HIV, HBV and syphilis and associated risk behaviours in male transvestites (Hijras) in Karachi, Pakistan. *International Journal of STD & AIDS*, 10, 300-304

Bastow, K. (1995). Prostitution and HIV/AIDS. *HIV/AIDS Policy & Law Newsletter*, 2(2), 1-5.

Belza, M. J. (2005). Risk of HIV infection among male sexworkers in Spain. *Sexually Transmitted Infections*, 81, 85-88.

Brussa, L. (1998). The TAMPEP project in Western Europe. In (K. Kempadoo & J. Doezema, Eds.), *Global sexworkers: Rights, resistance, and redefinition* (pp. 246-259). New York, NY and London, UK: Routledge.

Caldwell, G., Galster, S., & Steinzor, N. (1997). *Crime and servitude: An exposé of the traffic in women for prostitution from the Newly Independent States.* Washington: Global Survival Network.

Canadian HIV/AIDS Legal Network. (2005). *Sexworkers and HIV/AIDS: Stigma, discrimination and vulnerability. (Fact Sheet no. 2).* http://www.aidslaw.ca (accessed 12/26/2005).

Canadian Press (2004). Foreign women forced into sex trade: RCMP report. *Toronto Star*, A1 (December 6).

CDC (1987). Antibody to human immunodeficiency virus in female prostitutes. *Morbidity and Mortality Weekly Report*, 36, 157-161.

Chapkis, W. (1997). *Live Sex Acts: Women Performing Erotic Labor*. New York, NY: Routledge.

Doezema, J. (1999). Trafficking in myths? In (B.M. Dank & R. Refinetti, Eds.), S*ex Work & Sex Workers* (pp. 165-168). New Brunswick, NJ: Transaction Publishers.

Dreser, A., Caballero, M., Leyva, R., & Bronfman, M. (2002). The vulnerability to HIV/AIDS of migrant sexworkers in Central America and Mexico. *Research for Sex Work*, 5, 15-16.

Duddy, J. (2004). Expanding HIV treatment options for female sexworkers in Vancouver's Downtown Eastside. *Research for Sex Work*, 7, 23-25.

Elifson, K.W., Boles, J., & Sweat, M. (1993). Risk factors associated with HIV infection among male prostitutes. *American Journal of Public Health*, 83(1), 79-83.

Elifson, K.W., Boles, J., Posey, E., Sweat, M., Darrow, W., & Elsea, W. (1993). Male transvestite prostitutes and HIV risk. *American Journal of Public Health*, 83(2), 260-262.

Estcourt, C.S., Marks, C., Rohrsheim, R., Johnson, A.M., Donovan, B., & Mindel, A. (2000). HIV, sexually transmitted infections, and risk behaviours in male commercial sex workers in Sydney. *Sexually Transmitted Infections*, 76, 294-298.

EuroHIV (2003). *HIV/AIDS Surveillance in Europe: End-year Report 2002* (No. 68). Saint-Maurice: European Centre for the Epidemiological Monitoring of AIDS. Institut de Veille Santaire.

EuroHIV (2005). *HIV/AIDS Surveillance in Europe: End-year Report 2004* (No. 71). Saint-Maurice: European Centre for the Epidemiological Monitoring of AIDS. Institut de Veille Sanitaire.

EUROPAP (2000). *HIV infection: Screening, treatment and support*. European Network for HIV/STD Prevention in Prostitution. http://www.europap.net/ rep.html (accessed 11/1/2005).

EUROPAP (2001). *Final Report of the European Network for HIV-STD Prevention in Sex Work (Europap/Tampep 4), 1998-2000: Summary*. European Network for HIV/STD Prevention in Prostitution. http://www.europap.net (accessed 10/15/2005).

European Working Group on HIV Infection in Female Prostitutes (1993). HIV infection in European female sexworkers: Epidemiological link with use of petroleum-based lubricants. *AIDS*, 7, 401-408.

Family Health International (2005). *HIV/AIDS: Côte d'Ivoire Behavioral Surveillance Survey*. http://www.fhi.org/en/HIVAIDS/pub/Archive/bss/BSScotedivoire98.htm (accessed 12/27/2005).

Ghys, P.D., Diallo, M.O., Ettiegne-Traore, V., Kale, K., Tawil, O., Carael, M., Traore, M., Mah-bi, G., De Cock, K.M., Wiktor, S.Z., Laga, M., & Greenberg, A.E. (2002). Increase in condom use and decline in HIV and sexually transmitted disease among female sexworkers in Abijan, Côte d'Ivoire, 1991–1998. *AIDS*, 16, 251–258.

Gomes do Espirito Santo, M.E. & Etheredge, G.D. (2005). Male clients of brothel prostitutes as a bridge for HIV infection between high risk and low risk groups of women in Senegal. *Sexually Transmitted Infections*, 81, 342-344.

Green, S.T. & Goldberg, D.J. (1993). Female streetwalker-prostitutes in Glasgow: A descriptive study of their lifestyles. *AIDS Care*, 5(3), 321-335.

Hamers, F.F. & Downs, A.M. (2003). HIV in central and eastern Europe. *Lancet*, 361, 1035-1044.

Hawk, J. (1998). *Prevalence of HIV in sexworkers and risk to customers: A brief review.* http://www.worldsexguide.org/hiv.txt.html (accessed 10/16/2005).

Hughes, D. (2000). The "Natasha" trade: The transnational shadow market of trafficking in women. *Journal of International Affairs,* 53, 625-651.

Inciardi, J.A. & Surratt, H.L. (1997). Male transvestite sexworkers and HIV in Rio de Janeiro, Brazil. *Journal of Drug Issues,* 27(1), 135-146.

IOM (1998). *Information campaign against trafficking in women from Ukraine: Research report.* Geneva: International Organization for Migration.

IOM (2001). New IOM figures on the global scale of trafficking. International Organization for Migration's. *Trafficking in Migrants Quarterly Bulletin,* 23, 1-6.

IPEC (2002). *Every child counts: New global estimates on child labour.* International Programme on the Elimination of Child Labour. Geneva: International Labour Organization.

Leuridan, E., Wouters, K., Stalpaert, M., & Van Damme, P. (2005). Male sexworkers in Antwerp, Belgium: A descriptive study. *International Journal of STD & AIDS,* 16, 744-748.

MAP (2004). *AIDS in Asia: Face The Facts—A Comprehensive Analysis of the AIDS Epidemics in Asia.* Geneva: Monitoring the AIDS Pandemic Network.

Matteelli, A. & El-Hamad, I. (1996). Asylum seekers and clandestine populations. In (M. Haour-Knipe & R. Rector, Eds.), *Crossing borders: Migration, ethnicity and AIDS* (pp. 178-192). London and Bristol, PA: Taylor & Francis Ltd.

McClelland, S. (2001). *Inside the sex trade.* Maclean's, 21-25 (December 3).

McDonald, L. & Timoshkina, N. (2004). Examining service needs of trafficked women from the former Eastern Bloc: The Canadian case. *Journal of Social Work Research and Evaluation,* 5(2), 169-92.

McKeganey, N. & M. Barnard (1996). *Sex Work on the Streets: Prostitutes and Their Clients.* Buckingham: Open University Press.

McKeganey, N., Barnard, M., Leyland, A., Coote, I., & Follet, E. (1992) Female streetworking prostitution and HIV infection in Glasgow. *British Medical Journal,* 305, 801-804.

Miko, F.T. (2000). *Trafficking in Women and Children: The U.S and International Response. (Congressional Research Service Report 98-649-C, May 10).* http://www.usinfo.state.gov/topical/global/traffic/crs0510.htm (accessed 1/18/2002).

Ministry of Health and Family Welfare Bangladesh (2004). *HIV in Bangladesh: The present scenario.* Dhaka: Ministry of Health and Family Welfare.

Ministry of Health Pakistan, Department for International Development, & Family Health International (2005). *National study of reproductive tract and sexually transmitted infections: Survey of high-risk groups in Lahore and Karachi, 2005.* Karachi: Ministry of Health Pakistan.

Ministry of Health Viet Nam (2005). *HIV/AIDS estimates and projections 2005-2010.* Hanoi: General Department of Preventive Medicine and HIV/AIDS Control, Ministry of Health.

Morgan Thomas, R., Brussa, L., Munk, V., & Jiresová, K. (2006). Female migrant sexworkers: at risk in Europe. In (S. Matic, J.V. Lazarus, & M.C. Donoghoe, Eds.), *HIV/AIDS in Europe: Moving from death sentence to chronic disease management* (pp. 204-216). Copenhagen, Denmark: World Health Organization.

National AIDS Control Organization (2004). *State-Wise HIV Prevalence (1998-2003).* Delhi: Ministry of Health and Family Welfare.

National Center for HIV/AIDS, Dermatology and STIs (2004). *HIV Sentinel Surveillance (HSS) 2003: Trends, results, and estimates*. Phnom Penh: NCHADS.

O'Neill, R.A. (2000). *International Trafficking in Women to the United States: A Contemporary Manifestation of Slavery and Organized Crime*. An intelligence monograph, DCI Exceptional Analyst Program.

Pheterson, G. (1996). *The Prostitution Prism*. Amsterdam: Amsterdam University Press.

Pisani, E., Girault, P., Gultom, M., Sukartini, N., Kumalawati, J., Jazan, S., et al. (2004). HIV, syphilis infection, and sexual practices among transgenders, male sexworkers, and other men who have sex with men in Jakarta, Indonesia. *Sexually Transmitted Infections*, 80, 536-540.

Population Information Program (1996). People who move: New reproductive health focus. *Population Reports,* 24(3), 1-45.

RCMP (2004). *Environmental scan—June 2004*. Ottawa: Royal Canadian Mounted Police.

Riono, P. & Jazant, S. (2004). The current situation of the HIV/AIDS epidemic in Indonesia. *AIDS Education and Prevention*, 16(Suppl. A), 78-90.

Rodriguez-Arenas, A. (2002). Prostitution in Spain, health and policies. *Research for Sex Work*, 5, 8-10.

Robinson, L. & Rusinow, T. (2002). 'Like plastic that blows in the wind': Mobile sexworkers in southern Africa. *Research for Sex Work*, 5, 24-26.

Scarlet Alliance (2005). *National HIV Strategy: HIV and the Sex Industry*. http://www.scarletalliance.org.au/issues/hiv-strategy (accessed 12/26/2005).

Simkhada, P. (2002). Trafficking and HIV/AIDS: The case of Nepal. *Research for Sex Work,* 5, 27-28.

Simon, P.M., Morse, E.V., Osofsky, H.J., & Balson, P.M. (1994). HIV and young male street prostitutes: A brief report. *Journal of Adolescence*, 17, 193-197.

Spizzichino, L., Zaccarelli, M., Rezza, G., Ippolito, G., Antinori, A., & Gattari, P. (2001). HIV infection among foreign transsexual sexworkers in Rome: Prevalence, behavior patterns, and seroconversion rates. *Sexually Transmitted Diseases*, 28(7), 405-411.

Sudan National AIDS Control Program (2004). *Sex sellers situation analysis and behavioral survey: Results and discussions*. Khartoum: Sudan National AIDS Control Program.

TAMPEP (2004). *TAMPEP 6: Final report*. Amsterdam: Transnational AIDS/STD Prevention among Migrant Prostitutes in Europe Project.

Tchoudomirova, K., Domeika, M., & Mardh, P. A. (1997). Demographic data on prostitutes from Bulgaria—a recruitment country for international (migratory) prostitutes. *International Journal of STD & AIDS,* 8(3), 187-191.

Tomlinson, D.R., Hillman, R.J., Harris, J.R., & Taylor-Robinson, D. (1991). Screening for sexually transmitted diseases in London-based male prostitutes. *Genitourinary Medicine*, 67, 103-106.

Ukrainian AIDS Centre (2005). *HIV infection in Ukraine (Information Bulletin, 24)*. Kiev: Ukrainian AIDS Centre.

UN (2000). *Protocol to Prevent, Suppress and Punish Trafficking in Persons, Especially Women and Children, Supplementing the United Nations Convention against Transnational Organized Crime*. http://www.catwinternational.org/un_protocol.pdf (accessed 1/15/2001).

UNAIDS (2000). *Report on the global HIV/AIDS epidemic*. Geneva: Joint United Nations Programme on HIV/AIDS.

UNAIDS (2002). *Sex work and HIV/AIDS: UNAIDS technical update*. Geneva: Joint United Nations Programme on HIV/AIDS.

UNAIDS (2004). *2004 report on the global AIDS epidemic (4th global report)*. Geneva: Joint United Nations Programme on HIV/AIDS.

UNAIDS & WHO (2004). *AIDS epidemic update: December 2004*. Geneva: Joint United Nations Programme on HIV/AIDS.

UNAIDS & WHO (2005). *AIDS epidemic update: December 2005*. Geneva: Joint United Nations Programme on HIV/AIDS.

UNICEF (2005). *The State of the World's Children 2006*. New York, NY: United Nation Children's Fund.

UN-OCHA Integrated Regional Information Networks. (2005). *Ghana: Country profile: Assessment of the epidemiological situation, 2004*. http://www.plusnews.org/AIDS/ghana.asp (accessed 12/27/2005).

USDOS (2004). *Trafficking in persons report*. U.S. Department of State. http://www.state.gov/g/tip/rls/tiprpt/2004 (accessed 1/30/2005).

USDOS (2005). *Trafficking in persons report*. U.S. Department of State. http://www.state.gov/g/tip/rls/tiprpt/2005 (accessed 12/21/2005).

Van den Hoek, A., Yuliang, F., Dukers, N.H., Zhiheng, C., Jiangting, F., Lina, Z., & Xiuxing, Z. (2001). High prevalence of syphilis and other sexually transmitted diseases among sex workers in China: Potential for fast spread of HIV. *AIDS, 15,* 753-759.

Van der Helm, T. (2002). Migration and mobility of sexworkers in the Netherlands. *Research for Sex Work, 5,* 6-7.

Van Haastrecht, H.J., Fennema, J.S., Coutinho, R.A., van der Helm, T.C., Kint, J.A., & van den Hoek, J.A. (1993). HIV prevalence and risk behaviour among prostitutes and clients in Amsterdam: Migrants at increased risk for HIV infection. *Genitourinary Medicine, 69,* 251-256.

Verster, A., Davoli, M., Camposeragna, A., Valeri, C., & Perucci, C. A. (2001). Prevalence of HIV infection and risk behaviour among street prostitutes in Rome, 1997-1998. *AIDS Care, 13*(3), 367-372.

Wijers, M. & Lap-Chew, L. (Eds) (1997). *Trafficking in women, forced labour and slavery-like practices in marriage, domestic labour and prostitution: Summary*. http://www.inte.co.th/org/gaata/sum-irp.htm (accessed 9/29/1998).

Willis, B.M. & Levy, B.S. (2002). Child prostitution: Global health burden, research needs, and interventions. *Lancet, 359,* 1417-1422.

The World Bank Group (2003). *Bangladesh HIV/AIDS brief*. http://lnweb18.worldbank.org/sar/sa.nsf/Countries/Bangladesh/29D54DD8E1F82FCE85256DC0004BFFDA?OpenDocument (accessed 12/19/2005).

WHOROE (2004). *HIV infections epidemiology: Sentinel surveillance and risk factors: A comparative study in the Russian Federation, Azerbaijan and Republic of Moldova*. Copenhagen: World Health Organization Regional Office for Europe.

# Chapter 8

## Tracing the Diffusion of Infectious Diseases in the Transport Sector

YORGHOS APOSTOLOPOULOS, PH.D. AND
SEVIL SÖNMEZ, PH.D.

*". . . There can be no pause or let-up in the battle against HIV/AIDS. Every truck driver, taxi driver, bus operator, commuter, passenger, pilot, air steward and sea-farer can either be part of the problem or become part of the solution. . . . these movements can either continue to widen the spread of HIV/AIDS or become a powerful channel for disseminating the information, knowledge and understanding upon which effective prevention depends. . . ."*
Abdulah Omar, South African Minister of Transport, 2001

## Introduction

Despite notable differences in infrastructure and efficiency levels among transport sectors of industrialized and developing nations, technological advancements across different transport modes have contributed greatly to both socioeconomic development and accumulation of wealth. Efficient transport systems enable economies to develop optimal allocation of scarce resources, thereby maximizing wealth while securing the smooth operation of society at-large. In addition to its vital economic role, the transport sector carries indispensable social responsibilities vis-à-vis labor conditions, public health, and consequently, sustainable development.

While human biomass constitutes a sizeable fraction of the matter moved about the earth, most human mobility results from the planned transport of goods and services among different geographic points (EU, 2006). This combined movement has an ultimate impact on the jux-taposition of various species of oftentimes disparate ecosystems. While humans build road networks, tunnels, bridges, ports, railways, ferries, and supersonic planes that form effective means to traverse natural barriers to species spread, they often accelerate and even facilitate disease move-ment from one area to another. Mass processing and wide distribution networks further allow for the amplification and extensive dissemination of potential human microbes. Particularly in marginalized areas, transport milieux are highly conducive to risk-laden behavioral patterns and are

131

thus transformed into transmission settings and vectors of disease (Apostolopoulos, n.d.).

In the midst of the 2005-2006 fuel crisis, this chapter captures the transport sector in an era of intense competition and restructuring following the September 11 attacks. Wide geopolitical turmoil and subsequent demographic shifts in volatile regions along with the breakdown of public-health structures and environmental and ecological upheavals have contributed to an upsurge of pre-existing and the advent of emerging and re-emerging infectious diseases. This "anomaly" in the epidemiological transition poses additional threats to both the transport sector and humans, as wide dissemination of infectious pathogens remains an unintended but enormous consequence of transport. Within this context, this chapter places the transport sector firmly within the discourse of epidemiology and demography, and critically reviews its far-reaching role in the diffusion of disease— primarily of sexually transmitted (STIs) and bloodborne (BBIs) infections and secondarily of tuberculosis (TB), Severe Acute Respiratory Syndrome (SARS), avian influenza, and malaria. While all transport modes are reviewed, the chapter places particular emphasis on the trucking and maritime sectors in developing regions and presents new findings on trucking in the United States.

## Transport, Development, and Public Health

### Transport and Development

Socioeconomic development and public health represent essential forces of contemporary societies with the power to define human welfare. Within this context, transport functions as an intervening variable with the potential to affect both, by either hampering or accelerating growth that ultimately influences health. The transport sector—which physically moves humans, animals, goods, and services between different geographies—employs millions of workers, generates revenues, and consumes materials and services produced by other economic sectors. Not only does it provide vital links between centers of production and consumption, but the existence of adequate transport infrastructure and the provision of transport services are indispensable for the normal functioning of economic and sociocultural life and to the development of nations. Aggregate data indicate that the transport sector accounts for 5.3% of GDP in low-income and 6.8% in middle-income countries, while it ranges between 8-10% in the industrialized nations of North America and the European Union (EU) (BTS, 2006; EU, 2006).

The transport sector comprises a network of land (road, rail), water (sea, lakes, rivers), and air (civil aviation) modes, with streamlined intermodal connections at riverine-maritime ports and air-road-rail interfaces prevailing by the day (World Bank, 2006). It also includes subsectors that maintain and provide various services, such as forwarding, construction, fuel stations, truck- and bus-stops, border crossings, ports, bus and train terminals, and airports. In the post-WWII era, overall patterns and trends of travel and transport have exhibited marked changes. In the industrialized world, bus and rail travel have either remained relatively stable or have diminished while travel by car and air have increased; whereas, transport by bus and train has increased sharply in developing regions (BTS, 2006). Of EU's domestic land transport, passenger cars account for 81%, buses and coaches 9%, railway modes 7.5%, and powered two-wheelers the rest of total traveled miles (EU, 2006).

## Transport and Health Risks

Even though the transport sector has brought about a plethora of positive effects on the socioeconomic spheres of diverse communities, the correlation between the transport of people and goods and the propagation of disease has long been established (Hays, 2000). Health risks within the broad boundaries of transport range from the consequences of increased vehicle emissions (i.e., air pollution, asthma), traffic congestion (i.e., vehicle crashes and injuries, stress and mental health problems), and noise pollution (i.e., auditory disorders) to the ramifications of increased (i.e., inactivity, obesity, CHD) and decreased access to transport (i.e., transport wait time, maternal mortality, obstetric emergencies) (Frumkin, Frank, & Jackson, 2004; Marmot & Wilkinson, 2001).

The rapid geographic distribution of disease and its eventual ramifications of epidemic outbreaks represent some of the worst adverse consequences of transport growth (ILO, 2005). Overall, the transport sector has been linked with a multitude of airborne, foodborne, waterborne, bloodborne, and zoonotic disease risks (i.e., SARS, TB, malaria, avian influenza, STIs/HIV) (CDC, 2006). The inherent occupational risks of the transport sector render its workers as well as the populations they come into contact with particularly vulnerable to aquiring and spreading disease. Thus the dissemination of infectious diseases has far-reaching and complex implications not only for the transport sector but also for all sectors of economy and society. Transport appears to be the most affected economic sector in developing regions and as a result, STI/HIV outbreaks and epidemics have become serious barriers to development (World Bank, 2006).

Transport corridors, stopping places, and terminal points have proven to constitute prime vectors for STIs/HIV and associated risks (CSIR, 2004). These settings bring together transport services and construction and maintenance workers in temporary establishments where the absence of stable social networks is demonstrated with prevalent sexual multipartnering among non-regular partners (ILO, 2003). With about 80-90% of passengers and freight transported by road in East and Southern Africa, data show that mobility increases not only travelers' own STI/HIV risks but also that of their partners at home and of sexual partners encountered along transport corridors and at transport hubs (ILO, 2005b). Along Polish and Lithuanian borders, 42% of interviewed truckers reported engaging in commercial sex, 33% of whom without condoms (Kulis, Chawla, Kozierkiewicz, & Subata, 2004), and at about the same time, 50-fold HIV increases were recorded after the completion of the Kunming-Nanning highway in China (UNDP, 2001). In South Africa, 22% of transport workers were forecast to die of AIDS within five years while enormous economic impacts were anticipated, while in Thailand, HIV/AIDS related costs to the trucking sector were expected to surpass US$15 million just in 2000 (FHI, 2002). Despite the fact that railway tracks run along major road corridors in several African nations and Indian provinces, very limited research is available on the potential role of railways in disease spread.

Populations that are at the highest risk and also the most vulnerable fall under the following categories: (a) operators of transport services; (b) building and maintenance crews; (c) management professionals; (d) customers of transport services; (e) population segments that provide sex services in exchange for survival, safety, or resources; and (f) marginalized populations that the foregoing groups come into contact with. The first three categories, which constitute the core of the transport sector, include operators of buses, taxis, trucks, trains, boats, and airplanes, support personnel (i.e., loaders, vulcanizers, mechanics, and workers in roadside workshops), filling-station employees, infrastructure construction workers, supervisors and foremen, and other auxiliary employees. The last three categories represent those who use transport services or come into contact with transport employees, and include passengers, migrant laborers, itinerant traders, commercial sexworkers (street and brothel workers), reststop workers, lodge owners and attendants, residents of surrounding communities, local brew-sellers, barmaids, and their spouses as well as other sexual partners.

# Risk Vulnerability in the Road Sector of Developing Regions

## Sub-Saharan Africa and Southeast Asia: Different Settings, Same Scenarios

### Political Economy and Epidemiology

Sub-Saharan Africa (SSA), an enormous geographic area with numerous sociocultural differences but at least as many similarities, has been in a constant state of demographic flux in the post colonial era (IOM, 2003). A particularly gendered process by which men follow different routes and destinations than women, labor migration has been an important driving force in the culture and economy of SSA (Williams, Gouws, Lurie, & Crush, 2002). Interlinked customs and practices, such as patriarchy, gender relations, land tenure, and social customs (Schoepf, 2001) along with debt structural-adjustment policies (Stillwaggon, 2002) have fostered institutionalized circular (internal and crossborder) migration, which in turn has rendered people highly vulnerable and has deeply scarred the continent and its people (Synergy Project, 2002).

Propelled by socioeconomic marginalization, natural disasters and civil-military unrest, population mobility (facilitated by transport) has turned into the foremost factor fuelling HIV and associated epidemics (Apostolopoulos, n.d.). Just as severe malnutrition and multiple bacterial, viral, and parasitic infections have been predominant forces behind the unparalleled HIV epidemic—characterized by high prevalences, rapid spread, and uneven distribution and endemicity—the road sector has also consistently rendered populations highly vulnerable to STIs/HIV, TB, malaria, and other opportunistic infections (Caldwell, Caldwell, Anarfi, Ntozi, Orubuloye, Marck, Cosford, Colombo, & Hollings, 1999). The distribution of labor demand resulting in labor migration and family social structuring (IOM, 2003) has brought about prevalent multipartner sexual mixing and networking (Williams et al., 2002). Consequently, these and other factors have led to the current situation in SSA, which accounts for 60% of all HIV/AIDS cases in the world and the highest adult HIV/AIDS prevalence rates, estimated at 7.4% (UNAIDS, 2006).

Southeast Asia (SEA)[1] constitutes an equally large and diverse geographic area, where large population segments live in areas of pervasive poverty and maldevelopment (ADB, 2006). Equally pervasive is population mobility as internal (rural to urban) migration is gradually increasing with overall movement patterns involving high proportions of temporary migrants, and migration flows including significant numbers of youth and women (Guest, 1999). These "floating" populations, in search mainly of work, are highly vulnerable and oftentimes operate as bridges to the general population similar to other people at-risk (i.e., sexworkers, trafficked women, IDUs). Within such contexts, SEA is a collage of mini-epidemics displaying a considerable variation in scope and intensity. At the end of 2003, although adult HIV prevalences were estimated to be at most 0.9%, 4.1-9.6 million adults and children were living with HIV/AIDS (UNAIDS, 2006). India alone is second to South Africa in terms of the overall number of people living with HIV/AIDS, which was estimated to be about 5.1 million at the end of 2003 (UNAIDS, 2005). Epidemics in this region remain largely concentrated among intravenous drug-users (IDUs), men who have sex with men (MSM), sexworkers

---

[1] In this chapter, SEA refers to Pakistan, India, Nepal, Baglandesh, Myanmar, Thailand, Cambodia, Laos, Vietnam, Malaysia, and southern China.

and their clients, and the sexual partners of all these population segments (UNAIDS, 2006).

Road Construction and Transport Corridors

When roads, bridges, and other land-transport infrastructural works are built, they link low and high HIV prevalence villages and cities (UNDP, 2004). The impact of road construction on STI/HIV spread in a low prevalence area—comparing pre- and post-road construction and infrastructure improvement data—was recorded in the Mandalay-Muse highway that links Mandalay (Myanmar) via Muse (Myanmar) to Yunnan (China) (Hsu, 2001). Surveillance data reveal an overall increase of HIV prevalence among IDUs following the completion of the highway. Similar findings were reported during the highway construction project linking Kumming (Yunnan province, China) to Nanning (Guangxi province, China), as the overall documented HIV cases jumped from 10 to 525 within a three-year period (Kulis et al., 2004). Along the same lines, improvement works on National Highway One and Ho-Chi-Minh National Highway in Vietnam facilitated HIV spikes in Ha Noi and Hai Phong (UNDP, 2002).

Transport corridors in SSA are grouped into four sub-geographical regions. In western Africa, they are mostly vertical corridors connecting ports of higher STI/HIV prevalence countries of the south with land-locked lower-prevalence countries in the Sahel region, or horizontal corridors, connecting the capitals of coastal countries. Most notable are the Abidjan-Lagos, Bamako-Ouagadougou-Tema, Bamako-Ouagadougou-Niamey, Dakar-Bamako, and the Abidjan-Bamako corridors. In eastern Africa, major transport corridors connect land-locked countries to coastal ports in the Indian Ocean and the Red Sea, and they are the Djibouti-Galafi-Addis Ababa, Djibouti-Dewenle-Addis Ababa, Mombasa-Kampala-Kigali-Bujumbura-Goma, Dar es Salaam-Kigali-Bujumbura-Goma, and Dar es Salaam-Lusaka-Lilongwe/Blantyre corridors. The main corridors of central Africa include the Douala-Ndjamena-Bangui, Pointe Noire-Brazzaville-Bangui, and the Matadi-Kinshasa-Bangui. Finally, in southern Africa main corridors include the Durban-Lusaka-Lubumbashi (North-South), Beira-Harare-Lusaka-Lilongwe/Blantyre, Maputo Johannesburg, and Nacala-Lilongwe/Blantyre.

In the SEA region, transport corridors are grouped primarily into the Indian highway system (the largest in the world) and the ASEAN highway network, and secondarily into those crossing Pakistan, Afghanistan, Bangladesh, and Nepal. Within this division, and vital for transport and disease prevention, are the corridors of National Highway Six and Eight (China), National Roads One, Four and Five (Cambodia), Kolkota (India)-Patrapole-Benapole (Bangladesh), AH-01, AH-02, AH-03, and AH-14 (Myanmar), Kolkota-Birganj (Nepal), Peshwar (Pakistan)-Torkhum-Kabul (Afghanistan), and Quetta (Pakistan)-Spin Boldak-Kandahar (Afghanistan) (UNDP, 2004).

Truckers, Sexual Networks, and Bridging[2]

Truckers, who were implicated in the early geographic spread of HIV in SSA and later in SEA, are considered as regional core groups[3] in STI/HIV infection and transmission (Apostolopoulos, n.d.). Since 1983, when the Pasteur Institute identified HIV as the AIDS virus[4], numerous studies have tried to delineate how long-haul truckers have contributed to HIV spread in these regions. Findings from an exhaustive review, reported herein, cover 24 SSA nations—Benin, Burkina Faso, Cameroon, Congo, Ethiopia, Ghana, Guinea, Ivory Coast, Kenya, Lesotho, Malawi, Mali, Mozambique, Namibia, Niger, Nigeria, Rwanda, Senegal, South Africa, Swaziland, Tanzania, Togo, Zambia, and Zimbabwe—and 10 in SEA—Bangladesh, Cambodia, China, India, Myanmar, Nepal, Pakistan, Philippines, Thailand, and Vietnam.

Millions of truckers[5], their assistants, and their social and risk contacts have attracted extensive epidemiological attention and have been linked to STI/HIV transmission, while their mobility patterns have influenced the overall epidemiology of these diseases (Laukamm-Josten, Mwizarubi, Outwater, Mwaijonga, Valadez, Nyamwaya, Swai, Saidel, & Nyamuryekungé, 2000; Orubuloye, Caldwell, Caldwell, & Santow, 2001; Rao, Pilli, Rao, & Chalam, 1999). Although the "trucking hypothesis" (which suggests that truckers who frequent sexworkers on their routes across the Trans-Africa highway have spread the HIV-1 virus) lacks empirical support to single-handedly establish the magnitude of the epidemic in SSA (Hunt, 1996), it does however, corroborate the fact that when truckers travel, not only do they carry their genetic makeup, accumulated immunologic experience, and disease pathogens and vectors, but also their culture and capacity to introduce diseases into new regions (Apostolopoulos, n.d.). In fact, according to several studies, in 2001, 56% of long-haul truckers in the Kwa-Zulu/Natal midlands tested HIV positive (Ramjee & Gouws, 2002), while between 50 and 87% of Indian truckers were found to engage in risky sexual behaviors at "dhabas" (roadside hotels) (AVERT, 2006).

Truckers engage in vigorous sexual cultures around hotspots[6], the transient residents of which include poor, oftentimes young women from the rural

---

[2]When there is sexual mixing between high (core groups) and low (general population) STI-prevalence groups, these people serve as bridge populations.
[3]Core groups are defined as "small proportions of persons with an STI who are frequently infected with and transmit the disease, and who sustain the endemic and epidemic transmission of STIs" (Thomas & Tucker, 1996).
[4]While since 1959 scientists isolated what is believed to be the earliest known case of AIDS, suggesting that all AIDS viruses share a common African ancestor within the past 40-50 years, the term AIDS was not used until 1982.
[5]Eight million truckers and their assistants traverse the Indian subcontinent alone (IOM, 2005).
[6]Hotspots include, among others, trading centers, border posts/crossings, roadside settlements, squatter camps, truck depots, and other stops along truck routes that serve as homes to merchants, bar/restaurant owners and workers, young men who service the trucks, and sexworkers.

hinterlands (Synergy Project, 2002). Prevention experts believe that truck drivers play a major role in HIV spread in both SSA and SEA by importing HIV/STIs across borders and into rural communities and to people who were previously uninfected, thereby functioning as potent bridge populations (ILO, 2005). While there is extensive heterogeneity in work patterns and sexual cultures of truckers between countries, regions, and continents based on country size, religion, and culture, among others, risk behavioral patterns of trucking populations remain closely similar (Apostolopoulos, n.d.).

There are drivers who return home every one to two weeks, while others no more than once a year (Gibney, Saquib, & Metzger, 2003; Synergy Project, 2002). Long periods of separation from spouses and other regular sex partners give reason to drivers to engage in casual or transactional sex. In India, truckers engage consistently with large numbers of non-regular and usually commercial sex partners; in fact, they can have anywhere from 40-400 sex partners a year, depending on how much time and money they have on their hands (Synergy Project, 2002). In several predominantly Muslim SSA countries, quasi-polygamous patterns have been noted among truckers who have "serial" wives along their routes (Synergy Project, 2002), while others have "road wives" with whom they stay when traveling in certain directions (ILO, 2005). Commercial sexworkers are only part of the far-reaching sexual networks that exist at trucking-related hotspots. Both men and women who live and work around these settlements often have other regular sexual partners (in addition to their husbands and wives), while some trucker wives, who are left behind for months at a time, have other sexual partners of their own. Moreover, truckers frequently offer rides in exchange for sexual favors to itinerant market women traveling with their goods. Truck routes, therefore, operate as transmission settings that facilitate the travel of HIV from high- to low-prevalence areas along with trucks (Apostolopoulos, n.d.).

While heterosexual partnerships appear to be most prevalent, male truckers have also reported homosexual encounters on the road (Manjunath, Thappa, & Jaisankar, 2002). Truckers from Lahore, Pakistan who identify as Pathans (an ethnic group that accepts homosexuality) engage in regular sex transactions with other men (Agha, 2000). Nearly 50% of Pakistani, 25% of Brazilian, and 5-25% of Indian truckers report having had both oral and anal sex with other men but with erratic condom use (Synergy Project, 2002). It is worth noting here that most such homosexual transactions occur between drivers and crews—with clearly defined power differentials between operators and their assistants. In SSA, there is limited substance abuse involved in either homosexual or heterosexual transactions of truckers, while in SEA (India and Mekong region[7]), IDU has been recorded in both types of interactions (USAIDS, 2003; Zofeen, 2003a,b).

---

[7] The Mekong region derives its name from the river that runs through it and includes Myanmar, Thailand, Laos, Cambodia, Vietnam, and China's Yunan province.

In addition to truckers, several other commercial vehicle drivers and road transport populations are at high risk for STI/HIV infection. These populations include bus and taxi drivers as well as commuters using public-transportation (taxis, buses, and trains) predominantly in the Kwa-Zulu/ Natal, Gauteng, and Northern provinces in South Africa (Parker, Oyosi, Kelly & Fox, 2002), intra-city commercial bus drivers and motor-park attendants in Lagos, Nigeria (Ekanem, Afolabi, Nuga, & Adebajo, 2005), taxi drivers in Addis Ababa, Ethiopia (Taravella, 2005), commercial taxi and bus drivers in Ibadan, Nigeria (Akintola, 2001), motorcycle taxi drivers in Vietnam (FHI, 2006), and taxicab and tricycle drivers in the Philippines (Morisky, Nguyen, Ang, & Tiglao, 2005).

## Latin-American Truck Routes as Transmission Settings

### Demography and Epidemiology

Latin America, with Mesoamerica and South America as its two regions[8], is a diverse geographical entity with profound internal differences—demographic and epidemiological in nature, which are most visible in population mobility and disease risk. Civil-military strife, extreme poverty, and socioeconomic inequalities in Mesoamerica have produced constant crossborder movement within the region and towards the U.S. These sociodemographic factors along with larger economic imperatives—all deeply embedded in regional historical developments—have created caravans of refugees and other displaced populations, transport workers, sexworkers, merchants, truckers, sailors and portworkers, and other laborers (Population Council, 2006). In Mesoamerican migrant milieux, where institutional corruption, human trafficking, deportation, violence, and sex (transactional, survival, or non-consensual) are abundant, populations are highly vulnerable to disease (Bronfman, Leyva, & Negroni, 2002). On the other hand, South America with larger countries and enormous natural resources represents mostly internal, occupation-based mobility rather than crossborder movement.

With over 2.1 million HIV cases in Latin America and the Carribean basin combined, the STI/HIV epidemiology in Latin America is equally diverse across different geographies and demographies (UNAIDS, 2006). In South America, STIs/HIV are especially concentrated among IDUs and MSM— in fact, sex between men represents the predominant mode of transmission in Bolivia, Chile, Colombia, Equador, and Peru. While as South American nations with the highest HIV rates, HIV prevalences in Argentina and Brazil range around .5-.6%, infection levels among IDUs reach 60% in urban Brazilian centers and surpass 24% in some cases among MSM in Argentina (Fernandez, Kelly, Stevenson, Sitzler, Hurtado, Valdez, Vallejo, Somlai,

---

[8]Mesoamerica stretches from Mexico to Panama while South America spans from Colombia to Chile and Argentina.

Amirkanian, Benotsch, Brown, & Opgennorth, 2005). In Mesoamerica where HIV is transmitted predominantly via sex, IDU plays a lesser role, but HIV prevalence among female sexworkers ranges from about 1% in Nicaragua, 2% in Panama, 4% in El Salvador and 5% in Guatemala, to over 10% in Honduras (UNAIDS, 2006). Because developmental deficiencies in Mesoamerica frequently compel large numbers of people to migrate, which further fuels the epidemic, HIV is found mainly among marginalized populations. Recent surveillance data indicate that although sex between men is hidden, it is a powerful factor in the newly-emerging epidemics of Belize, Costa Rica, El Salvador, Nicaragua, and Panama (UNAIDS, 2006).

## Population Mobility, Truckers, and Disease

Epidemiological data indicate that within this volatile region characterized by constant movement, especially in Mesoamerica[9] some of the highest STI/HIV rates originate in areas where large populations on the move, with diverse origins, occupations and lengths of stay, converge. The most significant of these high-risk mobile populations are truckers, traders, sexworkers, employees of international organizations, and significant numbers of sailors who pass through such areas (Bronfman et al., 2002). A few examples of locations where they converge include Panama City's port, Mexico-Guatemala border towns, the Atlantic coast of Honduras, and Belize.

The foregoing begs the following questions: What are the conditions of transport corridors in Mesoamerica that render mobile populations vulnerable to STIs/HIV and associated diseases? Why are transport workers and their sexual partners particularly susceptible to these diseases, as compared to other professional groups? Part of the explanation lies in the fact that the broad risk environment includes transport corridors, nodes, and hubs as well as bars, brothels, and other related operations. Further, transport in Mesoamerica connects areas of high- and low-HIV prevalence, while busy transport routes, nodal points, and border crossings are associated with factors of transmission and higher than average prevalence (Bronfman et al., 2002; Bronfman, Negroni, & Kendall, 2002). Finally, transport workers experience elevated insecurity, have limited access to health services, and are vulnerable to harassment and extortion (often with police complicity) (Bronfman et al., 2002). Transport workers are not the only ones at risk; individuals who provide various services along transport corridors are also highly vulnerable to disease.

Transport, as a predominaly male sector, is also associated with peculiar notions of *machismo* (that is deeply embedded within Latin male culture), which often includes sexual relations on the road. Mesoamerican truckers have a reputation of being independent, aggressive, womanizing, macho men who consume large quantities of alcohol and engage in frequent sexual transactions with

---

[9] Four of the six highest HIV prevalence countries in the region—Belize, Honduras, Panama, and Guatemala—are located in Mesoamerica (USAID 2006).

multiple women on the road—which corroborates the prevalent "macho myth" (Bronfman et al., 2002). Extant studies corroborate the critical role of truckers in HIV spread in the region, especially through bridging and extensive sexual mixing among diverse, usually marginalized populations (Apostolopoulos, n.d.; Bronfman et al., 2002; Passador, Guirao, Pinto, et al., 1998).

The most comprehensive regional study was conducted at 11 transit stations (including crossborder stops, border ports, and seaports) in southern Mexico, Belize, Guatemala, El Salvador, Honduras, Nicaragua, Costa Rica, and Panama. Research results reveal that truckers (also referred to as land sailors) exhibit bisexual practices that do not contradict culturally defined machismo, drug use, practices involving casual and transactional sex, low condom-use, and frequent use of brothels, nightclubs, and other highway pickup places (Bronfman et al., 2002; Schifter, 2001). In some transit stations, reports indicate that over 60% of migrant women have forced sexual intercourse at some point of their travel.

In South America, the highest-risk transport workers operate along a highway corridor that connects Brazil, Paraguay, and Argentina. Argentinian truckers are known to engage in unsafe sexual practices with sexworkers, teenagers, and sometimes children, as young girls in the poorest northern regions often exchange unprotected sex for material resources (CDC, 2003). Brazilian truckers, on the other hand, who drive longer distances, are particularly vulnerable to risks due to their long waits at checkpoints to clear customs, which gives them time and opportunity for risky encounters (Population Council, 2006) and due to their extensive drug use (Silva, Greve, Yonamine, & Leyton, 2003). According to data collected in several Brazilian towns bordering Bolivia, Colombia, Peru, Argentina, Uruguay, and Paraguay as well as in the town of Santos, truckers form complex and risky sexual networks with multiple partners on the road (Lacerda, Gravato, McFarland, Rutherford, Iskrant, Stall, & Hearst, 1997; Lippman, Pulerwitz, Reingold, Chinaglia, Ogura, Hubbard, van Dam, & Diaz, 2004). In addition to truckers, three-wheeled motorcycle taxi-drivers, used heavily in public transport in Peru, play an important role in the spread of bacterial STIs (Paris, Gotuzzo, Goyzueta, Aramburu, Caceres, Crawford, Castellano, Vermund, & Hook, 2001). Motorcycle operators at a northeastern Amazon city were found to use the services of sexworkers and have other casual sex partners of both genders during their trips. In fact, findings reported high gonorrhea and chlamydia incidences along with low condom use.

## Eastern European and Central Asian Corridors: The Multiplier Effect

### Soviet Union Collapse and STI/HIV Explosion

Eastern Europe (EE) and Central Asia (CA) constitute diverse areas with notable sociocultural, economic, and topographic differences and extend from the Baltics and Ukraine in Eastern Europe to the central Asian states of Kazakhstan, Kyrgyzstan, and Tajikistan. The collapse of the Soviet Union, followed by an abrupt free-market transition, eliminated most social-safety mechanisms for millions of people, and fostered economic instability, unemployment upsurge, and westbound migration (ILO, 2005). As in SSA and SEA, circular migration became the driving force behind sex multipartnering and networking, as many migrant settings began to operate as sexual marketplaces rendering migrants vulnerable to sexual exploitation and numerous subsequent risks (Van Liemt, 2004). Sexwork and trafficking of women in particular continue to place migrants and their contacts in transit, destination, and home settings in highly risky situations (Limanowska, 2005).

The sexual and parenteral STI/HIV spread in EE/CA is believed to be getting out of control with a ninefold increase in HIV-positive cases since 1995 and 210,000 new infections recorded in 2005 alone (UNAIDS, 2006). The regional HIV epicenter—Belarus, Moldova, Russia, and Ukraine—continues to worsen with ripple effects felt by ever-larger segments of society, beyond IDUs and sexworkers. While the other EE/CA countries still have concentrated epidemics, they are rapidly expanding due to a high presence of HIV enabling factors (UNAIDS, 2006). In a recent speech, Peter Piot, UNAIDS Executive Director, stressed that while macrostructural antecedents drive HIV in the region (fueling both IDU and risky sex), it is crossborder migration that continues to shape both the patterns and distribution of HIV/STIs in the region (UNAIDS, 2005).

### Truckers in the Baltics and STI/HIV Risk

In Central Asia, several key transport corridors link broader regions and countries in the area that play an important role in disease spread by connecting high- and low-prevalence regions (Brushett & Osika, 2005). The northern corridor links Afghanistan to Russia through Kazakhstan, Kyrgyzstan, Tajikistan and Uzbekistan, while the south corridor links the Caucasus countries of Armenia, Azerbaijan, and Georgia via the Batumi/Poti-Baku and Batumi/Poti-Yerevan corridors (Brushett & Osika, 2005). Because drug and human trafficking prevail in the region, these corridors represent an area of special interest to public health specialists.

The Baltics—comprised of Poland, Latvia, Estonia, and Lithuania—stand at the crossroads of the main east-west and north-south transport corridors that link Former Soviet Union (FSU) and European Union (EU) countries. Baltic nations also neighbor Russia, Kaliningrad (Russian territory), Ukraine, Moldova and Belarus, where public-health conditions are rapidly deteriorating and STI/HIV rates are rapidly soaring (Benotsch, Somlai, Pinkerton, et al., 2004). In Russia and Ukraine alone, sexworker numbers are skyrocketing, condom use in the sex industry continues to be erratic, huge spikes are reported in syphilis alone, and IDU is on the upsurge (UNAIDS, 2006). Within this environment, Polish, Belarussian, Russian, Ukrainian, Moldovan, and Lithuanian truckers who cross the borders of these nations engage in regular casual sex on the road with random partners. Revealing data denote that over 60% of these truckers practice unprotected sex, even though they are aware of STI/HIV transmission risks (Kulis et al., 2004). Such findings denote that as transport networks of these regions improve and get integrated in the global market, so will the disease risks increase for transport workers at road transport relay-points, reststops, restaurants, vehicle repair-stations, and other locales where risk networks converge (Apostolopoulos, n.d.).

## Disease Risks Along U.S. Trucking Routes

### U.S. Truckers: Myths and Risks

Although the majority of industrialized nations rely mainly on railways for freight transport, in the U.S. the trucking sector constitutes the skeleton of the economy. Trucking comprises a sizeable part of the highway-services sector, which has over 55,000 facilities (4,500 of which are truckstops) and employs nearly 12 million truckers and 10 million other professionals (NATSO, 2005). From a health standpoint, truckstops[10] represent the most significant physical settings for truckers due to their policies, resources, and built environment characteristics with the potential to critically affect health (Apostolopoulos, Sönmez, & Kronenfeld, n.d.).

Popular culture has perpetuated the aura of "myth, danger, mystery, adventure, and manhood" for U.S. truckers, and has linked trucking to sexworkers and drugs, homosexual encounters at "pickle parks"[11], thieves and muggers, and highly sexualized conversations on Citizens Band (CB) radio (Ouellet, 1994)—further reinforcing the urban-cowboy legend. Truckers operate under stringent work conditions filled with stress and loneliness and in danger of traffic safety hazards (Solomon, Doucette, Garland, & McGinn, 2004). The vulnerability of truckers is further exacerbated by frequent relationship and physical-health problems as well as involvement in substance misuse and notorious gambling (Overdrive, 2002). Despite epidemiological links between a syphilis outbreak along a highway in the eastern U.S. and truckers, sexworkers, and drug use (Cook, Royce, Thomas, & Hanusa, 1999), little research has been carried out on truckers' risk interactions, their sexual mixing and drug use practices, or their elevated risks for disease acquisition and potential role in diffusion.

---

[10] Besides truckstops, trucking contexts and settings also include terminals, warehouses, and highway rest areas.
[11] Pickle parks are wooded, semi-public areas behind highway rest stops, known among truckers for incidents of homosexual activity.

# Trucker Networks, Substance Use, and Disease Risk

## Risk Milieux and Multimodal Populations

Trucking milieux are polymorphous settings with inextricable topographical, cultural, and psychosocial properties (Apostolopoulos, Sonmez, Kronenfeld, & Yang, 2006). Such contexts comprise interlinked entities with distinct sexual and drug cultures associated with spatial and temporal factors, types of risk exchanges and populations, and their position within broader risk geography (Apostolopoulos et al., 2006b). They mainly include truckstops and highway rest areas, various off-highway establishments that cater to truckers, highway adult bookstores, bars and nightclubs, striptease clubs, and mostly illegal brothels (Apostolopoulos et al., 2006b). Most risk exchanges unfold at truckstops (particularly those located in depressed urban areas), rest areas (more so when they are heavily wooded and have public toilets with stalls), and low-end motels (often close to adult clubs, sex stores, and bars, which do double duty as brothels). Since the late 1990s, truckers and truckchasers[12] have been exploiting the Internet to "hook up" in cyberspace and to arrange in-person meetings anywhere in the country. Thus, sexual encounters that might not have been feasible before are easier than ever to arrange.

The trucker typology of "highway cowboys," "old hands," "Christian truckers," and "old-married men" (Stratford, Ellerbrock, Akins, & Hall, 2000) was expanded on by ethnographies of truckers' multimodal risk networks (Apostolopoulos et al., 2006a). Findings reveal the existence of key players in these risk networks, best described as involved in supplying, consuming, or in some way facilitating risks: (1) *risk consumers* are truckers who are straight, gay, bisexual, or straight-identified MSM and who purchase and use illegal substances and sexual services; (2) *risk suppliers* provide or peddle illicit substances and sexual services and include female sexworkers[13], truckchasers and male sexworkers, and drug suppliers; (3) *intermediaries* facilitate transactions between consumers and suppliers and include pimps, polishers[14], lumpers[15], drug runners, and Internet webmasters and chatroom moderators who help to create virtual fora to bring together truckers and MSM;

---

[12] Truckchasers are men (gay, bisexual, or straight-identified MSM) who cruise for truckers in physical locations (i.e., rest areas, truckstops, bars, adult bookstores) and in cyberspace (i.e., Internet websites, chatrooms) with the intention to have sexual encounters.
[13] Sexworkers in trucking milieux are often called "lot lizards" (because they move from truck to truck in the parking lot and knock on doors of truck cabs to get truckers' attention) or CB prostitutes.
[14] Predominantly male transient/homeless persons, who buff and polish chrome details of trucks at or near truckstops.
[15] People who load or unload trucks and sometimes hitch rides with truckers for certain periods.

(4) *peripheral players* perform various tasks within the risk continuum and include female patrons of businesses that cater to truckers, "floating" migrant workers[16], hitchhikers, and other contacts at road settings; (5) *industry members* who serve various roles and include employees of trucking and shipping companies, truckstops, rest areas, and other highway settings; and (6) *relationship partners.*

## Sex and Drug Transactions on the Road

Empirical and anecdotal sources corroborate truckers' extensive sexual trans-actions with sexworkers and other women along U.S. highways and across the southern border in Mexican brothels (Hollister, 1999; Ouellet, 1994; Valdez, 2003). Sexual exchanges unfold primarily at truckstops where sex is solicited via CB-radio communication, via pimps and drug runners who provide women and drugs as "package deals," or by knocks on truck doors by women themselves and the actual sex takes place mostly in the cabs of trucks parked in the "party row"[17], at nearby motels, or in nearby wooded areas. Condom use is at best inconsistent, mainly due to truckers' incomplete understanding of potential risks and sexworkers' need for income expressed in the desire to have as many encounters as possible by going from one truck cab to the next. Research findings corroborate that truckers' risk-laden sexual encounters along their routes are often combined with substances that are used to relax or party during downtimes (alcohol, crack, cocaine, marijuana) or to stay awake during long drives (methamphetamines, speed) (Apostolopoulos et al., 2006a; Stratford et al., 2000). Various drugs are easily available around truck-stops and other trucking settings[18] and are frequently exchanged between truckers and sexworkers either as payment for sex or to use together during their encounters.

Most female sexworkers interviewed at truckstops were victims of various traumatic experiences (i.e., abuse, violence), homeless, addicted to drugs, and at great risk for STIs/HIV. Many women indicated that they came from socioeconomically depressed and densely populated urban areas, where they engaged in sex with members of other core groups (drug suppliers, pimps), thereby corroborating STI endemicity in these populations at risk (Apostolopoulos et al., 2006a,b). Life around truckstops further increases sexworkers' risks for physical, emotional, and sexual abuse as well as disease and social stigmatization. Nevertheless, many of these sexworkers remain at

---

[16] Usually transient and seasonal laborers who hustle around truckstops as they move to new jobs as they become available.

[17] Because trucks are parked in rows at truckstops, the last and least visible row is known as "party row" and is used by truckers who invite sexworkers into their cabs or others to use drugs or drink with them.

[18] Interviewed polishers and lumpers claim that 80-90% of truckers they interact with regularly use drugs.

truckstops because they feel safer than on the street, they assume that truckers have more money and can offer other resources such as rides, and some have repeat customers who are truckers. Sexworkers at truckstops are important members of truckers' risk networks and significantly influence the dissemination of STIs via truckers who bridge high- and low-STI prevalence groups and settings (Apostolopoulos et al., 2006a,b).

While truckers' heterosexual mixing is established, homosexual encounters have remained below the societal radar, primarily as a result of the hypermasculine and mostly homophobic nature of the trucking subculture. Sexual contacts between truckers and truckchasers often follow diverse cruising strategies and are characterized by carefully scripted interactions that depend on nonverbal communication and shared, but usually unarticulated, meanings[19] (Apostolopoulos et al., 2006a,b). Ethnographic research has revealed that truckchasers are often attracted to truckers who project a masculine image and represent the epitome of manhood as they perceive it (Apostolopoulos et al., 2006a,b). Homosexual encounters between truckers and truckchasers frequently occur in semipublic spaces such as highway rest-area bathrooms or stalls in adult bookstores (Apostolopoulos et al., 2006a,b). As revealed in interviews with truckchasers, safe-sex practices are often selective and defined by partners' "healthy appearance" and whether insertive or receptive sex is performed—which is closely related to perceptions of HIV/STI risks (Apostolopoulos et al., 2006a,b).

## Maritime Sector and HIV in Developing Regions

Millions of waterborne-transport workers handle over 90% of trade and a significant segment of travelers in seas, rivers and lakes around the world (EU, 2006). By default of their profession, sailors, mariners, seafarers, fishermen, motor-boat operators, workers on inland waterways, crew members, and port, harbor and dock workers, as well as boat passengers are highly vulnerable to HIV/STIs (WHO, 2004). Limited research[20] has been done on the potential role of these highly mobile populations—that remain away from home for protracted periods of time—as transmission pathways into the general population. The role of this population is even more critical in poverty-stricken areas where fishing and water transportation comprise survival activities for local communities (Wickramatillake, 1998).

---

[19] Initial contact ranges from truckchasers loitering in toilets at highway rest areas and tapping the brake-lights of their parked cars to various types of suggestive body language to get truckers' attention.
[20] Empirical studies have focused on Thailand, Myanmar, Vietnam, Cambodia, Laos, Ghana, Brazil, and Kiribati.

Waterborne crews face occupational (e.g., exposure to noxious agents, toxic or dangerous cargo, severe weather and climatic changes), health (e.g., injuries, depression, substance abuse, STIs), and psychosocial risks (e.g., separation and alienation from family and home, stress associated with shipboard living) on a regular basis (Wickramatillake, 1998; UNAIDS, 2005). Within such risk-filled environments, alcohol abuse, contact with sexworkers, poor knowledge of STIs, and unsafe sexual practices comprise key factors that contribute to elevated risks for STIs/HIV and disproportionately high infection rates (Binghay, 2005). As a result, waterborne workers oftentimes become STI transmitters into their own communities, particularly in small areas where locals are isolated, less mobile, and maintain an undeveloped commercial sex sector (WHO, 2004). One example is of the Mekong region, where it is estimated that 22% of seafarers are HIV infected (ILO, 2005).

## Seafarers in the Pacific and Southeast Asia

In the Micronesian island-state of Kiribati, high chlamydia prevalences were recorded among both trainee and experienced seafarers, while 85% of the syphilis cases were among experienced seafarers (WHO, 2004). There are parallels between the chlamydia prevalences among seafarers in Kiribati and truckers (10.2%) in China's Anhui province (WHO, 2001). The endemicity of chlamydia is of concern because most seafarers have regular female partners in Kiribati with whom they do not use condoms. It is likely that there is a significant rate of chlamydia transmission from seafarers to their partners who are at higher risk for STIs than the general population, as was the case with HIV infection in the same community. Moreover, despite a low .3% HIV seroprevalence, the STI picture suggests that seafarers are also vulnerable to the acquisition and rapid spread of HIV infection—supported by the fact that the high HSV-2 prevalence found reflects high levels of sexual activity by seafarers. In contrast, prevalence of nonviral STIs was lower than expected with no cases of gonorrhoea, and only nine cases of diagnosed syphilis. Low HIV rates can be explained by the low prevalence of bacterial STIs and low drug use (1.4%). Because these surveys did not test for chlamydia, gonorrhoea, or trichomoniasis in the general population, it is unclear if the risk behaviors are occurring in Kiribati at-large. Nevertheless, other studies (Synergy Project, 2002) suggest that itinerant men who have left behind wives and/or steady girlfriends demonstrate low condom use associated with increased STI/HIV transmission to their partners and the general community[21].

Epidemiological data from Vietnam corroborate analogous patterns. Factors influencing risk behaviors of seafarers in Haiphong (major city in

---

[21] A low acceptance of condoms was recorded in the study among seafarers for all sexual partners.

northern Vietnam) suggest that the "seafaring lifestyle" strongly determines conceptions of sexuality (Trang, 2002). Seafarers consider contacts with sex-workers or irregular partners a natural part of their occupation while their safe-sex practices (namely condom use) with sexworkers remain inconsistent and their knowledge of STIs/HIV remains unclear—which in turn lead to misconceptions regarding transmission routes. Similar behavioral patterns were also recorded in the HIV hotspot of Haiphong, among both fishermen and passenger-boat crewmembers (Trang, 2002). Irrespective of age or marital status, many fishermen in May Chai (docking area of fishing boats) and Binh dock visit sexworkers (with erratic condom-use patterns, despite easy access) even though they are not far from their wives as they live and work in the same town. In addition to frequenting sexworkers, many fishermen also have extramarital affairs along fishing routes, despite social disapproval, an'¹ share the view that condoms are not needed with mistresses because such relationships are based on love.

Fishing patterns, peer influences, sex industry, condom accessibility, and drug use play critical roles in fishermen's STI/HIV vulnerability in Kien Giang province, Vietnam (CARE, 2002). Because fishing involves heavy physical labor and keeps fishermen away from their homes for over three weeks each month, the men do not see their spouses for extended periods. As a result, during the week-long break when their boats are docked and fishermen get their pay, they engage in entertainment activities that often include commercial sex—readily available wherever the boats dock, and especially at popular karaoke bars in Haiphong and Cat Ba. Conversely, in the central region of Vietnam, there is some level of social pressure on fishermen to remain loyal to their wives, which deters the men from keeping mistresses but not from frequenting sexworkers. It is important to note that in this region condoms are also easily available (regardless of their regular use) and drug use is low among crews of fishing boats even though they are commonly used by locals.

Similar patterns were recorded in Thailand among fishermen working in commercial fishing trawlers (Entz, Prachuabmoh, van Griensven, & Soskolne, 2001). As with Vietnamese seafarers, Thai men also work under harsh conditions, staying out at sea for prolonged periods, thus remaining distant from their wives and families, with limited access to health care. When docked at ports, fishermen demonstrate risky sexual behaviors accompanied by excessive alcohol consumption—not surprisingly, 30% reported having had a current STI. Although STI/HIV rates have declined in Thailand per se due to aggressive government efforts, prevalences are rapidly increasing in the countries of origin of fishermen and boat crews (Entz et al., 2001).

## Seaport Workers in Western Africa and South America

Empirical works in Western Africa and South America indicate no major differences in patterns of risk behaviors among those working in the water as opposed to those who work by the water. Around the ports and harbors of

Ghana, women involved in informal economic activities (i.e., selling food), practice opportunistic transactional sex to supplement their income. Their clients include sailors, truckers, freight forwarders, various port employees, dock workers, and other food sellers and hawkers of various goods. Another HIV risk factor for the dockworkers is that many share occupation-protective items, such as gloves, boots, and helmets, and any accidents involving blood are opportunities for easy transmission (Okello & Ighure, 2004). Similarly, increased HIV rates of 7% have been recorded among sexworkers at Brazilian ports, whose clients are mainly dockworkers, sailors, and truckers (Hearst, Lacerda, Gravato, Hudes, & Stall, 1999; Lacerda, Stall, Gravato, Tellini, Hudes, & Hearst, 1996; Trevisol & da Silva, 2005).

## Air Transport and Disease

Approximately 60 million of the total 1.1 billion annual passengers of commercial airliners travel to developing areas of the world (EU, 2006). The enormous volume and speed of air travel along with the environment of the aircraft cabin facilitate the dissemination of infections that are endemic in developing regions to disparate geographic areas[22]. Both cargo and passenger aircrafts can become vectors of disease by transporting humans, mosquitoes, other insects, animals, and various animal products that, in turn, can transmit disease (DeHart, 2003).

Among infectious diseases that are easily transmittable via air travel, most important include avian influenza, TB, SARS, malaria, and west Nile fever (Mangili & Gendreau, 2005). Immediate transmission between passengers has occurred with TB and influenza, while vectors for yellow fever, malaria, and dengue have also been identified on aircrafts (Schuchat, 2005). Since 1946, a number of outbreaks of serious infectious diseases have been recorded aboard commercial airlines, with smallpox, SARS, influenza, TB, measles, and food poisoning among the most important ones (Herck, Castelli, Zuckerman, et al., 2004). Some of these diseases (i.e., influenza, SARS) are capable of causing even pandemics leading to high rates of morbidity and mortality, due to their ease of transmissibility among people, severity of the illness they cause, low level of immunity among populations, and ease and speed with which they travel (Toovey, Jamieson & Holloway, 2004).

Higher-risk populations of freight and passenger airplanes include pilots, flight attendants, cargo and cleaning personnel, other airplane and airport personnel, and passengers. As with truckers, rail conductors or mariners, the vulnerability of air-travel personnel to disease is intimately linked to the characteristics and environment of their occupational lifestyles. As road-transport

---

[22] Today it takes less than 24 hours to travel to almost anywhere around the world—a period that is shorter than the incubation period for most communicable diseases.

workers oftentimes have "road wives" and rail workers have "rail wives" with whom they stay and have sex when traveling certain routes, in a similar fashion, it is quite possible for airline pilots and crews to have similar arrangements with regular sexual partners in different cities (Apostolopoulos, n.d.). As with the road sector, hotspots for airline employees are locations away from home in which they stay for a day or longer.

## Surveillance and Interventions

Since the dawn of the HIV epidemic, the health ramifications of the transport sector have been treated as "collateral damage" associated with its many developmental benefits. But the elevated burden of the epidemic for humans and economies, particularly of developing regions, has given new emphasis to the acute need to develop and implement effective mitigation strategies. This is particularly imperative for those socioeconomically marginalized regions where STI/HIV rates have reached epidemic proportions not only among core risk populations but also among other vulnerable segments of the general population.

This overview has elaborated on how intertwined sociostructural, demographic, psychosocial, behavioral, and biological factors render transport populations vulnerable to disease risks. Road transport personnel (more so than rail or shipping) experience the longest and most serious border delays caused by bureaucratic inefficiencies or infrastructural problems that clog transport arteries and border crossings (ILO, 2005). The most notorious delays are experienced at Beitbridge (Zimbabwe-South Africa), Chirundu (Zambia-Zimbabwe), and Komatiapoort/Machipanda (Mozambique-other country) border crossings where truckers can be stuck for as long as several weeks. Consequently, hazards abound within these contexts, in which transport workers have frequent and easily-bought sexual contact with sexworkers along highways and border crossings and also maintain "road wives" with who they engage in risky sexual encounters.

As a result of its unique characteristics, the transport sector plays a critical role not only in the spread of STIs/HIV but also potentially in tackling disease spread (ILO, 2005). Just as its workforce is vulnerable to high risks for STI/HIV infection, it can also play a critical role in influencing the trend of such epidemics by serving as a social vector in disease transmission. This bidirectional relationship that the transport sector has with the STI/HIV epidemic can be instrumental in efforts to combat the epidemic and limit its impact. While prophylaxis, care, and treatment constitute the framework of interventions, the development of robust surveillance systems is fundamental to intervention strategies. Measures need to include comprehensive tracking of: (a) mobility patterns of transport workers; (b) HIV/STI knowledge, attitudes and behaviors of high-risk transport populations; (c) points and types of contact between transport populations and other high-risk core groups; (d) disease spikes and

Because these regions, in their effort to integrate into the world system of production and consumption, deal with millions of marginalized populations as well as increasing poverty and IDU rates, their transport sectors, which are anticipated to grow further, will only have adverse effects on their already generalized epidemics (Apostolopoulos, n.d.).

## References

Agha, S. (2000). Potential for HIV transmission among truck drivers in Pakistan. *AIDS*, 20, 2404-2406.

Apostolopoulos, Y. (n.d.). The "trucking hypothesis" revisited—long-haul trucking in Sub-Saharan Africa, India, the Mekong region and Mesoamerica, and STI/HIV diffusion (under review).

Apostolopoulos, Y., Sönmez, S., Kronenfeld, J., & Yang, S. (2006). Risk networks of truckers and STIs in North America: Drawing parallels with Sub-Saharan African and Indian cases. *International AIDS Conference*, Toronto, Ontario, Canada, August 13-18.

Apostolopoulos, Y., Sönmez, S., & Kronenfeld, J. (n.d.). Sexual mixing and drug exchanges of North American truckers (under review).

AVERT (2006). AIDS in India. http://www.avert.org/aidsindia.htm (accessed 7/4/06).

Benotsch, E.G., Somlai, A.M., Pinkerton, S.D., et al. (2004). Drug use and sexual risk behaviors among female Russian IDUs who exchange sex for money or drugs. *Intentional Journal of STD & AIDS*, 15, 343-347.

Binghay, V.C. (2005). Ensuring occupational health and safety for overseas Filipino seafarers. *International Society for Labor and Social Security Law* Regional Congress, Taipei, Taiwan, October 31-November 3.

Bronfman, M., Leyva, R., & Negroni, M.J. (2002). HIV prevention among truck drivers on Mexico's southern border. *Culture, Health & Sexuality*, 4, 475-488.

Bonfman, M., Leyva, R., Negroni, M.J., & Rueda, C.M. (2002). Mobile populations and HIV/AIDS in Central America and Mexico. *AIDS*, 16, S42-S49.

Brushett, S. and Osika, J.S. (2005). Lessons learned to date from HIV/AIDS transport corridor projects. Washington, D.C.: World Bank.

BTS (2006). Economic impact of transportation. http://www.bts.gov/programs/freight_transportation/html/transportation.html (accessed 4/5/2006).

Caldwell, J.C., Caldwell, P., Anarfi, J.K., Ntozi, J., Orubuloye, I.O., Marck, J., Cosford, W., Colombo, R., & Hollings, E. (Eds.) (1999). *Resistances to Behavioral Change to Reduce HIV/AIDS Infection in Predominantly Heterosexual Epidemics in Third World Countries*. Canberra: Australian National University.

CARE (2002). Seafarers, their sex partners, and HIV/AIDS/STD in Kien Giang province, Vietnam: CARE Vietnam.

CDC (2003). Argentine, Brazilian Truck Drivers at HIV Risk. http://www.cdcnpin.org/scripts/display/NewsDisplay.asp?NewsNbr=37449 (accessed 5/8/2006).

Cook, R., Royce, R.A., Thomas, J.C., & Hanusa, B.H. (1999). What's driving an epidemic? The spread of syphilis along an interstate highway in rural North Carolina. *American Journal of Public Health*, 89, 369-73.

CSIR (2004). A scoping study on community responses to HIV/AIDS along the transport corridors and areas of intense transport operations—Kenya, Tanzania, and Zimbabwe. Pretoria, South Africa: Council for Scientific and Industrial Research.

DeHart, R.L. (2003). Health issues of air travel. *Annual Reviews of Public Health*, 24, 133-151.

Ekanem, E.E., Afolabi, B.M., Nuga, A.O., & Adebajo, S.B. (2005). Sexual behavior, HIV-related knowledge, and condom use by intra-city commercial bus drivers and motor-park attendants in Lagos, Nigeria. *African Journal of Reproductive Health*, 9, 78-87.

Entz, A., Prachuabmoh, V., van Griensven, F., & Soskolne, V. (2001). STD history, self treatment, and healthcare behaviors among fishermen in the Gulf of Thailand and the Andaman Sea. *Sexually Transmitted Infections*, 77, 436-440.

EU (2006). Energy and transport in figures, 2005. Brussles, European Commission.

Fernandez, M.I., Kelly, J.A., Stevenson, L.Y., Sitzler, C.A., Hurtado, J., Valdez, C., Vallejo, F., Somlai, A.M., Amirkanian, Y.A., Benotsch, E.G., Brown, K.D., & Opgennorth, K.M. (2005). HIV prevention programs of nongovernmental organizations in Latin America and the Caribbean: The Global AIDS Intervention Network project. *Pan American Journal of Public Health*, 17, 154-162.

FHI (2006). Men's interventions: Peer education by motorcycle taxi drivers in Vietnam. http://www.fhi.org/en/HIVAIDS/country/VietNam/res_VietNamTaxi.htm (accessed 3/20/2006).

Gibney, L., Saquib, N., & Metzger, J. (2003). Behavioral risk factors for STD/HIV transmission in Bangladesh's trucking industry. *Social Science & Medicine*, 56, 1411-24.

Herck, K.V., Castelli, F., Zuckerman, J., et al. (2004). Knowledge, attitudes, and practices in travel-related infectious diseases: The European aiport survey. *Journal of Travel Medicine*, 11, 3-8.

Hollister, J. (1999). A highway rest area as a socially reproducible site. In (W.L. Leap, Ed.) *Public Sex, Gay Space*, New York, NY: Columbia University Press.

Hsu, L.N. (2001). Building an alliance with transport sector in HIV vulnerability reduction. Bangkok: UNDP.

Hunt, C.W. (1996). Social vs. biological: Theories on the transmission of AIDS in Africa. *Social Science & Medicine*, 42, 1283-1296.

ILO (2005a). *HIV/AIDS in the Transport Sector of Southern African Countries*. Geneva: International Labor Organization.

ILO (2005b). *HIV/AIDS and Work: Guidelines for the Transport Sector*. Geneva: International Labor Organization.

ILO (2003). *HIV/AIDS Prevention in the Transport and Informal Sectors of 11 African Countries—Botswana, Ghana, Lesotho, Malawi, Mozambique, Namibia, South African, Swaziland, Tanzania, Uganda, Zimbabwe*. Pretoria, South Africa: International Labor Organization.

IOM (2005). *HIV and Mobile Workers: A Review of Risks and Programs among Truckers in West Africa*. Geneva: International Organization for Migration & UNAIDS.

Kulis, M., Chawla, M., Kozierkiewicz, A., & Subata, E. (2004). *Truck Drivers and Casual Sex: An Inquiry into the Potential Spread of HIV/AIDS in the Baltic Region*. Washington, D.C.: World Bank.

Lacerda, R., Gravato, N., McFarland, W., Rutherford, G., Iskrant, K., Stall, R., & Hearst, N. (1997). Truck drivers in Brazil: Prevalence of HIV and other STIs, risk behavior, and potential for spread of infection. *AIDS*, 11, S15-S19.

Lacerda, R., Stall, R., Gravato, N., Tellini, R., Hudes, E.S., & Hearst, N. (1996). HIV infection and risk behaviors among male portworkers in Santos, Brazil. *American Journal of Public Health*, 86(8), 1158-1160.

Hearst, N., Lacerda, R., Gravato, N., Hudes, E.S., & Stall, R. (1999). Reducing AIDS risk among portworkers in Santos, Brazil. *American Journal of Public Health*, 89(1), 76-78.

Laukamm-Josten, U., Mwizarubi, B.K., Outwater, A., Mwaijonga, C.L., Valadez, J.J., Nyamwaya, D., Swai, R., Saidel, T., & Nyamuryekungé, K. (2000). Preventing HIV infection through peer education and condom promotion among truck drivers and their sexual partners in Tanzania, 1990-93. *AIDS Care*, 12, 27-40.

Lippman, S.A., Pulerwitz, J., Reingold, A., Chinaglia, M., Ogura, C., Hubbard, A., van Dam, J., & Diaz, J. (2004). Mobility and sexual partnerships of truck drivers in southern Brazil. *International AIDS Conference*, Bangkok, July 11-16.

Mangili, A. & Gendreau, M.A. (2005). Transmission of infectious diseases during commercial air travel. *Lancet*, 365, 989-996.

Manjunath, J.V., Thappa, D.M., & Jaisankar, T.J. (2002). STDs and sexual lifestyles of long-distance truck drivers: A clinico-epidemiologic study in south India. *International Journal of STD & AIDS*, 13, 612-617.

Morisky, D.E., Nguyen, C., Ang, A., & Tiglao, T.V. (2005). HIV prevention among the male population: Results of a peer education program for taxicab and tricycle drivers in the Philippines. *Health Education & Behavior*, 32, 57-68.

NATAC (2003). HIV/AIDS Policy and Strategic Framework of Action for the Transport Sector in Malawi. Lilongwe, Malawi: National Transport Sector HIV/AIDS Committee.

Okello, F.O. & Ighure, J. (2004). HIV/AIDS and the workplace—A qualitative assessment of the Ghana port and harbor communities for an HIV/AIDS workplace program. Cambridge, MA: Abt Associates.

Orubuloye, I.O., Caldwell, J.C., Caldwell, P., & Santow, G. (Eds.) (2001). *Sexual Networking and AIDS in Sub-Saharan Africa: Behavioral Research and the Social Context*. Canberra: National Australian University.

*Overdrive* (2002). When trouble knocks. September, pp. 28-47.

Ouellet, L.J. (1994). *Pedal to the Metal: The Work Lives of Truckers*. Philadelphia, PA: Temple University Press.

Paris, M., Gotuzzo, E., Goyzueta, G., Aramburu, J., Caceres, C.F., Crawford, D., Castellano, T., Vermund, S.H., & Hook, E.W. (2001). Motorcycle taxi drivers and STIs in a Peruvian Amazon City. *Sexually Transmitted Diseases*, 28, 11-13.

Parker, W., Oyosi, S., Kelly, K., & Fox, S. (2002). On the Move: The responses of public transport commuters to HIV/AIDS in South Africa. Pretoria, Department of Health, Center for AIDS Development, Research and Evaluation.

Passador, L.H., Guirao, J.L., Pinto, T.C., et al. (1998). Pe no Breque—Prevention of STD/HIV among truck drivers in the city of Sao Paulo, Brazil. *International Conference on AIDS*, Geneva, June 28-July 3.

Population Council (2006). An unfinished development agenda. http://www.popcouncil.org/pdfs/LACbrochure_6-06.pdf (accessed 6/5/2006).

Rao, K.S., Pilli, R.D., Rao, A.S., & Chalam, P.S. (1999). Sexual lifestyle of long-distance lorry drivers in India: Questionnaire survey. *British Medical Journal*, 318, 162-163.

Ramjee, G. & Gouws, E. (2002). Prevalence of HIV among truck drivers visiting sexworkers in KwaZulu-Natal, South Africa. *Sexually Transmitted Diseases*, 29, 44-49.

Schifter, J. (2001). *Latino Truck Driver Trade: Sex and HIV in Central America*. Binghamton, Haworth Hispanic/Latino Press.

Schuchat, A. (2005). CDC efforts to prevent pandemics by air travel. Statement before the U.S. House of Representatives, Committee on Transportation and Infrastructure. www.hhs.gov.us/asl/testify/t050422.html (accessed 2/23/2006).

Solomon, A.J., Doucette, J.T., Garland, E., & McGinn, T. (2004). Healthcare and the long haul: Long distance truck drivers—A medically underserved population. *American Journal of Industrial Medicine*, 46, 463-71.

Sorensen, W.C. (2003). Using mixed methodology to assess high-risk sexual behavior and adult stage among Bolivian truckers. University of New Orleans, USA: Doctoral Dissertation.

Stratford, D., Ellerbrock, T.V., Akins, J.K., & Hall, H.L. (2000). Highway cowboys, old hands, and Christian truckers: Risk behavior for HIV infection among long-haul truckers in Florida. *Social Science & Medicine*, 50, 737-749.

Synergy Project (2002). *Putting on the Brakes: Preventing HIV Transmission along Truck Routes*. Seattle, WA: University of Washington.

Taravella S. (2005). Driving HIV away: Helping taxi drivers protect themselves and others. Arlington, VA: FHI.

Thomas, J.C. & Tucker, M.J. (1996). The development and use of the concept of a sexually transmitted disease core. *Journal of Infectious Diseases*, 174 (Suppl 2), S134–S143.

Toovey, S., Jamieson, A., & Holloway, M. (2004). Travelers' knowledge, attitudes and practices on the prevention of infectious diseases: Results from a study at Johannesburg International Airport. *Journal of Travel Medicine*, 11, 16-22.

Trang, N.Q. (2002). Seafarers and HIV vulnerability: A study of fishermen and passenger-boat crewmembers in Haiphong, Vietnam. Haiphong: World Vision.

Trevisol, F.S. & da Silva, M.V. (2005). HIV frequency among female sexworkers in Imbituba, Santa Catarina, Brazil. *Brazilian Journal of Infectious Diseases*, 9, 500-505.

Ubaidullah, M. (2004). Social vaccine for HIV prevention: A study on truck drivers in south India. *Social Work in Health Care*, 39, 399-414.

UNAIDS (2005). Profiling the maritime industry and responses to HIV and drug use among seafarers in Cambodia, Myanmar, Thailand, and Vietnam. Bangkok: Seafarers Research Team.

UNDP (2000). Reduction of HIV vulnerability within the land transport sector: Towards a public policy framework for addressing HIV/AIDS in the transport sector. Bangkok: UNDP, UNAIDS and UNESCAP.

USAID (2005). *Transport Sector in Southern Africa—AIDS Brief for Sectoral Planners and Managers*. Pretoria, South Africa.

Valdez, A. (2002). *Sexworkers in Border Regions Potential Source for HIV/AIDS Spread*. http://www.uh.edu/admin/media/nr/2002/122002/valdezaids12022002.htm, 12/03.

Wickramatillake, H.D. (1998). *Infectious Diseases among Seafarers*. Seafarers International Research Center, Cardiff University, UK.

Williams, B., Gouws, E., Lurie, M., & Crush, J. (2002). *Spaces of Vulnerability: Migration and HIV/AIDS in South Africa*. Kingston, Queen's University.

World Bank (2006). Working with road contractors on HIV/AIDS prevention in Ethiopia. Africa Transport—Technical note. Addis Ababa: World Bank.

World Bank (2006). *Development Report*. Washington, D.C.: World Bank.

WHO (2004). Prevalance surveys of STIs among seafarers and women attending antenatal clinics in Kiribati. Manilla: World Health Organization.

WHO (2001). *STI/HIV Prevalence of Sexually Transmitted Infections among Female Sexworkers and Truck Drivers in China, 1999-2000*. Manila: World Health Organization.

Zofeen, E. (2003a). *Pakistan: Highways of Vulnerability*. www.youandaids.org (accessed 8/12/2006).

Zofeen, E. (2003b). *Pakistan: Truckers' Sexual Behavior a Risky Journey to HIV/AIDS*. www.aegis.org (accessed 2/23/2006).

# Part III
## Forced Migration: A Public Health Catastrophe

# Chapter 9

# War, Refugees, Migration, and Public Health: Do Infectious Diseases Matter?

FREDERICK M. BURKLE, JR., M.D., M.P.H.

## Introduction

This chapter addresses the various ways in which increasing world conflict, war, refugees, population migration, and the political and developmental inequities of these factors influence risk to infectious disease. There are many parallel factors occurring on the global front that may adversely affect capacity of public health to respond and protect the population it serves. Political violence, civil war, ethnic and religious conflicts, and in particular, the generation of millions of refugees by forced migration are obvious factors that are changing the balance between human beings and microorganisms (Pirages, Runci, & Sprinkle, 2001). Competing with public health's capacity to mitigate the effects of forced displacement are demographic and ecological factors such as increased population growth and density, urban migration and urbanization, failures of governance and the protection of public health infrastructures, human invasion of the habitats of animals and arthropods, and population induced environmental change.

Furthermore, because of post 9/11 preoccupation and anxiety with what advanced biotechnology easily provides to the arsenal of militaries and to those singularly disposed to wreck havoc on an unwary population for political purposes, most of these new disease outbreaks are first thought to have been the result of a deliberate release of an infectious agent. Indeed, whether these bioevents, accidental or deliberate, result in risk to populations locally, nationally, regionally or internationally lies squarely on the capacity of public health and a nation-state's capacity to ensure public health viability. However, public health can no longer be narrowly confined to aspects of preventive healthcare. Increasingly 'public health' is understood in the context of multidisciplinary and multi-sector capacities of governance and political will, economics, judiciary, public safety, quality of public health utilities, health security, agriculture, communication, transportation, education and training, and other capacities that allow a village, town, city, and nation-states to functionally protect its citizens (Burkle, 1999).

Current wars, internal conflict, refugees, migration, and the consequential worry over the spread of infectious disease have synonymously become, right or wrong, a catalyst to what some fear is either a prelude to a downward trend or eventual worldwide collapse of public health as we know it (Doyle, 2004; Glasser, 2004). Additional questions arise as to the relationship, if any, with the emergence or re-emergence of at least 40 infectious diseases, as well as an unprecedented increase of once-controlled and now antibiotic resistant infections, all in less than one decade (Heymann & Rodier, 1998, 2004; Paluzzi & Farmer, 2004). Any infectious disease emerging locally has immediate global ramifications. This is occurring in a world where the generous predictions of a decade ago of an emerging global economy have failed to emerge, but a state of global health is here to stay. As such, issues of war, conflict, migration, politics and whether they significantly impact global concerns of infectious disease are worth exploring.

## War and Internal Conflict

War has always been, and still remains, the prototype for understanding public health's dependency on societal order and the harsh consequences that occur when society witnesses its own physical, social, and cultural destruction. War and disease have accounted for a major proportion of human suffering and death. In the American Civil War, an estimated 660,000 deaths of soldiers resulted from pneumonia, typhoid, dysentery, and malaria causing a 2-year extension of the war. These diseases became known as the "third army" (Connolly & Heymann, 2002).

The United Nations Charter, drafted in 1945, was written with one thing in mind: *to end cross border wars*. Little appreciation was given at the time to Charter language which guaranteed that what occurred within borders of a nation-state were inviolable under laws of national sovereignty (UN Charter, 1945). Yet, since the end of the Cold War, 95% of all major conflicts have been internal nation-state wars, raising grave concern in the world community that the UN Charter is outmoded and fails to adequately address war provoked by political conflicts in sovereign nation-states. Indeed, no legal document exists that will undeniably enforce outside protection of nation-state innocent lives. (Burkle, 1999). By the end of the 20th century more people were killed by their own country than from cross border forces. Unfortunately, human rights and international law abuses by sovereign nations against their citizens have led to unthinkable ethnic cleansing and genocide, terms that largely characterize war at the beginning of the 21st century. These internal armed conflicts, otherwise commonly referred to as complex emergencies (CEs) or complex political disasters (Toole, Waldman, & Zwi, 2001; Zwi & Uglade, 1991) are now the most common human-induced disaster. CEs are further defined as "situations affecting large civilian populations which usually involve a combination of factors including war or civil strife, food shortages, and population displacement." (Toole, et al., 2001). The definition carries a lethal mix of poverty, racism, ignorance, oppression, religious fundamentalism, and cultural incompatibilities that contribute inextricably to inequities in access to and availability of healthcare, food, water, sanitation, shelter, and fuel for basic heating and cooking. Despite the obvious violence and deaths caused by weaponry in these CEs, it is infectious diseases alone that cause up to 70% of all deaths (Connolly & Heymann, 2002). This will occur, not only from declining public health protections, but also from the consequences of mass migration of populations fleeing the conflict.

# Refugees

Refugees are defined as people who flee their country to escape war or persecution. Refugees, who by definition cross sovereign borders, enjoy the immediate protections under international law afforded by the UNHCR (United Nations High Commissioner for Refugees) under the 1951 Convention on Refugees. This law protects them from being sent back home to unsafe areas and confers to them the rights for food, shelter and clothing, employment, and protection in the courts (Refugee International, 2002). However, the reality is too often that they will live in marginal and unsanitary camps that are large, crowded, lack clean water, sufficient food, or health services. Refugee camps are public health anomalies and as such are ideal locations for the propagation and spread of disease and are serious health risks to the population.

Camps may afford temporary protection but crowded camps, with poor environmental protections and increased density of populations, promote the spread of infectious disease. There are diminishing public health infrastructure problems in camps that exceed 25,000 people (Cosgrave, 1996). Fleeing the mass slaughter in Rwanda, refugees in neighboring Zaire found little solace when the crude mortality rates exceeded 60 times the population baseline, primarily from epidemics of uncontrolled cholera and dysentery especially when camp populations swelled rapidly to a population of over 300,000 lacking even the rudiments of public health infrastructure and protections. (CDC/MMWR, 1991; CDC/MMWR, 1993; CDC/ MMWR, 1996).

Despite declining incidence of CEs, refugee camps are still being built and populated. Refugees steadily increased during the 1980s to almost 20 million in 1990, mostly within Africa, Asia, and the Middle East (Toole et al., 2001; Prothero, 1987, 1994). In South Asia alone, some 35 to 40 million crossed international borders (Pirages et al., 2001). Over three million long-term refugees languish today in camps in Gaza, West Bank, and other areas of the Middle East (Refugees International, 2002).

Since the Cold War era, state-centric geopolitical efforts aim to prevent, rather than welcome, people from crossing political borders to seek safety. Refugees may bring many political, economic, and health concerns including real or rumored infectious diseases and fears that permanent refugees will threaten social cohesion in the host nation (Hugo, 1997). The UN has been forced to provide an alternative system using 'UN protectorates, preventive zones, and safe havens,' that assume temporary facilities and rapid repatriation (Hyndman, 1999).

## Internally Displaced Populations

Internally displaced populations (IDPs) are defined as those who have fled the conflict but remain within the borders of the country. Technically, IDPs remain the responsibility of their own country even though they find themselves persecuted by the government in power. They do not enjoy the legal protections afforded under international law to refugees. The UN with the objective to expand rights, protections, and services for all internally displaced populations is currently addressing these contradictory treatments. In the meantime, severely deplorable conditions affect IDPs, chance of survival (Refugees International, 2002). The larger numbers of IDPs over refugees are difficult to measure but ranged between 27 and 32 million in 1999. Political interference in IDP protection still occurs, as it has in Western Sudan, where NGOs and UN agencies continue to struggle with the Sudanese government to recognize a UN Security Council Resolution that allows protective access to camps under threat from rebel factions.

Political violence, destroyed health facilities, infrastructure, and disruption of food security led to forced IDP migration with many finding themselves in even worse environments, such as hostile mountain slopes or desolate deserts (Toole, et al., 2001). Not unusual, adult males often remained behind to care for animals and land, or to fight, leaving the IDP women and children to fend for themselves. High mortality occurs immediately following migration when relief efforts have not yet begun. Like refugees, the causes of death are generally preventable common infectious diseases such as measles, diarrhea, malaria, cholera, dysentery, and acute respiratory infections (Burkholder & Toole, 1995).

IDP mortality rates are frequently 7 to 10 times the baseline population. Unaccompanied minors and orphans, without critical protections afforded by adult supervision number in the tens of thousands (Toole et al., 2001; CDC/MMWR, 1991) resulting in mortality rates 100 to 800 times the baseline. A cluster survey study, performed in hostile territory of Eastern Congo among rapidly moving IDPs, found that at least 2.5 million excess deaths occurred within a 4-month period. Only 10% of these deaths were from war-related trauma; 90% were from preventable infectious diseases (diarrheal dehydration and malaria) and malnutrition (Roberts, 2001).

# Epidemiological Models of Complex Emergencies

Seventy-one countries have internal conflict situations severe enough to warrant placement on a Crisis Watch List where conditions are assessed monthly for deterioration or improvement (International Crisis Group, 2005). Studies performed over the last 20 years of evolving complex emergencies in Africa, Asia, Middle East, and Eastern Europe have suggested that at least three distinct epidemiological models exist: *developing country* (e.g., primarily seen in Africa and Asian countries such as Somali, Angola, Rwanda, East Timor), *chronic* or *smoldering country* (e.g., Sudan, Haiti, Israel-Palestine), and *developed country* (e.g., Former Yugoslavia, Iraq, Macedonia, Kosovo). These epidemiologically described models are helpful in illustrating to policy level decision-makers the impact of conflict on civilian populations and public health infrastructure, but are also useful in planning for humanitarian interventions if and when they occur. Non-governmental aid organizations and UN agencies usually have, by legal mandate, an ongoing presence in crisis prone countries. These interventions are often designed to mitigate the severe consequences on the most vulnerable populations (women, children, elderly, disabled). If a wider assistance intervention occurs, it takes the form of a larger multi-sectoral, multidisciplinary, and multinational humanitarian model of intervention under UN Security Council Resolution political authority.

## Developing Country Model

Living in a developing country does matter when it comes to vulnerability to infectious diseases. Overall, more people are affected by disasters where there is a rapid population increase and rapid unplanned development, particularly in urban areas. Where high human development (HHD) occurs, averages of 44 people are killed per disaster event, whereas in countries of low human development (LHD), averages of 300 people are killed per event (Walter, 2004) and governance easily falters with increasing violence and declining public health services that these disasters often bring (Zwi & Uglade, 1989).

This model, common to Africa and Asia, provides an acute phase health profile of moderate to severe malnutrition, outbreaks of communicable diseases, high crude mortality rates, high case fatality rates, and the virtual absence of functionally protective public health infrastructure (Burkholder & Toole, 1995; Toole et al., 2001). Countries in crisis, all with high endemic disease burdens, claim 75% of all reported epidemics of the 1990s. (Toole et al., 2001). Infectious diseases that kill so many are, for the most part, no different from those endemic bacteria, viruses, and parasites that prevail in non-emergency conditions. If we learn anything from CEs, it is that once the pre-conflict protective public health infrastructure lid is removed, the endemic diseases, given the opportunity, will become epidemic (Toole et al., 2001; Toole & Waldman, 1990, 1997).

Countries are also more likely to suffer famine and few have occurred that were not human induced or catalyzed the onset of CEs. Severe malnutrition, often referred to as protein energy malnutrition (PEM), is characterized by malnutrition, micronutrient deficiencies (in particular Vitamin A, C, and B6), and secondary infections. A PEM induced state of immunodeficiency is to blame for the frequent complications of secondary infections that account for the majority of deaths. High case fatality rates occur from simple childhood diseases such as measles, upper respiratory infections, diarrhea, and vaccine preventable diseases. Mortality and morbidity rates from measles can be greatly improved with the emergency use of low cost measles vaccine and Vitamin A supplements (Burkle, 1999; Burkholder & Toole, 1995; Toole et al., 2001). The objective of humanitarian assistance is to decline these consequences by provision of food, water, sanitation, and shelter, a Health Information System (HIS), diarrheal disease control, immunization programs, basic curative care, and maternal and child health care, among other primary care essential programs (CDC/MMWR, 1992).

## Chronic or Smoldering Country Model

In all chronic, smoldering country models there are too few public health resources to defend an epidemic outbreak. Countries must rely on outside resources. Sudan, which has been at war since 1955, has a health profile of chronically malnourished children who know only a culture of violence and have little access to healthcare or education. Reproductive health and safe birthing remain an unknown luxury for most of the population. In 2003, an acute internal war resulted in over 70,000 deaths and 1.2 million internally displaced non-Arabs fleeing to the Darfur region in western Sudan. Mortality rates from acute traumatic small arms and machete-induced violence were 16 to 18 times the population baseline. Once the internal population fled to makeshift camps in the western region the deaths from rebel violence diminished but deaths from preventable diseases predictably escalated (Depoortere, Checchi, Broillet, Minetti, Gayraud, Briet, Pahl, Defourney, Tatay, & Brown, 2004).

In Haiti, disease demographics, except for HIV/AIDS, are similar to that seen in the U.S. in the early 1900s. Haiti represents, for outside aid organizations, both a chronic developmental emergency as well as an acute emergency situation. Chronically poor public health infrastructure, massive environmental problems (i.e., severe deforestation), along with high population density and acute and chronic outbreaks of preventable disease are commonplace (Farmer, 2004; Regan, 2004).

There are marked differences between the availability and access to health services seen in Israel and the occupied zones of the Palestinian West Bank and Gaza refugee camps. Initial mortality and nutritional indices were similar to those seen in Somalia and Bangladesh (Bennett, 2002). Once these studies were made public, the UN, which has oversight responsibility for refugees in these occupied zones, increased and improved their aid capacity but like other chronic CEs these health indices fluctuate depending upon political and conflict conditions.

## Developed Country Model

Before the onset of internal conflicts, countries such as Iraq, the Former Yugoslavia, Macedonia, and Kosovo had relatively healthy populations with demographic profiles similar to Western countries. With war, the relatively low prevalence of malnutrition among children and infants were superseded by under nutrition and untreated chronic diseases (e.g., hypertension, diabetes, chronic heart diseases) among the elderly who could not flee the conflict and were later unable to access food, health care, and pharmaceuticals. High mortality rates were primarily from trauma from advanced weaponry (Spiegel & Salama, 2000). In contrast to the previous two models, few outbreaks and no epidemics occurred due to dedicated attempts by the humanitarian community to keep the rudiments of the public health system functioning and encouragement of the educated population to maintain daily hygiene and hand washing practices.

After the first Persian Gulf War in 1991, for 71 days Baghdad and other cities throughout Iraq suffered loss of electricity, refrigeration, and disruption of water and sewage pipes from bombing (CDC/MMWR, 1991). Within two weeks, Baghdad, which had not seen a case of endemic cholera in over 20 years, experienced an outbreak. In the prolonged violence that has plagued Iraq since the beginning of the 2003 war, insecurity and social disorder have accounted for failure to return function to clinical and public health facilities. Only a semblance of a national surveillance system exists, preventing confirmation as to the status of a pre-war gradual rise in malaria, leishmaniasis, tuberculosis (TB), and cholera cases (Burkle & Noji, 2004). A 2004 UN and Iraq Ministry of Health rapid nutrition assessment study confined to Baghdad showed that 7.7% of children under the age of five were suffering from acute malnutrition, compared to 2002's figure of 4% (Office of the Coordinator for Humanitarian Affairs, 2004). In 2005, higher than expected cost of protecting workers against insurgents attacks (about 25 cents of every reconstruction dollar now pays for security) has severely limited original plans for public health utility infrastructure repair, and rising security costs led to budget cuts by occupying forces for crucial water treatment plants, sewage networks, and power grids.

# Public Health and Infectious Disease

## State Capacity

Each nation-state strives to maintain continuity of government. This can be measured by how bioevents negatively affect a state's capacity (SC) by creating political, economic, and social instability. Price-Smith defines SC as a country's capacity to maximize its stability in exerting de facto control and protecting its population from infectious agents, both accidental and deliberate (1998). He demonstrated that public health is a major driver of SC, in that a strong positive correlation exists between health, and in particular, infectious disease control (Price-Smith, 1998).

An objective of terrorism is to compromise SC and embarrass the government in power by revealing its political, social, public health, and economic weaknesses (Burkle, 2002). Developed countries possess internal levels of SC in the form of economic resources, human capital, infrastructural investments, and scientific capability (Price-Smith & Daly, 2004). Such countries have had success in responding to epidemics such as SARS and HIV/AIDS. Countries in crisis, especially developing ones, have low SC levels primarily due to poor governance, which leads to decline in public health capacity. Zimbabwe is cited as an example where HIV/AIDS, in particular, has destabilized the government by exacting an increasingly larger toll on the country's economic productivity, political capacity, its life expectancy, and capacity of the police and military security forces (Price-Smith & Daly, 2004). Declining SC can open a failing nation-state to internal violence. The term 'health security' has historical basis in CEs, the threat of bioterrorism, and newly emerging and re-emergent diseases. All have in common the threat to destroy a significant proportion of the population. Infectious disease, in particular, may in fact contribute to societal destabilization and to chronic low-intensity internal violence, and in extreme cases, it may accelerate the processes that lead to state failure (Fourie & Schonteich, 2001, Price-Smith, 1999, 2002). For countries in crisis, HIV/AIDS and TB programs fail quickly (UNAIDS, 2004). TB programs are forced to taper the availability of medications leading quickly to the emergence of drug-resistance and increased opportunities for communicability.

Historically, no country has acted fast enough or done enough to mitigate the consequences of HIV/AIDS or TB. In the U.S., cutbacks in essential program funding at the state levels have threatened public health by curtailing efforts to combat disease, such as TB. Ironically, some cutbacks are attributed to diversion of funding resources to fight bioterrorism (Dolye, 2004).

Both Uganda and Thailand are cited as examples of countries that may suffer in public health capacity, but through good governance and use of simple public health measures have 'mobilized civil society' to reduce behaviors (e.g., unsafe sex) that increase the risk of transmission of disease (Price-Smith & Daly, 2004). Although major epidemics were averted in most developed country model CEs, lessons learned from humanitarian missions in Africa, the Balkans, and other developing countries forced healthcare workers to plan for outbreaks, especially enteric diseases, when the water and sanitation systems were disrupted, and to perform more stringent scrutiny on refugees entering the U.K. from these regions (Black & Healing, 1993).

An argument against use of politically driven economic sanctions, commonly used to control internal conflict within rogue sovereign countries, is that sanctions may contribute to decline in health standards (Toole, Galson, & Brady, 1993). Unfortunately, with time and inattention, all CE epidemiological models steadily decline in SC and health security. With a continuum of protracted social and political conflict, the model boundaries blur and eventually all represent catastrophic public health emergencies (e.g., Chechnya, Liberia, Gaza, Sudan, Haiti) that require continual outside assistance to survive.

## Mobility and Urbanization

There is much historical evidence of the spread of disease through human mobility (Prothero, 1977, 1987; Siem, 1997). In spite of medical advances and international health measures, there is still much cause for concern. Today, there is now more mobility, redistribution of populations across the developing world, and massive rural-urban movements than ever before. (Carballo & Nerukar, 2001; Cookson, Carballo, Nolan, Keystone, & Jong, 2001). Most movement comes from the Third World and the majority are the consequence of fleeing violence and economic collapse.

The urbanized proportion of the world's population has grown from 5% to 50% in the last two centuries and is still rising (McMichael, Kjellstrom, & Smith, 2001) In Africa, high rates of urban growth and rural-to-urban movement resulted in almost 67% of the population now living in cities. It is predicted, by 2012 to 15, the world will experience more people living in urban settings than rural. It is most worrisome that by the year 2015 there could be at least 26 urban areas (mega cities) of 10 million inhabitants, or more, all but four being in developing countries (Pirages et al., 2001) without complementary economic development and public health infrastructure protection (Prothero, 1987, 1994). By 2025, Asia's population is expected to contain half the world's people, more than half of whom will live in cities. Unlike much of the industrialized world, where urbanization followed industrialization, urbanization and industrialization have largely taken place independently. According to the Asian Development Bank, 13 of the 15 most polluted cities are already in the Asia-Pacific region, where some rivers carry up to three to four times the average world's levels of fecal pollutants (Brower & Chalk, 2003).

Urban migrant populations tend to be young adult males escaping conflict or rural poverty. Women, many widowed with 2 to 5 children, who first resisted migration from rural villages, were forced to migrate to urban areas to flee disease, rape, and seek support services and protection. Factors associated with infectious disease, HIV/AIDS and other sexually transmitted disease transmission, are directly related to population migration, disruption of rural families, urbanization, social disruption, poor medical services, declining economy, low social status of women, and prostitution for means of survival. Population mobility, as a whole, has also contributed to the transmission of malaria and prejudiced programs for control and eradication of malaria, TB, and HIV/AIDS (Quinn, 1995).

As a consequence of urbanization, the crude population density increased on an average greater than 100% in every country where data was available (Quinn, 1995). Consequently, outside humanitarian assistance is slowly moving to the urban environment, however little is known and few people are trained in how to defend a collapsing urban public health system. Most of the problems with infectivity in densely crowded settings such as refugee camps and cities arise through contamination of the environment by permanent excretors, such as livestock and humans, in particular young children who defecate everywhere and anywhere, and generate an inexhaustible reservoir for contamination of the soil, water, and urban dwellings (Toole et al., 2001). Researchers claim that 'risk for the health of humans' due to symptomatic and non-symptomatic carriers of infectious agents and permanent excretors has 'dramatically increased' with refugees, urbanized crowding, and international tourism (Smith, 2001).

## International Migration

Although international migrants only represent 4.5% of the world's population, they remain a challenge especially on the potential impact on a host countries' health (Santoro, Visona, Pusterla, & Vigevani, 2000). Refugees resettling in their new country carry a significant burden of infectious diseases because of exposure in their countries of origin and circumstances of their migration. The death rate of newly arrived refugees was estimated to be 30 times the death rate in their country of origin. During a two year study period, 156 asylum seekers in the Netherlands died, 15 from infectious disease (Koppenaal, Bos, & Broer, 2003). Among migrants to Italy, mostly from the Former Yugoslavia and Africa, 8.2% were admitted to hospital in 1998 for infectious diseases (Santoro et al., 2000). Ten thousand refugees to Sweden, primarily from the Former Yugoslavia, Africa, Asia, and Iraq showed high prevalence of hepatitis B, TB and HIV (Christenson, 1995), and TB prevalence rates for refugee populations reaching Australia were 157/100,000 as compared to incidence in Australia of 4.93/100,000 population (King & Vodicka, 2001).

Overseas screening of refugees is required, but it inadequately assesses infectious diseases. Negative results may occur in overseas screening so there is a need to monitor the infectious disease prevalence and the effectiveness of overseas screening by on-arrival screening (Barnett, 2004). Entry screening protocols exist for TB, hepatitis B, intestinal and other parasites, and updating immunizations, as well as tests for malaria, HIV, and sexually transmitted diseases. Researchers caution that war-related outbreaks of diphtheria, now surfacing in Central Asia, and drug-resistant TB in Russia require greater public health 'vigilance' (Christenson, 1995).

## Emerging and Re-emerging Diseases

Emerging infectious diseases are those due to newly identified and previously unknown infections that cause public health problems either locally or internationally. Many emerging diseases are thought to be due to a closer contact of humans with their reservoir in nature, with a jump of the infectious agent from animal to human across the species barrier (e.g., avian influenza).

Legitimate concerns exist that prolonged war or smoldering conflict places economic drain on nation-states leading to conditions ripe for the emergence of new diseases. The world's burden of disease disproportionably affects the people of Sub-Saharan Africa that represents 10% of the total population but 26% of the total fatal and non-fatal health outcomes (Bloom, 2001; Michaud, Murray, & Murray & Lopez, 1996). At the beginning of 2003, only two countries in Sub-Saharan Africa were polio-endemic. However, in 2004 at the height of political turmoil, a tragic setback occurred in Sudan when, after three polio-free years, new cases were confirmed. Asia, with overcrowding, few resources, and lacking the political will to keep up with public health infrastructure demands, have had epidemics of cholera, typhoid fever, rabies, and plague posing major public health problems. Newly emerging infectious diseases such as Nipah virus, avian influenza and enterovirus 71 infections have also caused significant epidemics (Western Pacific Regional Organization, 2003).

Emerging infectious diseases pose a significant but unappreciated threat to public health. Infectious disease terminology referring to 'regional' or 'tropical' diseases no longer has basis in fact. Using a political-ecology framework, studies have examined the relationship between the geographies of exile and refugee movements and the associated implications for newly emerging and re-emerging infectious diseases. This research examined four main themes: examination of the geography of the refugee crisis, disruption of health services, breeding of disease in refugee camps, and creation of an optimal environment for emergence and spread of disease due to the chaotic nature of war and violence. Researchers concluded that once an infectious disease is out in the public, rapid diffusion, despite political boundaries, is likely. Secondly, they concluded that there is great potential for more virulent diseases than cholera, dysentery, Ebola and others endemically known to emerge (Kalipeni & Oppong, 1998). Additional human behavior changes brought about by 'poverty, war, population growth, migration, and urban decay' contribute to the emergence of viral and rickettsial diseases (Smith, 2001). For example dengue, often the result of vectors inhabiting standing water in uncollected urban trash, has emerged as a unique economic indicator of decaying urban infrastructure, prompting closer scrutiny by economists and public health authorities alike (Economist Editorial, 1998).

Factors such as unwarranted and too frequent antibiotic prescriptions, low vaccination rates among the elderly, and continuous exposure to small amounts of antimicrobials in the food supply contribute to resistance patterns among common pathogenic bacteria (e.g., *E. Coli, Klebsiella, Pseudomonas, Staphylococcus*) of up to 36% (Gums, 2002). In developing countries where antibiotic usage in often uncontrolled, contributing factors leading to inadequate infectious disease management include:

- lack of infectious disease expertise,
- lack of national infectious disease programs,
- lack of education and training,
- lack of a secure supply of equipment and supplies (e.g., syringes, soap, gloves),
- lack of surveillance,
- lack of an emergency preparedness program, and
- lack of coordination at all management levels.

Universal and common fears of infectious contamination by plagues and pestilence, first occurring from refugees and immigrants, and now from bioterrorism, can provoke much community anxiety and underscore the crucial role of rapidly mobilized health information systems and population education as a priority in the management of all outbreaks. Disaster planners recognize that vulnerable populations (those more at risk of becoming victims of a disaster) include refugees and recent immigrants unfamiliar with the host country's language and often influenced by their own cultural interpretations of disease. This takes many forms; 'delusions of fatal contagion' have even appeared in Southeast Asian Hmong refugees who, familiar with the deadly consequences of severe infectious disease outbreaks in their former country, presented to healthcare providers with signs of severe depression. This and other examples underscore the need to understand the multicultural interpretations of disease and death and to accurately portray these risks to any society, especially the identified vulnerable populations (Westermeyer, Lyfoung, Wahmanholm, & Westermeyer, 1989).

Throughout history, certain infectious diseases always provoked great anxiety. During a plague (*Yersinia Pestis*) epidemic in war ravaged Viet Nam in 1968, (Burkle, 1973) fear caused a rapid halt to the fighting and a virtual standstill to any social and commercial activity in towns and surrounding villages. Whereas a few patients developed expected resistance to common Third World antibiotics such as Sulfa, new western antibiotics and simple but effective public health measures, unchanged since the 16th century, such as rat control measures, isolation, and quarantine easily controlled the disease spread. It was only decades later, after the end of the Cold War in the early 1990s, that disclosures of clandestine Soviet Union research on developing plague (*Yersinia Pestis*) as a bioweapon in 1963, five years before the Viet Nam epidemic, in which a *Yersinia Pestis* microorganism was made resistant to 16 different antibiotics. Scientific advancements have altered forever both the playing field and the manner in which we consider infectious outbreaks. One can only contemplate how the 1968 epidemic in Viet Nam would have faired if a deliberate, biologically altered, and antibiotic resistant plague, secretly available at the time, had been unleashed on an unsuspecting and highly vulnerable population.

In September 1994 the "very rumor of plague" in Surat, India prompted a frenetic exodus from the city of more than 300,000 refugees. Neighboring countries of Pakistan, Bangladesh, Nepal, and China rapidly closed their borders to both trade and travel from India (Price-Smith, 2002). The Bombay stock exchange plunged and soon after countries "began to restrict imports from India and impounded goods in quarantine." Physicians who fled the area were forced to return under a threat of legal prosecution (Price-Smith, 2002). To complicate issues further, the Centers for Disease Control and Prevention (CDC) reported that the strain of the *Yersinia Pestis* microorganism was an "unknown and presumably new strain." Indian authorities, falsely interpreting this information as possibly representing a bioweapon accused rebel militants of procuring the microorganism to manufacture an epidemic (Price-Smith, 2002). These scenarios emphasize the crucial importance of maintaining a timely and accurate health information system, from credible health authorities, at every level of the government and the public. The World Health Organization's (WHO) experience in the SARS epidemic found that a priority challenge for governments is to "move fast and decisively to communicate incredibly well to the public" (Heymann & Rodier, 2004).

## Reflecting on Risks and Myths

### Infectious Diseases Without Borders

In the last three decades, there has been a global explosion of infectious diseases which public health experts call 'unique in human history.' The recent SARS outbreak was not an isolated incident. Despite public health measures, some diseases, such as West Nile Fever, have spread rapidly across the U.S. in a matter of a few years and is now found in all continental states. News of these 'infectious diseases without boundaries' is focused on avian influenza (H5N1) which is not a new disease but an old one that is undergoing antigenic shifts to new subtypes that is highly pathogenic among poultry. The natural asymptomatic carrier, it appears, is the waterfowl (aquatic ducks and geese) with capacity to transmit this virus to other migratory birds, chickens, pigs, domestic cats, tigers, and leopards (H5N1 is 100% fatal to chickens). Viruses infect the respiratory and intestinal tracts of birds and then shed in respiratory secretions and feces. Human infections are extremely uncommon and usually associated with direct contact with sick poultry outbreaks occurring on small-scale and backyard farms. Human fatality rates are about 51% but human-to-human transmission has not yet been confirmed (WHO, 2005).

The longer H5N1 remains on the local level, the greater the opportunity for it to mutate to a human pathogenic form. It is crucial to provide economic incentives to small farmers to ensure early reporting and culling of infected birds and chickens, especially in Asian, African, and Middle Eastern economies which depend on flocks for survival.

The world community is preparing for the potential mutation of such a strain or a reassortment of such a strain with the human influenza virus. The current H5N1 will need to mutate if it is to become highly pathogenic to humans. Any *clusters of human cases* might represent the beginning of an epidemic. Action would be quick and decisive with (WHO, 2005):

- rapid mobilization of health and veterinary resources,
- culling of birds,
- investigation of the nature of transmission and whether it represents human-to-human transmission or co-exposure,
- stockpiling of and scaling up of pandemic vaccine production and/or anti-virals to reduce the fatality rate among the general population and to protect key-workers and cullers,
- increased vigilance through active surveillance and early case reporting, and,
- support of countries in rapid investigation and containment activities (WHO, 2005)

It is critical to vaccinate for seasonal Influenza A to avoid the potential of co-infection of H5N1 with the human avian strain in the same individual (WHO, 2005). Currently, only 40 countries have some kind of preparedness plan, including access to or plans to produce vaccines. As a global health problem, solutions will be global.

## Ground Truth

In general, infectious disease medical problems are generally common rather than exotic and pose little risk to public health. Other infectious diseases, except for malaria where vectors remain, do not pose a significant threat to public health given their low prevalence and/or low infectivity in the new environment. The historical plagues and other epidemics killed many people but far more survived than succumbed. Death rates were rarely more than 30% (Smith, 2001). They occurred during times when poor public health infrastructure was the norm. Inferences here suggest that survival rates today, with improved technology, vaccines, and public health infrastructure, would result in much less morbidity and mortality. Unfortunately, the inequities brought about by an uneven world development and increasing war and conflict allows us to witness, all too often, environments in the developing world that shamefully remain too close in poverty, malnourishment, and decay to conditions of centuries past.

Although our attention is easily drawn to bioterrorism threats and the formidable alterations in the biological and genetic makeup of microorganisms, the major barrier to significant reduction in infectious disease is poverty leading to poor public health infrastructure (Heymann & Rodier, 1998). All infectious disease outbreaks draw increasing attention to principles of infection control, outbreak investigation, personal hygiene, and public health infrastructure capacity, as they should. Whereas most developed countries enjoy a surveillance system, these systems often lack an early warning component and do not provide the information necessary for a rapid response.

The direction for countries is to turn to active surveillance systems that mitigate misdiagnosis and increase both sensitivity and specificity of investigative diagnosis through improved laboratories and detection devices. When it comes to making a rapid diagnosis of an infectious disease, clinicians remain constrained by expensive and poorly distributed diagnostic testing technologies such as polymerase chain reaction (PCR). In a matter of a few years, RNA/DNA microarray diagnostic chips will allow rapid real time accurate diagnosis of infectious agents from available bodily fluids having unprecedented impact on how medical and public health care is practiced worldwide. However, anything so powerful as this technology should face scrutiny for the potential it has to be a military weapon or political tool. This statement is not farfetched. A *New York Times* editorial blasted scientists for publishing the full genome findings of the 1918 influenza virus on the Internet in the GenBank database, claiming that the genome is essentially the design of a weapon of mass destruction far worse than an atomic bomb (Kurzweil & Joy, 2005). This article prompted a debate on fear-mongering versus need for even more scientific censorship (*New York Times*, 2005). Clearly, public health must take precedence over politics. Such advanced technology has the opportunity to disrupt inequities in both surveillance and response, ensuring in many situations that endemic disease will indeed remain endemic. However, with a pattern, over two decades of increasing political interference and influence on public health (Burkle, 2002; Kaufmann, Meltzer, & Schmid, 2000) there remains a strong risk that this technology will be misused.

The WHO, recognizing that strengthening the public health and public health surveillance is the most effective way to prepare for accidental or deliberate bioevents, has urged:

- Priorities in nation-state disease-surveillance plans must be complementary to regional and global disease-surveillance mechanisms for collaboration of rapid analysis and sharing of surveillance data of international concern.
- Collaboration and mutual support to enhance national capacity in field epidemiology, laboratory diagnoses, and case management.
- To treat any deliberate local bioevent (and chemical and radio-nuclear events) as a global public health threat and to respond to such a threat by sharing expertise, supplies and resources in order to rapidly contain the event and mitigate its effect (WHO, 2002).

## Global Health and the World Health Organization

At a recent National Disaster Management Conference, a lecture was presented subtitled, "SARS, the Best Thing Since Sliced Bread!" (Burkle, 2004). The lecture was not typically what was heard at medical conferences during the height of the SARS epidemic but challenged the audience to focus more on looking at disasters as one means of defining the existing public health and exposing its vulnerabilities. Now that SARS is over, what did the world learn and what did it need to change?

The SARS epidemic was similar for many countries, as all disasters seem to be, but was critically different in that this was a global disaster demanding each country to use its resources, not only to mitigate the effects on its own population, but to ensure that it did not spread within and across borders. This disaster opened eyes on how a bioevent, deliberate or accidental, would impact societies which were now more at risk because of increased density of populations and easy access to global travel. SARS spread, impressively, from a rural area of China to 40 countries within 10 days. SARS transmissibility was moderately high with an attack rate of about 24% and a disease mortality rate between 5.6% and 18.2% (WHO, 2003) that fluctuated depending on country and age, with WHO emphasizing that SARS is particularly dangerous for the elderly where mortality rates are over 50%. Comparatively, Ebola has a disease fatality rate of 36% to 88%, smallpox 30%, and bubonic plague 15.4% (WHO, 2003).

In the pre-SARS era, WHO relied on countries to report outbreaks of communicable diseases and to organize their own surveillance systems, if they existed at all. This awareness placed any semblance of a global health community in question. WHO existed as a passive but expert technical organization who offered its expertise to countries that were in need. WHO did not have the authority to force an outbreak investigation, could not compel itself on to a sovereign country unless requested, and then had only "advice and limited resources" to offer (Heymann & Rodier, 2004). WHO, when faced with rumors and unsubstantiated evidence of an epidemic of global importance, as it did in China during the early days of the SARS outbreak, offered their services. In fact, China refused, and when they did allow WHO presence, they hid the patients from the WHO assessment team.

Recognizing a pending catastrophe, the World Health Ministers representing UN member states gave unprecedented authority, through new International Health Regulations, to WHO to act and intervene even without sovereign state permission, actions which proved instrumental in controlling the SARS epidemic. WHO's actions included collaboration with Canada's Global Public Health Information Network (GPHIN) that digitally searched for any hints of potential outbreaks, and the WHO Global Outbreak Alert and Response Network (GOARN) which provided technical, operational, and political assistance to governments at all levels. Countries must now report any disease outbreak of "international concern." Moreover, through

International Health Regulations (IHR), WHO now has authority to coordinate response to any infectious disease that is a threat to international public health. These roles apply to both accidental and deliberate outbreaks allowing WHO to verify outbreaks based on any available "official or non-official information" (Heymann & Rodier, 2004) and attempts to maximize security against the international spread of disease with minimum interference to sovereignty, travel and trade" (Merianos & Peiris, 2005).

As this chapter has indicated, WHO and the post-SARS environment must still rely on local expertise to identify sentinel cases, but WHO teams are now able to arrive early and assist. WHO provides a "decision instrument" of criteria for sovereign countries to use in determining whether an unexpected or unusual public health event within its territory, irrespective of origin or source, constitutes a public health emergency of international concern and require WHO notification (Merianos & Peiris, 2005). Criteria include (Heymann & Rodier, 2004):

- Mortality and morbidity,
- Is the event unusual or unexpected?,
- Its potential to lead to a major public health effect,
- Whether external assistance is needed to detect, investigate, respond and control the outbreak,
- Potential for international spread, and
- Potential for risk to international travel or trade.

These criteria clearly define new elements of what Price-Smith initially referred to as 'state capacity' (1998), but also sets a precedence that global health responsibilities exist before nation-state sovereignty and political will to do otherwise. IHRs will be expected to address these issues and the central authority of WHO will be expected to act on them (Fidler, 1996, 1998). The global public health lessons learned during the SARS epidemic must serve as the sentinel alarm for a stronger WHO authority with clear guidelines for improved local, national, and regional capacity to deal with infectious disease investigation and control within migrating populations and nation-states whether at peace, war, or conflict.

## References

Barnett, E.D. (2004). Infectious disease screening for refugees resettled in the United States. *Clinical Infectious Diseases*, 39(6), 833-841.

Bennet, J. (2002). In Palestinian children, signs of increasing malnutrition, *New York Times*, July 26: Section A: 326.

Black, M.E. & Healing, T.D. (1993). Communicable diseases in former Yugoslavia and in refugees arriving in the United Kingdom. *Communicable Disease Report CDR Review*, 3(6), R87-R90.

Burkholder, B.T. & Toole, M.J. (1995). Evolution of complex emergencies. *Lancet*, 346, 1012-1015.

Burkle, F. M. (1999). Lessons learnt and future expectations of complex emergencies. *British Medical Journal*, 319, 422-426.

Burkle, F.M. (1973). Plague as seen in South Vietnamese children: A chronicle of observations and treatment under adverse conditions. *Clinical Pediatrics*, 12(5), 291-298.

Burkle, F.M. (2002). Mass casualty management of a large-scale bioterrorist event: an epidemiological approach that shapes triage decisions. *Emergency Medical Clinics of North America*, 20, 409-436.

Burkle, F.M. (2004). Grasping Public Health Emergencies: What we have learned from the SARS epidemic or SARS, The best thing since sliced bread. *Presentation, National Disaster Management System Annual Conference*, Dallas, TX, April 18-20.

Burkle, F.M. & Hayden, R. (2001) The concept of assisted management of large-scale disasters by horizontal organizations. *Prehospital and Disaster Medicine*, 16, 128-137.

Burkle, F.M. & Noji, E.K. (2004). War and politics in the 2003 war with Iraq: Lessons learned. *Lancet*, 364(9442), 1371-75.

Brower J. & Chalk, P. (2003). The Global Threat of New and Reemerging Infectious Diseases: Reconciling US National Security and Public Health Policy. *Rand*, Santa Monica, CA. pp. 20-24.

Carballo, M. & Nerukar, A. (2001). Migration, refugees, and health risks. *Emerging Infectious Diseases*; 7(3) Supplement http://www.cdc.gov/ncidod/EID/vol7no3_supp/carballo.htm (accessed 11/19/2004).

CDC (1991). International notes public health consequences of acute displacement of Iraqi citizens-March-May, 1991. *Morbidity Mortality Weekly Report*. July 5, 40(26), 443-446.

CDC (1993). Nutrition and mortality assessment-Southern Sudan, March 1993. *Morbidity Mortality Weekly Report*. April 30, 42(16), 304-308.

CDC (1993). Status of public health-Bosnia and Herzegovina-August-September, 1993. *Morbidity Mortality Weekly Report*. December 24, 42(50), 979-982.

CDC (1996). Morbidity and mortality surveillance in Rwandan refugees-Burundi and Zaire, 1994. *Morbidity Mortality Weekly Report*. February 9, 45(5), 104-107.

Christenson, B. (1995). Panorama of infections among refugees-the lack of epidemics from the east. *Nordicum Meditteraneum*, 110(2), 40-41.

Connolly, M.A. & Heymann, D.L. (2002). Deadly comrades: War and infectious diseases. *Lancet*. Dec, 360 Suppl, s23-s24.

Cookson, S.T., Carballo, M., Nolan, C.M., Keystone, J.S., & Jong, E. C. (2001). Migrating populations: A closer view of who, why, and so what. *Emerging Infectious Diseases*, 7(3) Supplement, 551.

Cosgrave, J. Refugee density and dependence: Practical implications of camp size. *Disasters*. 1996 Sep, 20(3), 261-270.

Depoortere, E., Checchi, F., Broillet, F., Minetti, A., Gayraud, O., Briet, V., Pahl, J., Defourney, I., Tatay, M., & Brown, V. (2004). Violence and mortality in West Dafur, Sudan (2003-04), Epidemiological evidence from four surveys. *Lancet*, 364(9442), 1315-1320.

Doyle, R. (2004). Getting sicker: State budget constraints threaten public health. *Scientific American*; Nov: 15.

*Economist* (1998). Dengue fever. A man-made disease. *Editorial*, 2, 21.

Farmer, P. (2004). Political violence and public health in Haiti. *New England Journal of Medicine*, 350(15), 1483-1486.

Fidler, D.P. (1996). Globalization, international law, and emerging infectious diseases. *Emerging Infectious Diseases*, 2(2), 77-84.

Fidler, D.P. (1998). Legal issues associated with antimicrobial drug resistance. *Emerging Infectious Diseases*, 4(2), 169-177.

Fourie, P. & Schonteich, M. (2001). Africa's new security threat: HIV/AIDS and human security in Southern Africa. *African Security Review*, 10(4), 29-57.

Glasser, R.J. (2004). We are not immune: Influenza, SARS and the collapse of public health. *Harpers Magazine*, Essay, July, 35-42.

Gums, J.G. (2002). Assessing the impact of antimicrobial resistance. *American Journal of Health-System Pharmacy*. April 15, 59 (Suppl 3), S4-S6.

Heymann, D.L. & Rodier, G.R. (1998). Global surveillance of communicable diseases. *Emerging Infectious Diseases*, 4(3). http://www.cdc.gov/ncidod/eid/vol4no3/heymann.htm (accessed 11/7/2004).

Heymann, D.L. & Rodier, G.R. (2004). Politics of global epidemics. *The Brown Journal of World Affairs*, X(II), 185-196.

Hugo, G. (1997). Asia and the Pacific on the move: workers and refugees, a challenge to nation states. *Asia Pacific Viewpoint*, 38(3), 267.

Hyndman, J. (1999). A post-Cold War geography of forced migration in Kenya and Somalia. *The Professional Geographer*, 51(1), 104.

International Crisis Group (2005). Crisis Watch List. http://www.icg.org (accessed 5/1/2005).

Kalipeni, E. & Oppong, J. (1998). The refugee crisis in Africa and implications for health and disease: a political ecology approach. *Social Science and Medicine*, 46(12), 1637-1653.

Kaufmann, A.F., Meltzer, M.I., & Schmid, G.P. (2000). The economic impact of a bioterrorist attack: Are prevention and post attack intervention programs justifiable? *Emerging Infectious Diseases*. http://www.cdc.gov/ncidod/EID/vol3no2/kaufman.htm (accessed 6/1/2001).

King, K. & Vodioka, P. (2001). Screening for conditions of public health importance in people arriving in Australia by boat without authority. *The Medical Journal of Australia*, 175, 600-602.

Koppenaal, H., Bos, C.A., & Broer, J. (2003). High mortality due to infectious diseases and unnatural causes among asylum seekers in the Netherlands, 1998-1999. *Ned Tijdschr Geneeskd*, 147(9), 391-395.

Kurzweil, R., & Joy, B. (2005). Recipe for Destruction. New York Times, Op-Ed Contributors, http://www.nytimes.com/2005/10/17/opinion/17kurzweiljoy.html?th=&emc=th&pagewa (accessed 10/17/2005).

McMichael, A.J., Kjellstrom, T., & Smith, K.R. (2001). Environmental Health. In M.H. Merson, R.E. Black, & A.J. Mills, (Eds.), *International Public Health: Diseases, Programs, Systems, and Policies*. Aspen Publishers, Maryland, pp. 379-434.

Merianos, A., & Peiris, M. (2005). International Health Regulations: 2005. *Lancet*, October 8-14, 366(9493), 1249-1251.

Michaud, C.M., Murray, C.J.L., & Bloom, B.R. (2001). Burden of disease-implications for future research. *Journal of American Medical Association*, 285, 553-539.

Murray, C.J.L. & Lopez, A.D. (1996). Estimating causes of death: New methods and global and regional applications for 1990. In (C.J.L. Murray & A.D. Lopez, Eds.) *The Global Burden of Disease: A Comprehensive Assessment of Mortality and Disability from Diseases, Injuries, and Risk Factors in 1990 and Projected to 2020*. Boston: Harvard University Press, pp. 118-200.

*New York Times* (2005). Turning the Flu into a Weapon (6 Letters). Letters to the Editor. October 20: A26.

Office of the Coordinator of Humanitarian Affairs (2004). Iraq: Child malnutrition increasing in the south. *UNOCHA Iraq Crisis News*, United Nations, New York. http://www.irinnews.org/report.asp?reportID=40923&SelectRegion=Iraq (accessed 11/21/2004).

Paluzzui, J. & Farmer, P. (2004). A tale of two viruses: Social response to AIDS and SARS. *The Brown Journal of World Affairs*, X (II), 199-206.

Pirages, D.C., Runci, P.J., & Sprinkle, R.H. (2001). Human populations in the shared environment. In (J.L. Aron & J.A. Patz, Eds.), *Ecosystem Change and Public Health*, pp. 165-183. Baltimore, MD: The Johns Hopkins University Press.

Price-Smith, A.T. (1998). Wilson's bridge: A consilient methodology for analysis of complex biological-political relationships. Program on Health and Global Affairs, University of Toronto: *Center for International Studies working paper* No. 1998-8; November: 2-43.

Price-Smith, A.T. (1999). Ghosts of Kigali: Infectious disease and global stability in the coming century. *International Journal*, 54(3), 426-442.

Price-Smith, A.T. (2002). The Health of Nations: Infectious disease, environmental change, and their effects on national security and development. *Massachusetts Institute of Technology Press*, pp. 117-140.

Price-Smith, A.T. & Daly, J.L. (2004). Downward spiral: HIV/AIDS, state capacity, and political conflict in Zimbabwe. United States Institute of Peace, Washington, D.C. *Peaceworks*, 53, 5-15.

Prothero, R.M. (1977). Disease and mobility: a neglected factor in epidemiology. *International Journal of Epidemiology*, 6(3), 259-267.

Prothero, R.M. (1987). Populations on the move. *Third World Quarterly*, 9(4), 282-310.

Prothero, R.M. (1994). Forced movements of populations and health hazards in tropical Africa. *International Journal of Epidemiology*, 23(4), 657-664.

Quinn, T.C. (1995). Population migration and the spread of types 1 and 2 human immunodeficiency viruses. Infectious Diseases in an age of change: The impact of human ecology and behavior on disease transmission. National Academy of Sciences. http://books.nap.edu/books/0309051363/html/77.html (accessed 11/11/ 2004).

Refugees International (2002). More effort needed to protect internally displaced. Washington, D.C. http://www.refugeesinternational.org/content/article/detail/1461/ (accessed 11/19/2004).

Regan, J. (2004). Flood-hit struggles to manage health disaster: International agencies are helping clean up, but health workers warn of long-term disease risks. *Lancet*, 363(9424), 1880.

Roberts, L. (2001). Mortality in Eastern Democratic Republic of Congo: Results from eleven mortality surveys. Health Unit, International Rescue Committee. New York, NY: *Final Draft*.

Santoro, D., Visona, R., Pusterla, L., & Vigevani, G.M. (2000). Migrants' admissions to hospital: a retrospective study in Como: 1994 to 1998. *Journal of Travel Medicine*, 7(6), 300-303.

Siem, H. (1997). Migration and health-the international perspective. *Schweiz Rundsch Med Prax*, 86(19), 788-793.

Smith, H. (2001). Dangerous pathogens 2000: An overview of the international conference. *Journal of Applied Microbiology*, 91(4), 621-623.

Spiegel, P.B. & Salama, P. (2000). War and mortality in Kosovo, 1998-99: An epidemiological testimony. *Lancet*, 357(9257), 2204-2209.

Toole, M.J. & Waldman, R.J. (1990). Prevention of excess mortality in refugee and displaced populations in developing countries. *Journal of American Medical Association*, 263, 3296-3302.

Toole, M.J. & Waldman, R.J. (1997). The public health aspects of complex emergencies and refugee situations. *Annual Review of Public Health*, 18, 283-312.

Toole, M.J., Galson, S., & Brady, W. (1993). Are war and public health compatible? *Lancet*, 341(8854), 1193-1196.

Toole, M.J., Waldman, R.J., & Zwi, A.B. (2001).Complex humanitarian emergencies. In (M.H. Merson, R.E. Black, & A.J. Mills, Eds.), *International Public Health: Diseases, Programs, Systems, and Policies*, pp. 439-510. Maryland: Aspen Publishers.

UNAIDS (2004). Report on the global AIDS epidemic: Focus-AIDS and conflict: a growing problem worldwide. Geneva: pp. 175-181. http://www.unaids.org/bangkok2004/GAR2004_html/GAR2004_00_en.htm (accessed 11/21/2004).

UN Charter (1945). http://www.un.org/aboutun/charter/unflag.htm (accessed 12/4/2004).

Walter, J. (Ed.) (2004). *Disaster data: Key trends and statistics. World Disaster Report-2004*. International Federation of Red Cross and Red Crescent Societies, Geneva. http://www.ifrc.org/publicat/wdr2004/chapter8.asp (accessed 11/19/2004).

Westermeyer, J., Lyfoung, T., Wahmanholm, K., & Westermeyer, M. (1989). Delusions of fatal contagion among refugee patients. *Psychosomatics*, 30(4), 374-382.

WPRO (2003). Combating Communicable Diseases: Focus on Communicable Diseases Surveillance and Response, Western Pacific Regional Organization, Chapter 5, pp. 61-66. http://www.wpro.who.int/themes_focuses/theme/special/t1special.asp (accessed 11/11/2004).

WHO (2002). *Global Public Health Response to the Deliberate Use of Biological and Chemical Agents, and Radio-nuclear Attacks to Cause Harm. 109th Session*: EB109.R5, Agenda item 3.13, January 17, 2002, 1-3.

WHO (2003). *WHO Report on SARS Case-Fatality Ratio*. http://www.who.int/csr/sarsarchive/2003_05_07a/en/ (accessed 11/11/2004).

WHO (2005). *News Teleconference on Avian Influenza and Human Pandemic Influenza. WHO Transcript*, 17 October WHO Headquarters, Geneva, Switzerland, 13h00 GMT.

Zwi, A. & Uglade, A. (1989). Towards an epidemiology of political violence in the Third World. *Social Science of Medicine*, 29(7), 633-642.

# Chapter 10

## Natural Disasters, Climate Change, and the Health of Mobile Populations

Jonathan D. Mayer, Ph.D.

## Introduction

One approach to understanding how humans and the environment interact to produce conditions of health and disease is that of the human ecology of disease (Meade & Earickson, 2005). Basic to this approach is an understanding of the ways in which behavior, culture, population, environment, and biology all interact in what Krieger (1994) has termed the "web of causation." For example, to understand why malaria occurs in a particular place at a particular time, one must not only understand the vector biology of the relevant anopheline species, but also understand the distribution of population, anopheline habitats, and human behaviors that bring people into contact with the vector. Moreover, one must understand the behaviors and their cultural underpinnings that underlie peoples' daily travel patterns, which dictate movement that make populations susceptible to anopheline feeding behavior. A specific example is that of the increase of schistosomiasis upriver from the Akosombo Dam (Volta River Dam) in Ghana following completion of the dam in the mid 1960s. The ecological and behavioral patterns were already appropriate for schistosomiasis transmission prior to the completion of the dam, so schistosomiasis was endemic in this area. After completion of the dam, and the ensuing creation of the largest human-made lake in the world, ecological and behavioral conditions were even more ideal for the transmission of schistosomiasis. The area bounding the lake increased tremendously, and more people, many of whom were displaced by the dam, had contact with Lake Akosombo, which was the most obvious source of water for drinking, bathing, laundering, fishing, and other activities. As a result, the prevalence of schistosomiasis increased, as did other diseases, such as onchocerciasis.

To take this example one step further, the human ecology of disease may also encompass the political decisions of development projects such as the Akosombo Dam. The dam was constructed in order to provide hydroelectric power for both industry and population in Ghana, and specifically to power the aluminum industry—indeed, one particular aluminum plant—in Ghana.

181

The decision to build the dam, which was largely a political decision, had unintended but significant health consequences. The approach that appreciates the political origins of diseases through mediating causes of landscape modification and altered patterns of human-pathogen contact can be termed the "political ecology of disease" (Mayer, 1996, 2000).

Natural disasters are among the major causes of migration, and particularly of involuntary migration. As a result, there has been a long tradition of scholarship in a number of interrelated disciplines that analyze the effects of natural disasters on migration. Disasters frequently make communities uninhabitable, or are responsible for intolerable economic, social, and health conditions. This is what happened as a result of Hurricane Katrina, which struck New Orleans, Louisiana on August 29, 2005. In the case of Hurricane Katrina, a major metropolitan area became virtually devoid of its population within two weeks due to forced migration.

Natural disasters can have significant implications for local and regional health conditions. While the systematic study of the health implications of disasters is relatively new, significant knowledge has been developed in disaster epidemiology and related fields. The health effects of disasters are best understood through an ecological approach, for mortality and morbidity result through altered patterns between pathogens and humans in the case of infectious diseases, or between humans and the built or natural environment more generally, in the case of non-infectious diseases. Political decisions that are made prior to the disaster, or during the disaster, frequently alter these patterns, so the political ecologic approach is also relevant.

The ecological approach is equally useful in understanding some of the actual and anticipated effects of global environmental change. Global environmental change refers most popularly to global climate change, but also to other environmental changes including environmental degradation, pollution, overgrazing, deforestation, desertification, and a host of other factors that affect human populations; many of these have actual or anticipated health effects. Thus, this chapter is, at once, a chapter on the human ecology of disease, and a chapter on how the environment affects human health, using the examples of natural disasters and global climate change.

# Impact of Natural Hazards and Disasters on Health

## Introduction to Natural Hazards and Disasters

As Tobin and Montz (1997) observe, the terminology of natural hazards research has sometimes suffered from imprecision, and this has created unnecessary confusion. Natural hazards are the result of an extreme event, which is usually a geophysical event, such as an earthquake, tsunami, or hurricane, interacting with a vulnerable human population. A hazard is an issue of probability, and is defined as the potential for an extreme natural event acting on a human system. For example, the conditions in New Orleans for years prior to Hurricane Katrina could be regarded as hazardous, because of defects in the city's levies, inadequate disaster response plans, and concentrated poverty. As the hurricane approached, the probability of the hazard becoming a disaster increased. A disaster refers to a hazard once it has occurred and impacted the human system. It is no longer a matter of probability, but one of certainty. A hazard—an issue of potential—has already disrupted and stressed the normal functioning of a region. Once Hurricane Katrina struck New Orleans, it became a disaster. For a hazard to become transformed into a disaster, it must, in some way, overwhelm the coping capacities of the social system:

*"Whilst physical phenomena are necessary for the production of natural hazard, their translation into risk and potential for disaster is contingent upon human exposure and a lack of capacity to cope. . . ."*

(Pelling, 2003, p. 4)

This is a good description of what occurred during and following Hurricane Katrina's landfall. There are numerous taxonomies of disasters, and many discussions of disasters begin with a typology of disasters, including suddenness of onset, time of persistence of disaster (long or short), geographical extent of the disaster (localized or widespread), and severity of the disaster. Severity may be measured in terms of morbidity of mortality, some metric of property damage, or an analysis of social disruption. Disasters may also be classified in terms of the purely geophysical features of the disaster, an approach which is usually of greatest interest to earth scientists.

A significant proportion of the earth's population is affected by natural hazards. Abramovitz (2001) estimated that 20-25% of the population was affected by hazards in the 1970s and 1980s. The social effect of disasters is increasing, which is due to the concentration of populations in disaster-prone regions, and to population growth itself (Kondratyev, Krapivin, & Phillips, 2002).

Vulnerability

Vulnerability is a concept that is crucial to understanding the social and health impacts of disasters. Vulnerability is, in part, a product of a population's location relative to areas of geophysical risk, such as in the Asian tsunami of December 26, 2004, where residence on the coastal floodplain led to the greatest risk of mortality, destruction, and displacement. In the case of earthquakes, location in an area or great seismic activity leads to increased vulnerability. But vulnerability is also a product of social conditions. Social class, for example, frequently predisposes the impoverished to living in poorly constructed shacks in shantytowns or squatter settlements with poor resistance to flooding, earthquakes, and windstorms. Thus, disasters are the product of both nature and social relations (Oliver-Smith, 2004) The social dimensions of vulnerability are a major focus of interdisciplinary research, and this work concentrates on culture, poverty, location, political ecology, distribution of political power, inequity, land use policies, and environmental degradation (Noji, 1997). Finally, risk is a unifying concept that has tied together the diverse approaches to natural disasters. Both qualitatively and quantitatively, risk is the product of vulnerability, and the probability of occurrence of a disaster. As such risk is the product of both natural and social factors. The concentration of poverty in New Orleans, with its deficient flood protection infrastructure, made the city's population especially vulnerable to the effects of a major hurricane and flood.

Though there is anecdotal evidence of migrants being at increased risk of morbidity and mortality from natural hazards, there has been no systematic review of the sparse literature on this subject; Wisner (2003) cites a number of examples. Groups whose members have been victims of genocide are frequent refugees, and live in areas of cities that are vulnerable to natural hazards. In Los Angeles, there are several thousand indigenous Mayans from Guatemala who speak neither Spanish nor English, and are refugees from the genocide of the Civil War of the late 1990s. These people are at risk of infectious and noninfectious disease, and they are also highly vulnerable to the earthquakes common to Southern California.

## Health Effects of Natural Disasters

Disaster epidemiology is a comparatively new subfield in epidemiology, yet it is undeniable that one of the major effects of disasters is the resulting morbidity and mortality. For example, while there are no accurate estimates of the direct mortality from the 2005 Asian tsunami, it is clear that mortality, due mostly to traumatic injuries and drowning, exceeded 150,000; this qualifies the tsunami as one of the worst natural disasters in history (Bloom, 2005). Interestingly, and for reasons that are not fully understood, the predicted longer term health effects of the tsunami, such as increased transmission of malaria and dengue fever, have not been realized, although there have been very localized outbreaks of cholera and other diarrheal diseases, particularly in Indonesia.

In general, health effects constitute some of the most significant effects of natural disasters. Sometimes this is due to direct mortality from trauma, with the mechanism of injury depending upon the type of disaster. Mortality and morbidity are exacerbated by localized destruction of healthcare facilities, transportation infrastructure, and communications systems. For example, Hurricane Katrina destroyed much of the health and public health infrastructure of New Orleans in a very brief period, necessitating air and ground evacuation of critically ill patients to relatively distant locations. Some of these were as near as Baton Rouge, Louisiana, and others as far as Houston, Texas, and major medical centers in the northeastern U.S. In the days immediately following Katrina's landfall, most medical treatment was carried out locally in makeshift facilities because the transportation infrastructure connecting New Orleans with the rest of the U.S. had been severely compromised and New Orleans had functionally become an isolated island.

Infectious diseases that occur weeks or even months after the disaster can be significant sources of mortality and morbidity. Locally, the poor are most subject to the consequences of disasters. For example, in the case of Hurricane Katrina, New Orleans' African-American residents, who constitute 69% of the city's population, and the poor, who constitute 23% of the population, both suffered disproportionately severe consequences of the disaster (Quinn, 2006).

Following major floods in tropical areas, the ecological conditions are often appropriate for the transmission of vectorborne diseases such as dengue and malaria (National Research Council, 2003; Toole, 1997). This is because the conditions can be ideal for the reproduction of anopheline or *aedes spp*. The distribution of population, which brings people into contact with vectors, makes people vulnerable to the resulting diseases. In addition, recent attention has been devoted to the psychosocial consequences of disaster, including posttraumatic stress disorder (PTSD), other anxiety disorders, and affective disorders including depression (Benin, 1985; Noji, 1997).

The vulnerability to infectious diseases following disasters is greatest in the most impoverished areas of the world (National Research Council, 2003; Toole, 1997). Indeed, it is useful to view both *populations* and *places* as being vulnerable. Though the two are intertwined, place-related vulnerability simultaneously considers the populations associated with place as well as the local ecological conditions. Thus, refugee-camp-associated sexually transmitted infections (STIs) are associated with place only insofar as a large group of assembled, vulnerable people had to collect somewhere, and STIs and HIV/AIDS are frequently associated with refugee camps (Salama & Dondero, 2001). Disasters are a common reason for displacement and forced relocation. If the same population were to be affected by a large outbreak of *Plasmodium falciparum* with both a high prevalence rate and a high case-fatality ratio, then the place itself would be vulnerable, because the local ecology, combined with a dense concentration of people, would have been appropriate for the reproduction of the relevant anopheline species, and for the chain of transmission. Moreover, assuming that the refugee camp had not been located arbitrarily, but was strategically placed as a result of political and economic decisions, the political ecologic framework would be entirely appropriate in the analysis of the malaria outbreak.

Population displacement, with population frequently residing in refugee camps, is a common result of natural disasters in vulnerable and poor populations. Migration may be over long or short distances and refugee camps typically have high population densities, and this creates appropriate ecological conditions for the transmission of respiratory and enteric diseases. Kalipeni and Oppong (1998) have noted increased transmission of cholera in refugee camps, while other researchers have documented increased transmission rates of TB, including multiple drug resistant TB (MDRTB) (Rutta, Kipingili, Lukonge, Assefa, Mitsilale, & Rwechungura, 2001).

While the focus of this book is on infectious diseases, it is worth noting that the long term health effects of disasters are not limited only to infectious and communicable disease. For example, numerous studies suggest that there is an increase in myocardial infarctions following severe earthquakes. This finding has been replicated in several cultural contexts using several epidemiologic study designs (Ogawa, Tsuji, Shiono, & Hisamichi, 2000; Tsai, Lung, & Wang, 2004). The 1994 Northridge earthquake in California was associated with number of out-of-hospital cardiac arrests (Leor, Poole, & Kloner, 1996). The putative pathophysiologic mechanism was a stress response in which the hypothalamic-pituitary-adrenal (HPA) axis had become activated, resulting in increased levels of serum cortisol, epinephrine, and norepinephrine. This could result in increased platelet aggregability and blood viscosity, as well as cardiac rate variations. Although this is at the frontier of research, this mechanism could result in increased rates of myocardial infarction as well as fatal cardiac arrhythmias, all as a result of the tremendous stress of the extreme geophysical event. The sudden stress-cardiac disease link needs intensive research, and the role of events such as earthquakes in this cascade needs to be linked to the initiating stress, since it is the stressor.

The psychosocial effects of disasters have also been appreciated; this is anticipated since the individual and social stress of these traumatic events can be significant. Social networks are frequently disrupted and family members and friends may die or be severely injured. One review of natural disasters found that nearly 70% of those interviewed suffered from symptoms of PTSD in a series of 160 disasters occurring between 1981and 2001 (Norris, Friedman, & Watson, 2002) and another study in Mexico following severe flooding found a high rate of PTSD and significant comorbidity with depressive disorder (Norris, Murphy, Baker, & Perilla, 2004).

There is no direct evidence of increased rates of non-infectious disease in migrants or refugees following disasters. Based upon evidence in analogous situations, however, this might be expected, and it is certainly testable. Similarly, the evidence concerning psychiatric disorders in victims of natural disasters has not concentrated specifically on refugees; however, it would be both expected and testable that rates of PTSD, major depressive disorders, and perhaps exacerbation of schizophrenia would be increased in those who have been forced to relocate due to natural disasters.

Those who are displaced due to environmental events have been termed, in several papers, as "environmentally-displaced peoples" (Charnley, 1997). These groups have also been called "environmental refugees." Analysis of the ecological causes of migration is a field that is relatively unexplored, at least in comparison to other causes of migration, such as the familiar "push" factors such as poor economic opportunities at the origin, or, in the cause of involuntary migration, political repression, despotism, and other factors. "Pull factors" traditionally include the perception of greater economic opportunities at the destination, greater cultural, religious, and political freedom, and other attractions.

Unfortunately, whereas studies of environmental refugees have explored the consequences of migration for ecological sustainability and ecological degradation, as well as the social effects on groups that migrate, the health effects of environmental refugees remain virtually unexplored. For example, Charnley (1997) examines migration and ecosystem change in Tanzania, but the health effects are not even addressed. Understanding is better in the context of natural hazards, but even in this case, the health effects are understood mostly with respect to the short term—the direct mortality, and the medium term—the ensuing epidemics of cholera, malaria, and dengue due to altered ecological conditions and crowded living conditions of refugee camps following the disaster and the longer term implications remain unknown. What is needed are long term, prospective cohort studies, but the logistics of conducting such studies, particularly in poor countries where the infrastructures may be poor for conducting cohort studies, can be overwhelming. The effects of Hurricane Katrina on environmental refugees and the resulting health effects presents us with an opportunity to increase our understanding of disasters on the long-term health of environmental refugees.

## Climate Change, Population, and Health

### Introduction to Climate Change

The Intergovernmental Panel on Climate Change (IPCC) estimated that the mean global temperature could increase by as much as 5.5°C by 2010. This influential panel, which is sponsored jointly by the United Nations Environment Program (UNEP) and the World Meteorological Organization, issued their most recent report in 2001 (IPCC, 2001), their fourth assessment report will be released in 2007. Although the figure cited above was the IPCC's mathematically modeled "high" scenario, it illustrates the fact that there is considerable, and, in the past decade, nearly universal consensus in the scientific community that global warming is a real phenomenon, and that the warming that the global community is now facing is more than just "normal" climatic variation. Moreover, there is also consensus that the majority of the past century's warming is due to human activity, or represents so called "anthropogenic" climate change. Activities such as industrialization, fossil fuel use, transportation, and urbanization all add greenhouse gasses to the atmosphere, whereas deforestation eliminates the major $CO_2$ sink which serves to eliminate this greenhouse gas.

Predicting future climate change is difficult and is not limited to predicting temperature change, which is frequently forgotten or unknown by the public, the policy community, and even by the scientific community. Climatic variables include rainfall, humidity, wind magnitude and direction, weather severity, periodicity variables, and other variables. Modeling future climates is very difficult because it requires both temporal and geographical specificity at high levels of resolution, and requires "coupling" of ocean, land, and atmospheric systems, since they all interact. This makes prediction computationally intensive and extensive. But in addition, climate systems require the simultaneous consideration of interacting nonlinear equations with multiple feedback loops. Systems that are based upon nonlinear equations are exquisitely sensitive to initial conditions, which make end-state conditions highly variant. Because of this, prediction of climate conditions decades in the future is difficult at best. Despite this difficulty, the IPCC predictions represent the best existing scientific estimates.

Climate Change and Health

What are the consequences of global climate change scenarios for populations, and, in particular, for the health of populations? There is much speculation (e.g., Patz, McGeehan, Bernard, Ebi, Epstein, Reiter, Romico, Rose, Samet, & Trtjan, 2001) that climate change—these authors really mean global warming—"will" allow anopheline and aedes vectors to move northwards and southwards and will therefore cause malaria, dengue, and other vectorborne diseases to move into more temperate regions. The speculation suggests, logically, from this assumption that the prevalence rates of many vectorborne diseases will increase significantly, and based upon the assumption that higher temperatures are more conducive to vector breeding. While the speculation is based upon reasonable scientific principles established in medical entomology and environmental health, there is little evidence that climate change already has resulted in the redistribution of vectors and especially in the diseases that result from these vectors. The ongoing debate is complex.

The National Academy of Sciences formed a committee jointly with the Institute of Medicine in 1999, of which the author was a member, to address the issue of how climate variability would affect infectious disease. The committee, titled "Committee on Climate, Ecosystems, Infectious Diseases, and Human Health," was much more cautious in its conclusions after examining all of the evidence. Indeed, the committee observed that the level of understanding of disease-climate relationships is at an early stage, and that a predictive epidemiology in this area has yet to be developed (National Research Council, 2001). Among the key findings were:

- Modeling studies must be interpreted circumspectly. Associative studies that find correlation between climate variation and disease do not account for causation.
- Future impacts of climate change are uncertain. Climate change may impact some infectious diseases, but the evidence is unclear. Human adaptation may negate negative impacts, as may public health measures, ranging from surveillance to vector control. In addition, housing

design, including screens, use of bednets, or air conditioning may exert significant mitigating effects.

- Technical advances in modeling, such as the advent of geographical information systems (GIS) and remote sensing may improve the predictive capacities of infectious disease epidemiology (National Research Council, 2001).

It is thus very difficult to predict accurately the effect of climate change on populations, and even more difficult to construct linkages between climate change and mobile populations or refugee populations. Thus, it appears premature to conclude that global warming will necessarily lead to either an increased range of vectorborne disease, or that the prevalence of specific vectorborne diseases will either increase or decrease, because the predictive science is not yet mature enough to allow such prediction. For example, there is an ongoing and vibrant debate concerning the extent to which global warming accounts for recent increases in malaria in the East African Highlands, with a number of well recognized and highly credible scientists denying such a link (Hay, Rogers, Randolph, Stern, Cox, Shanks, & Snow, 2002; Reiter, Thomas, Atkinson, Hay, Randolph, Rogers, Shank, Snow, & Spielman, 2004; Rogers & Randolph, 2000), and other equally well known and credible scientists arguing that the former group is misinterpreting the evidence (Patz, Hulme, Rosenzweig, Mitchell, Goldberg, Githeko, Lele, McMichael, & Le Sueur, 2002).

In the face of uncertainty the "precautionary principle" whereby mitigation and prevention should be invoked if situations have potentially negative environmental consequences, the environment is fragile. But in the case of malaria, for example, it appears that climate change as a whole, rather than global warming in isolation, will result in increased precipitation in many areas—precipitation that may flood anopheline breeding sites, and perhaps decrease the prevalence of malaria. Rogers and Randolph (2000) combined empirical data and a global circulation model and concluded that malaria will decrease in many areas in Africa where it is now highly prevalent—largely as a result of increased precipitation.

## El Niño Southern Oscillation (ENSO) and Health

Much of the evidence of the effects of climate change is indirect rather than predictive, and comes from studies of the health effects of the El Niño Southern Oscillation (ENSO) phenomenon (e.g., Kovats, Bouma, Hajat, Worrell, & Haunes, 2003). This is because the rapid temperature and precipitation changes that occur under ENSO conditions are thought by many to serve as a surrogate or a "natural experiment" for global climate change. The experiment is far from perfect, because the weather changes that occur during ENSO years are short-term and relatively localized and do not replicate the gradual climate change that is global that the "ENSO experiment" supposedly simulates. Thus, humans and their institutions do not have a chance to predict, mitigate, and adapt to change under ENSO scenarios. Nonetheless, in the absence of adequate predictive epidemiology and conclusive empirical evidence, the evidence during ENSO years from areas of the world that are warmer and wetter than usual suggests that these conditions are associated with increased rates of malaria and dengue. Moreover, there is evidence that ENSO years are associated with an increase in extreme weather events and associated natural disasters. Thus, there appears to be a link between global climate change and those natural disasters that are associated with weather and climate, such as tropical cyclones, heavy rainfall, and flooding. Finally, there is some evidence that ENSO years may be associated with drought in other areas of the world (National Research Council, 2001).

Climate Change and Sea-Level Rise

A very significant characteristic of climate change that is firmly established is that of sea level rise. As the IPCC wrote in 2001, "Although the severity of the threat will vary regionally, sea level rise of the magnitude currently projected . . . is expected to have disproportionately great effects on the social and economic development of many small island states (IPCC, 2001b, p. 855)." The IPCC's estimate is that the mean sea level rise will be 5 mm per year, with a range of 2-9 mm per year (IPCC, 2001b). This is a consequence of global mean temperature increases, and more specifically, of temperature increases in the Arctic and Antarctic regions, and, to a lesser extent, in glacial regions elsewhere. These temperature increases have already resulted in measurable polar icecap melting, and in glacial retreat due to melting. Climate change scenarios predict even mean sea level rise, but climate change scenarios predict more significant increases in the future. This will create environmental refugees—most notably in countries that are below or close to sea level in developing regions such as Bangladesh or in the Pacific atolls.

One of the consequences of sea level rise in Bangladesh will be the flooding of agriculturally productive land in densely settled areas. This would result in both the loss of fisheries and of rice production, as well as the creation of population displacement (Nelson, 2003). It is unclear how rapidly the flooding, loss of agricultural land, and population displacement would take, since sea level rise is a gradual process. Presumably, this would allow the government of Bangladesh, perhaps with multilateral assistance, to mitigate some of the effects of the sea level rise, and possibly to construct planned communities that would have living conditions that would be superior to those of refugee camps that are constructed following unexpected natural disasters. It is even conceivable that dikes and levies could be constructed along that coast of Bangladesh, though this would be quite costly. Prevention, or, if that fails, mitigation, require planning, cooperation, funding, and foresight, and there is no assurance that the positive adaptation scenario would be realized. Analogously, the breach of the levies in New Orleans during a hurricane such as Katrina had been predicted for years, but this resulted in inaction, despite a realization of the dire consequences of the levies' being breached. The location of the specific breaches had even been anticipated, yet short-term thinking and denial dominated. There is no assurance that the situation will be any different with sea level rise. It is similarly difficult to state definitively what the health impacts will be of displacement that will follow sea level rise. Bangladesh is a country of particular concern since it is located at the confluence of three major rivers, and has one of the 10 highest population densities in the world. In fact, the vast majority of the land area—80%—lies within the Ganges River Delta (Broadus, 2001) and most of the country is near or at sea level (Dore & Etkin, 2003). Disasters that have already occurred in Bangladesh in the past 20 years, such as flooding from monsoon rains, have demonstrated that inhabitants of the country, and its infrastructure, exhibit extreme vulnerability, largely due to the amplifying effects of poverty. Broadus (2001) estimates that approximately 5% of the population would be displaced by flooding due to sea-level rise within the predicted limits of the IPCC, although this is qualified by the fact that future population densities during this century will increase, thus compounding the difficulties of prediction. Though 5% of the rice cultivation would be directly affected by sea level rise, if saltwater affects the groundwater, as much as 85% of the agricultural production of Bangladesh could be affected (Broadus, 2001). Much of this, however, could be mitigated by the construction of seawalls, levies, and dykes. Another country that will be severely affected by sea-level rise is Egypt. The Nile Delta and Nile River Basin contain a significant proportion of Egypt's population. It has been estimated that 12% to 15% of the country's arable land will be flooded and 14% of Egypt's population might be displaced, thereby creating a large number of environmental refugees (Broadus, 2001). Whether the spread of infectious diarrheal and respiratory diseases would be a consequence of this displacement would depend largely upon the living conditions into which the refugees move, and the rapidity of displacement. Planned, gradual movement would be far less subject to infectious and transmissible disease outbreaks than would sudden, forced migration.

The IPCC, in their 2001 assessment, devoted an entire chapter to the effects of climate change on small island states (Nurse & Sem, 2001). Particularly noteworthy will be the increased vulnerability of population and infrastructure due to the increasing severity and frequency of tropical cyclones. In the longer run in the next century we will see the effects of sea-level rise on population and land use in Pacific atolls and the low limestone islands in the Caribbean—effects of such a magnitude that all social and economic sectors in these nations would be disrupted (Nurse & Sem, 2001). Some of the smaller islands, and particularly the Pacific atoll sovereignties, may simply cease to exist as physical entities, and therefore sea level rise would also affect the global political system, at least on a small scale. It would eliminate sovereign nations such as Kiribati, the Maldives, the Marshall Islands, and Tuvalu. While sea-level rise is presumably happening slowly enough that the only direct mortality is from natural hazards, it will probably result in out-migration from low-lying islands to other locations, and relocation of population from coastal areas, where people are now concentrated in most island states, to areas of the islands that are farther from the coast (Barnett & Adger, 2003). The IPCC did note, however, that many island states have significant adaptive capacities, and that government land use policies can mitigate the effects of sea-level rise.

The health effects of natural disasters, as we have seen, are significant; however, the health effects of planned displacement in anticipation of a "natural" event with decades of warning and with planned mitigation, as well as individual psychological and collective adaptive responses is unpredictable. Some of this will be determined by how displacement will be handled by the Bangladeshi government—will it be a problem that will be ignored until it turns into a disaster, or will it be treated as a planned series of resettlements? Will there be planned agricultural change and relocation? These are some of the unknown yet crucial questions that must be answered. One might certainly speculate that the human and landscape ecologies in Bangladesh under flooding scenarios secondary to sea level rise would be appropriate for increases in malaria and dengue, because the stagnant water and other pools would facilitate vector breeding. However, the accuracy of this generalization depends very much upon the actual ensuing conditions and the local geographies.

## Conclusion

Humans and the environment are in constant and dynamic interaction; part of this interaction includes environmental sources of disease, as well as human-amplified sources of environmentally caused or mediated disease. In the case of natural disasters, there are both direct and indirect sources of morbidity and mortality, particularly when the disaster has overwhelmed the coping capacities of human systems. This was the case with the South Asia (Kashmir-Pakistan) earthquake of 2005. In the case of more gradual environmental change, such as global climate change, health effects are more subtle, and their assessment is therefore more difficult, with the evidence being difficult to discern. Modeling can be extremely difficult because of the complexities of dealing with coupled earth-atmosphere-ocean physical systems, and then putting these in the context of both biological and social systems.

The resulting effects on human health in the cases of both natural hazards and global climate change have some of their sources in human activities themselves, in much the same way as the schistosomiasis following the completion of the Akosombo Dam had its origin in human activity, as much as in biological disease ecology. Thus, the political ecology of global climate change is such that human modification of the earth in terms of land use change, use of fossil fuels, and industrialization, is indirectly causing any increases in vectorborne disease as well as sea-level rise. In the case of natural hazards, increased vulnerability is partly the result of human decisions, since people or groups either choose or are forced, to relocate to precarious locations. Thus, while people appear to be the passive subjects of nature, it is clear that this is an oversimplification. This oversimplification can become tragic quite rapidly, and can result in great unnecessary human suffering, disease, and death.

## References

Abramovitz, J. (2001). *Unnatural Disasters*. Worldwatch Paper 158. Washington, DC: Worldwatch Institute.

Barnett, J. & Adger, W.N. (2003). Climate dangers and atoll countries. *Climatic Change*, 61, 321-337.

Benin, L. (1985). *Medical Consequences of Disasters*. Berlin: Springer-Verlag.

Bloom, S. (2005). Tsunami threats: the long and short of it. *The Journal of Clinical Investigation*, 115, 481-482.

Broadus, J.M. (2001). Sea-level rise and the Bangladesh and Nile deltas. In (J.X. Kasperson & R.E. Kasperson, Eds.), *Global Environmental Risk* (pp. 353-372). London, UK: Earthscan Publications.

Charnley, S. (1997). Environmentally-displaced peoples and the cascade effect: Lessons from Tanzania. *Human Ecology*, 25, 593-618.

Dore, M.H.I. & Etkin, D. (2003). Natural disasters, adaptive capacity and development in the twenty first century. In (M. Pelling, Ed.), *Natural Disasters and Development in a Globalizing World* (pp. 75-91). London, UK: Routledge.

Hay, S.I., Rogers, D.J., Randolph, S.E., Stern, D.I., Cox, J., Shanks, G.D., & Snow, R.W. (2002). Hot topic or hot air? Climate change and malaria resurgence in East African highlands. *Trends in Parasitology*, 18, 530-534.

Intergovernmental Panel on Climate Change (2001a). *Climate change 2001: Synthesis report. A contribution of working groups I, II, and III to the Third Assessment Report of the Intergovernmental Panel on Climate Change*. R.T. Watson and the Core Writing Team (Eds.), Cambridge, UK: Cambridge University Press.

Intergovernmental Panel on Climate Change (2001b). *Climate change 2001: Impacts, adaptation, and vulnerability*. R.T. Watson and the Core Writing Team (Eds.). Cambridge, UK: Cambridge University Press.

Kondratyev, K.Y., Krapivin, V.F., & Phillips, G.W. (2001). *Global Environmental Change: Modelling and Monitoring*. Berlin, Germany: Springer-Verlag.

Kovats, R.S., Bouma, M.J., Hajat, S., Worrell, E., & Haines, A. (2003), El Niño and health. *The Lancet*, 362, 481-489.

Krieger, N. (1994). Epidemiology and the web of causation: has anyone seen the spider?" *Social Science and Medicine*, 39, 887-903.

Leor, J., Poole, W.K., & Kloner, R.A. (1996). Sudden cardiac death triggered by an earthquake. *New England Journal of Medicine*, 334, 413-419.

Meade, M.S. & Earickson, R.J. (2005). *Medical Geography*. New York, NY: Guilford Press.

National Research Council (2001). *Under the Weather: Climate, Ecosystems, and Infectious Disease*. Washington, DC: National Academy Press.

National Research Council (2003). *Malaria Control During Mass Population Movements and Natural Disasters*. Washington, DC: National Academy Press.

Nelson, D.I. (2003). Health impact assessment of climate change in Bangladesh. *Environmental Impact Assessment Review*, 23, 323-341.

Noji, E. (1997). *The Public Health Consequences of Disasters*: New York, NY: Oxford University Press.

Norris, F., Friedman, M., & Watson, P. (2002). 60,000 disaster victims speak: Part II: summary and implications of disaster mental health research. *Psychchiatry*, 65, 240-260.

Norris, F.H., Murphy, A.D., Baker, C.K., & Perilla, J.L. (2004). Postdisaster PTSD over four waves of a panel study of Mexico's 1999 flood. *Journal of Traumatic Stress*, 17, 283-292.

Nurse, L. & Sem, G. (2001). Small island states. In (J. McCarthy, O. Canziani, N. Leary, D. Dokken, & K. White, Eds.). *Climate Change 2001: Impacts, Adaptation, and Vulnerability*. Cambridge, MA: Cambridge, Cambridge University Press.

Ogawa, K., Tsuji, I., Shiono, K. & Hisamichi, S. (2000). Increased acute myocardial infarction mortality following the 1995 Great Hanshin-Awaji earthquake in Japan. *International Journal of Epidemiology*, 29, 445-455.

Oliver-Smith, A. (2004) Theorizing vulnerability in a globalized world: a political ecological perspective. In (G. Bankoff, G. Frerks, & D. Hilhorst, Eds.), *Mapping Vulnerability: Disasters, Development and People*. Sterling, VA: Earthscan.

Oppong, J. & Kalipeni, E. (1998). The refugee crisis in Africa and implications for health and disease: a political ecology approach. *Social Science and Medicine*, 46, 1637-1653.

Patz, J.A., McGeehin M.A., Bernard S.M., Ebi, K.L., Epstein, P.R., Grambsch, A., Gubler, D.J., Reiter, P., Romieu, I., Rose, J.B., Samet, J.M. & Trtanj, J. (2001). The potential health impacts of climate variability and change for the United States. Executive summary of the report of the health sector of the U.S. National Assessment. *Journal of Environmental Health*, 64, 20-28.

Patz, J.A., Hulme, M., Rosenzweig, C., Mitchell, T.D., Goldberg, R.A., Githeko, A.K., Lele, S., McMichael, A.J. & Le Sueur, D. (2002). Climate change: Regional warming and malaria resurgence. *Nature*, 420, 627-628.

Pelling, M. (2003). Paradigms of risk. In (M. Pelling, Ed.), *Natural Disasters and Development in a Globalizing World*. London, UK: Routledge.

Quinn, S.C. (2006). Hurricane Katrina: a social and public health disaster. *American Journal of Public Health*, 96, 2.

Reiter, P., Thomas, C. J. Atkinson, P.M. Hay, S.I., Randolph, S.E., Rogers, D.J., Shanks, G.D., Snow, R.W., & Spielman, A. (2004) Global warming and malaria: a call for accuracy. *The Lancet Infectious Diseases*, 4, 323-324.

Rogers, D.J. & Randolph, S.E. (2000). The global spread of malaria in a future, warmer world. *Science*, 289, 1763-1766.

Rutta, E., Kipngili, R., Lunkonge, H., Assefa, S., Mitisilale, E., & Rwechungura, S. (2001). Treatment outcome among Rwandan and Burundian refugees with smear-positive tuberculosis in Ngara, Tanzania. *International Journal of Tuberculosis and Lung Diseases*, 5, 628-632.

Salama, P. & Dondero, T.J. (2001). HIV surveillance in complex emergencies. *AIDS*, 15, S4-S12.

Tobin, G.A. & Montz, B.E. (1997). *Natural Hazards: Explanation and Integration*. New York, NY: The Guilford Press.

Toole, M.J. (1997). Communicable diseases and disease control. In (E. Noji, Ed.). *The Public Health Consequences of Disasters* (pp. 79-100). New York, NY: Oxford University Press.

Tsai, C.H., Lung, F.W., & Wang, S.Y. (2004). The 1999 Ji-Ji (Taiwan) earthquake as a trigger for acute myocardial infarction. *Psychosomatics*, 45, 477-482.

Wisner, B. (2003). Changes in capitalism and global shifts in the distribution of hazard and vulnerability. In (M. Pelling, Ed.), *Natural Disasters and Development in a Globalizing World* (pp. 43-56). London, UK: Routledge.

# Part IV
## Leisure Migration and Health Concerns: A Paradox or Inevitability?

# Chapter 11

## Casual Sex in the Sun Makes the Holiday: Young Tourists' Perspectives

EUGENIA WICKENS, PH.D. AND
SEVIL SÖNMEZ, PH.D.

## Introduction

Sexually transmitted infections (STIs), including HIV, is a major health issue with respect to international travel. According to the World Health Organization (WHO), HIV/AIDS–associated illnesses have caused the deaths of over 20 million people since 1981 and an estimated 39 million or more cases had occurred worldwide by the end of 2004. Moreover, an estimated 5 million new HIV infections occurred worldwide in 2004 alone, which represent approximately 14,000 new infections each day.

Although the majority of all AIDS cases occur in developing countries, current predictions make grim reading particularly when HIV-infection rates are expected to continue climbing in many Western countries. For instance, an estimated 50,000 people were living with HIV within the U.K. by the end of 2002 while the number was predicted to increase by 25% the following year (Health Protection Agency, U.K, 2002), with the fastest growth rate in new HIV infections among young people 18 to 30 years old (Meikle, 2002). Currently the warning from the Public Health Laboratory Service (PHLS) is that there is an urgent need to restart efforts to educate young travelers about safe sex, including the use of condoms (Meikle, 2002, p. 2). PHLS officials indicated that they:

"...were very concerned last year when we saw a record number of new HIV diagnoses, but these latest figures are even more disturbing. We now appear to be seeing more than twice as many new HIV diagnoses each year than we were at the end of the 1990s"

(Meikle, 2002, p. 2)

The fastest growth rate in cases of HIV infection is found among young people traveling and on holiday. Concern about young people's hedonistic behavior is voiced by many commentators (e.g., Bellis, Hughes, Thomson, & Bennett, 2004). Research clearly indicates that hedonistic holidays pose sexual health risks.

This chapter explores the health risk behaviors of young tourists with a review of current literature followed by examples from authors' own research studies involving youth travelers from Britain and the U.S. (Apostolopoulos, Sönmez, & Yu 2002; Sönmez, Apostolopoulos, Yu, Yang, Yu, & Matilla 2006; Wickens, 1997, 2002) and concludes that young tourists not only represent a significant risk group in terms of sexual health but must be targeted by effective preventive intervention strategies to positively impact their sexual choices and behaviors and to control the spread of STIs/HIV.

## Mass Tourism

The evolution of travel and tourism shows that while people, including young adults, have traveled around the world for centuries, mass tourism is a relatively recent phenomenon. Before the end of WWII, foreign travel was a luxury available only to the privileged few; however, in the last 50 years, the nature of this pleasure industry has changed dramatically (Boorstin, 1964; Bruner, 1991; MacCannell, 1976; Urry, 1991). Rising living standards in many Western societies have made pleasure travel a possibility even for young travelers. In particular, the development of mass air transport and the continued expansion of low cost air travel have led to the creation of inexpensive package holidays. The advent of holidays at bargain prices together with the growth of global communications via the Internet have contributed to the 'democratization of travel,' with large numbers of young people visiting a wide range of holiday destinations (Ryan & Hall, 2001; Urry, 1991), led by Australia, U.S.A., Thailand, Goa, Spain, Cyprus and Greece.

### Youth Travel: A Growing Market Segment

The youth travel market has grown significantly particularly over the past two decades and is now considered to be the fastest growing segment of the travel market. According to the World Tourism Organization (WTO), it now accounts for 25% per cent of all international tourist trips and continues to grow into a highly lucrative business (Richards & Wilson, 2003). The increase of this market segment is supported by global demographic trends that indicate the growth of the youth population in many Western countries along with the growth of the ageing population. Furthermore, the youth travel market has been stimulated by the popularity of backpacking, adventure tourism packages, and higher rates of participation in overseas study programs (Richards & Wilson, 2003). Reports indicate that young tourists originating mainly from Western countries, including Australia, Britain, France, Germany and the U.S. are now traveling farther from home, prefer sun and beach holidays (Richards & Wilson, 2003), and frequently include casual sex in their travel expectations and experiences.

## Tourism as a Leisure Activity

As a phenomenon, tourism has been approached from a variety of disciplinary perspectives, including sociology, geography, psychology, anthropology, and economics and has also been the subject of a number of multidisciplinary studies (Burns & Holden, 1995). Extant literature presents tourism as a freely chosen leisure activity with an emphasis on the traveler's autonomy in decision making. A defining characteristic of leisure is that it involves change as something different from one's normal routines and obligations of day-to-day living. Tourism is also linked with the widely held belief that the essence of leisure is its comparative freedom from societal constraints and occurs during genuine free time (Shields, 1992).

## Advertising Hedonistic Holidays

In the literature, youth travel has been treated in terms of its impacts on host destinations, experiences and motives of youth travelers, their health-risk intentions and behaviors, demand and supply, and the role of advertising in the selling of hedonistic holidays (e.g., Herold, Maticka-Tyndale, & Mewhinney, 1998; Josiam, Hobson, Dietrich, & Smeaton, 1998; Maticka-Tyndale 2003; Maticka-Tyndale & Herold 1997, 1999; Maticka-Tyndale, Herold, & Mewhinney 1998; Maticka-Tyndale, Herold, & Opperman, 2003; Mewhinney, Herold & Maticka-Tyndale, 1995; Smith & Rosenthal, 1997; Apostolopoulos et al., 2002; Sönmez et al., 2006). Research suggests that advertisements for hedonistic holidays that stress the availability of alcohol and sex are instrumental in influencing travelers' decisions in the selection of 'sun and fun' destinations. For example, tourists are sold images of Greece as a destination governed by the 'Four Ss' of sun, sea, sand, and sex (Wickens, 1997).

Several studies document how destinations (e.g., Paris, Amsterdam, Thailand, and Gambia) are promoted as 'playgrounds' and how tour operators use photographic images in their promotional materials to create a sense of heightened sexual anticipation (Mewhinney et al., 1995; Ryan & Hall, 2001). Thailand is one such destination, marketed by tour operators primarily for its sex clubs, sex shows, countless topless beaches, and the promise of finding an exotic sex partner. Researchers have written specifically about the flow of youth travelers to Bali and Thailand for the purposes of engaging in casual sex and the role of advertising in selling sex tourism (Ryan & Hall, 2001).

# The Holiday Behavior of Travelers: Some Generalizations

The centrality of sex in tourists' experiences was identified in early studies on international travel and tourist behavior (e.g., Lett, 1983; Wagner, 1977). Reporting on the sexual encounters of tourists and their experience in Gambia, Wagner (1977) applied Turner's (1973) concepts of 'communitas' and 'anti-structure,' in the attempt to explain the playful and permissive behavior of Scandinavian female tourists. A key finding of this early work is that female tourists indulge in 'spontaneous communitas' type of behavior and experience freedom, carefree fun, and casual sex.

Likewise, in a study of charter yacht tourism in the Caribbean, further evidence was provided that tourists often indulge in unlimited hedonism and casual sex, thereby experiencing Turner's (1973) spontaneous communitas (Lett, 1983). It was suggested that the hedonistic behaviors of tourists revitalize and prepare them for their return to their structured, everyday lives and the "ludic and liminoid license provide a temporary release from, but not a permanent alternative to, everyday life" (Lett, 1983, p. 54). From his study of American tourists and their holiday pursuits, Lett concluded that they "begin to play at the moment they abandon the restrictions and requirements of everyday life and enter vacation time" (ibid, p. 43). Lett also revealed that while tourists play with rules of everyday life, particularly those applicable to social relationships, personal indulgence, and sexual behavior—some female tourists reported 'increased sexual appetites' in the British Virgin Islands, while male tourists boasted of their 'increased virility.' Participants in Lett's research appear to share the belief that "sex with strangers is part of the collective fantasy of an adventurous holiday."

One of the main thrusts of this early work on tourist behavior is that travelers experience a 'liminal' or 'non-ordinary' world during their holidays that liberate and enable them to indulge in pleasurable pursuits. Holiday resorts are viewed as playgrounds where tourists can enjoy the experience of 'liminality' while summer holidays away from home are seen as analogous to a 'sacred journey.' In other words, the travel experience is a 'rite of passage' and one to be distinguished from the 'profane' experience of everyday and viewed as the 'sacred' experience of the holiday atmosphere in another place. Travel away from home functions as the rite of recreation and is marked by a beginning, a series of events along the way, and an end or a return to the ordinary home environment. From this perspective, it is understandable for tourists to behave differently from 'ordinary life.'

The notions of liminality and communitas have informed the majority of studies of tourist behavior. Several researchers reporting on tourists' hedonistic and self-indulgent lifestyles have argued that tourist resorts are 'liminal' spaces that provide the hedonistic tourist with opportunities to step outside of social conventions (Ryan & Kinder, 1996; Shields, 1992). While liminality describes the sense of in between-ness involving a temporary loss of social bearings, 'liminal space' refers to an area where "strict social conventions are relaxed under the exigencies of travel and of relative anonymity and freedom from community scrutiny" (Shields, 1992, p. 50), whereas tourists are viewed as "free of all constraints. . .to do as one pleases, to dress . . .celebrate and feast. . .they break the fetters of everyday rules. . .have-a-good-time ideology and the tomorrow-we-shall-be gone-again attitude sets the tone" (Krippendorf, 1987, p. 33). This perspective of tourism echoes others' views of it as an escape from everyday life into a free area—a notion that is isomorphic with the concept of 'liminal space.'

## Youth Travelers

A number of studies that examined the health risk behaviors of young tourists in vacation settings have found high levels of casual sex and alcohol consumption among young Britton and New Zealander vacationers, U.S. and Canadian spring breakers, and Australian "schoolies" (Apostolopoulos et al., 2002; Clark & Clift 1996; Eiser & Ford, 1995; Ford & Eiser, 1996; Herold et al., 1998; Hennink, Cooper, & Diamond 2000; Josiam et al., 1998; Maticka-Tyndale et al., 1998, 2003; Maticka-Tyndale & Herold 1997, 1999; Mewhinney et al., 1995; Ryan & Robertson 1997; Ryan & Martin, 2001; Sönmez et al., 2006). Not only was travel found to increase the probability of sexual activity, but young travelers were found to equate vacation-time with loosening of one's sense of responsibility while offering opportunities for sexual activity— or a time when anything is permissible (Carter, 1997). Substance use and risky sexual behaviors were found among young vacationers at higher rates than in their non-vacation environments. These high-risk behaviors were linked to the 'situational disinhibition' experienced by tourists in settings that encourage sexual and emotional transience as well as liminality. Risky behaviors in vacation settings were also associated with situational factors (what the vacation setting entails), tourists' expectations of certain types of experiences, social context (peer group), and risky leisure choices (casual sex and excessive drinking), as well as behavioral intentions for casual sex and excessive drinking.

Studies with Canadian and American beachfront vacationers have reported incidence rates for sex with new partners the day of meeting that range from 15% to 24% for males and from 13% to 21% for females (Josiam et al., 1998; Maticka-Tyndale et al., 1998). In addition, intentions, prior experience with casual sex, influences by one's peers, and facilitating situational conditions emerged as critical factors in explaining risky sexual behaviors (Maticka-Tyndale et al., 1998; Maticka-Tyndale & Herold, 1997, 1999).

In a study of U.S. spring breakers, students from two universities were administered pre- and post-spring break surveys designed to understand their behavioral intentions prior to spring break as well as their actual vacation behaviors. Opportunities for drinking, for trying drugs, and for having sex were among the most significant vacation motives, and in fact, destination choice was based on each location's potential for drinking and sexual opportunities. Significant numbers of student travelers expressed their intentions to drink, get drunk, experiment sexually, and have sex with someone they met on vacation and the majority of spring breakers expected to be in a 'break-loose,' 'have fun' mood. Students reported making pacts with their friends to get drunk, to have sex with someone new, and to experiment with drugs on vacation. Furthermore, attitudes toward casual sex, personal normative beliefs, situational expectations, and pacts emerged as significant predictors of intentions to engage in casual sex. Upon returning home, about one third of respondents reported having casual sex, while a majority reported irregular condom use. More specifically, substantial numbers of spring breakers got drunk, had three or more drinks in one sitting, had sex as a result of drinking, and had sex with a partner that they knew less than one week, while most 'rarely or never used a condom.' Given that the traditional spring break environment facilitates alcohol bingeing and casual sex, young adults clearly participate in activities and behaviors that they may not otherwise engage in—which may make it easier to engage in such risk behaviors in subsequent vacations when opportunities present themselves.

Similar findings were reported by Maticka-Tyndale and associates (2003) from their study of 'schoolies.' Each year, thousands of high school seniors or graduates travel with their friends to the Australian Gold Coast in early December in order to experience an adult-free, fun-time holiday. Similar to U.S. spring breakers, male 'schoolies' reported having sex with strangers during their holiday experience.

The themes of casual sex, bingeing and how touristic spaces such as beach resorts provide young people with the ideal conditions for suspending social codes of behavior are corroborated by a number of researchers. Some scholars have suggested that young people's hedonistic lifestyles—indulgence in casual sex and excessive alcohol consumption—have already been established at home and are simply replicated in vacation settings (Smith & Rosenthal, 1997). According to this perspective, it is young people's routine behaviors and lifestyles that influence their sexual behaviors during vacations, rather than the holiday setting. Although the debate continues, social analysts agree that having sex with a stranger during vacation is often the expectation and experience of many young tourists (Apostolopoulos et al., 2002, Maticka-Tyndale et al., 1998, 2003; Sönmez et al., 2006; Wickens, 1997).

## Sexual Risk-taking

Research reveals that young tourists not only indulge in casual sex when on vacation but are also willing to take sexual risks (Abdullah, Fielding, & Hedley, 1998; Apostolopoulos et al., 2002; Bellis et al., 2004; Maticka-Tyndale et al., 2003; Sönmez et al., 2006; Vorakitphokatorn, Pulerwitz, & Cash, 1998). A survey study of the sexual behaviors of British tourists visiting Ibiza (Spain) provides further evidence that substantial numbers of young people have sex with people they meet while abroad and also that having sex abroad is often associated with the use of illicit drugs (Bellis et al., 2004). This study corroborates results of research on U.S. spring breakers which provide evidence that youth travelers also participate in excessive drinking and experimenting with illicit drugs in addition to demonstrating unsafe sexual practices (Apostolopoulos et al., 2002; Sönmez et al., 2006). Young adults frequently place themselves in risky situations that result in the acquisition of STIs/HIV.

In more extreme situations, young travelers' engagement in risk behaviors leads not only to loss of health but the tragic loss of life. In fact, young male travelers, placed in a category of 'risk-takers,' have been associated with dangerous activities that include excessive alcohol use, drug use, physical risk-taking (e.g., jumping from hotel balconies), as well as driving while intoxicated leading to fatal accidents (Pizam, Reichel, & Uriely, 2002). One investigation found a correlation between travelers' likelihood of getting involved in high-risk sexual activities with how far away from their normal environments they were vacationing (Abdullah et al., 1998). The findings of this study of tourists departing from Hong Kong—that male travelers are more likely to have unprotected sex with a stranger and thus more likely to place themselves at greater risk for STIs—support findings of other studies that male travelers are more likely to have casual sex during their vacations (Daniels, Kelly, Nelson, & Barton, 1992; Maticka-Tyndale et al., 1998). In contrast, a study of tourists in Chalkidiki, Greece provides evidence that young female tourists seek opportunities for exploring their sexuality while on vacation (Wickens 1994; 1997). To borrow a phrase from Giddens (1992, p. 77) "a search for a fix governs the sexual behavior" of both female and male tourists.

## Young Tourists: A Case Study from Greece

Chalkidiki in Northern Greece is a well-established destination that regularly attracts British, Austrian, and German package travelers. Semi-structured interviews were conducted with 286 English speaking travelers at various sites, including tavernas, cafes, and bars. Interview questions covered a wide range of issues including tourists' holiday activities, their views of Chalkidiki as a tourist destination, and issues concerning travel and health, as well as tourist attitudes toward unprotected sex and drug use. Data were clustered in order to identify tourist types suggested by Wickens (2002) with particular attention paid to the category of tourist identified as a 'raver.'

In their conversations, young tourists (ravers) emphasized the possibilities offered by Chalkidiki for sensual and hedonistic pleasures and reported that they selected Chalkidiki as their holiday destination due to its low cost, sun, beach, and nightlife and identified 'getting a suntan,' 'having sex,' and 'getting drunk' as common motives. Interviews also revealed that the anonymity and relative freedom from social constraints ravers experienced in Chalkidiki were conducive to the suspension of customary rules of moral conduct. Common statements made by respondents to this effect include: *"you can do everything you want to, you can be silly, you can go topless or bra-less, nobody bothers you," "you feel less restricted here, because you're away from home," "you feel free to do whatever you want to, because not everyone knows each other," "there is no need to conform to expectations," "no one controls what you do and what you should do," "no one criticizes you for your behavior," "in every respect you're free, no one knows us here and there is no pressure on us to conform. . . above all there is no police."* Ravers' perceptions of Chalkidiki as a place offering opportunities to do as one pleases and *"to have sex in a hot climate"* are illustrated further:

*". . .I think because of the hot climate. . .and people are less inhibited. . .and so people tend to look at each other in bars and perhaps, weigh each other up. And I think people always behave differently when they are away from home, rather than at home. . .when they go to a bar or a disco-they can talk to somebody else, and if they fancy this person, because they have lost their inhibitions, they think 'wow' I'll go to bed with this person. . .yes a lot of people come here for the sun, sea and sex, but well I do that alright."*

(Male raver, Age 20)

A common theme to emerge from the interviews is that 'sex makes the holiday.' Seeking out sexual liaisons with strangers and indulging in sexual activities on the beach were typical examples of hedonistic behavior demonstrated by Chalkidiki's young tourists:

*"Oh yeah. . .we came here with the idea of having sex. . .it makes the holiday. . .partly because of the climate, the resort, the beach. . .I think a lot of us are here for this reason."*

(Female raver, Age 19)

*"Yes, this is one of the reasons for this holiday. . .not the only reason. . .it serves its purpose. . .you can dream to yourself about it, through the winter. . .it makes the holidays . . .no problem finding a man. . .Greek men always volunteer for sex. . .when they are chatting you up, they would give you flowers and things. . .no I wouldn't do this at home, never, ever, ever. You have your reputation to think about."*

(Female raver, Age 19)

It is undeniable that the pursuit of such adventures leads ravers to take risks with their health. A useful perspective on tourist risk-taking was provided by Goffman's notion of 'action space.' He uses the term 'action' to refer to "the activities that are consequential, problematic and undertaken for what is felt to be their own sake" (Goffman, 1967, p. 185). In his analysis of the world of gambling in Las Vegas, he identifies casinos, pool halls, and amusement parks, as prototypical 'action spaces'—such spaces, dedicated to pleasure, thrills, and excitement allow individuals to experience the adventures denied to them in their everyday life. He goes on to argue that 'players' in a casino are in search of 'action' and take instantaneous risks, by putting their money in jeopardy, in order to get 'a piece of it.' According to Goffman, winning a game is a secondary consideration for players; they are primarily concerned with the intensity of the action. As he rightly points out, action (in his sense of the term) can also be found in other areas of life: track racing, where drivers experience a 'slight danger' to life, and taking drugs such as LSD, where the experimenter uses 'his mind as the equipment for action.'

Action spaces such as discos, bars, and holiday resorts provide the individual with the opportunity to experience 'fancy milling,' which refers to the relaxed and uninhibited participation with others, in an action space, with the consequent exposure of oneself to risks and uncertainties. Goffman argues that "the mere presence in a large, tightly packed gathering of revelling persons can bring not only the excitement that crowds generate, but also the uncertainty of not quite knowing what might happen next, the possibility of flirtations, which can themselves lead to relationship formation" (1967, p. 197). Such spaces provide opportunities for "sexual or courtship action: that is, the initiation of a sexual affair with the unacquainted" (Goffman, 1967, p. 210). Moreover, the novelty of a new sexual partner is a thrill, especially if the stranger is of "another race, color or creed" (Balint, in Goffman, 1967, p. 197). The argument is taken further by suggesting that there are 'special times and places' set aside in society for 'role reversals,' for opening oneself up to risks in the pursuit of thrills and adventures, normally denied to us in everyday mundane and routinized life: "On one side are the safe and silent places, the home, the well-regulated role in business. . .on the other are all those activities that generate expression, requiring the individual to lay himself on the line and place himself in jeopardy during a passing moment" (Goffman, 1967, p. 268). More importantly, the defining characteristics of all thrills are a "mixture of fear, pleasure and confident hope in face of external danger. . .the danger will pass and that one will be able to return unharmed to safety" (Balint, in Goffman, 1967, pp. 196-7). Thus, action spaces reaffirm, by opposing, the security and the reality of our everyday 'serious life.'

This theoretical perspective is applicable to Chalkidiki's touristic space. Voluntary risks undertaken by tourist 'players' in their quest for thrills are not explained by the notion of 'liminality' alone; the relative anonymity and freedom from community scrutiny, which characterize a liminal touristic space, is enhanced by fancy milling in action spaces. The study found that ravers were not only in search of 'sexual action' but were also willing to take risks in 'getting a piece of it.' Ravers often engage in unprotected sexual activities, often with multiple partners, gambling their health in the quest for thrills (Wickens, 1994, 1997).

## Sexual Scripts and Risks

The literature often portrays young single males as the most likely to be involved in sexual relationships while abroad and more likely to report having unprotected sex with new partners (Abdullah et al., 1998; Daniels et al., 1992; Pizam, 2002). Results from the Chalkidiki study indicate, however, that there is no reason to believe that men are more or less sexually opportunistic than women. As Giddens powerfully argues, the pursuit of sexual pleasure is no longer the province of men alone. Sex plays an important part in the lives of both men and women: "Women want love, men want sex. . .men's appetite for sex, with as many partners as possible, would simply be a defining characteristic of their masculinity. Yet this hoary old observation. . .could be turned around. Women want sex? Yes, for the first time women. . .seek out sexual pleasure as a basic component of their lives and their relationships." (1992, p. 66). Furthermore, women are no longer frightened of being seen as flirtatious and seek opportunities for exploring their sexuality with multiple partners. Sexual experiences are now more freely available than ever before and we live in a culture where sexual signs are everywhere (Giddens, 1992). Female ravers demonstrate these changes:

*"Without the emotional baggage of love, I enjoyed the lust in the brief sexual liaison I had with Kosta. I met him in a bar. . .he sent a drink across to me. . .and we ended up in bed. No, I didn't experience any emotional pain when we parted a few days later."*

(Female raver, Age 22)

Fancy milling in Chalkidiki's action spaces allowed this raver to be a willing participant in the sexual pleasures made accessible by a two week, packaged celebration of the 'here and now.' Discos, bars, nightclubs, and tavernas provide opportunities for initiating sexual affairs with either a Greek *kamaki[1]* or another tourist. Conversations were initiated with questions such as *"where do you come from?"* or *"what are you doing tonight?"* Sexual propositions such as *"look at what my mum has bought me"* (indicating a packet of condoms to her potential sexual partner) or *"I've got to use all of them up, before I go home"* were also observed in Chalkidiki (Wickens, 1997).

Male ravers were found to favor a rather direct approach; for example, they followed an opening question, such as *"would you like to go out with me"* with explicit propositions, such as *"let's have fun"* or *"I'll give you a night you'll never forget."* Greek men adopted similar approaches when playing their 'national sport of being a *kamaki* using some of the following lines to start conversations: *"you are so beautiful, you can't possibly be here on your own"* or *"hello, gorgeous, are you doing anything tonight?"* or *"you take me back to your room and we have good sex."* In those situations where verbal communication is impossible, the linguaphone of the body was used to send its sexual signals:

*"You don't have to talk—I think the way somebody touches you and looks at you, means . . .you know. . .things might happen. . .eye contact, a lot can be said from eye contact, you just have to look at somebody's eyes and you know exactly what. . .yes I enjoy sexual pleasures, touching and feeling and being close to somebody. It progresses as the evening goes on and you feel from the way they touch you, you know. . ."*

(Female raver, Age 23)

Another common theme to emerge from conversations with ravers was the availability of 'one night bonks'—or the relative ease of meeting someone to have sex with for one night:

*"That would be the main place. . .the beach or maybe in the sea. There is a lot of midnight swimming. . .I think a lot of it happens on the beach, you can hear the voices. Some of them would take cameras down and take pictures. Especially a favorite one is of five or six people having sex maybe in the sea and totally naked and they would have their picture taken totally naked."*

(Male raver, Age 20)

---

[1] Kamaki is a harpoon which is used by fishermen to catch octopus. As in fishing, Greek men known as *kamakis* use their skills to seduce female tourists.

According to the above respondent, *"this sort of thing happens all around the Mediterranean, certainly the south of France and Spain. . . .it's partly the sun and the sea and the holiday atmosphere."*

Although young travelers seek out sexual opportunities, neither male nor female ravers were found to take seriously the medical advice about STI/HIV risks but both were clearly willing to enter into transient sexual relationships without using condoms. In fact, both male and female young adults reported indulging in unprotected sex, particularly when they were under the influence of alcohol. When study participants were asked about the possibility of getting AIDS, they reported: *"You don't think of AIDS when you are drunk," "the brain doesn't work well after having lots of alcohol,"* or *"I have a bigger risk of getting hit by a car in Chalkidiki than catching AIDS."* According to one study participant, unprotected sex was not only associated with "getting drunk" but also with taking a drug known as 'a love dove' (also known as Ecstasy):

*"People call it a love dove because it makes you a lot friendlier. It produces a feeling of euphoria and makes you more confident to go and ask somebody to dance with you or to ask somebody to have sex with you. Most people bring their own stuff, no one gets checked at the airport."*

(Male raver, Age 20)

In fact, nearly half of the ravers admitted to drug use, such as cannabis, while on holiday in Chalkidiki. One respondent reported that young tourists also experiment with acid:

*"Some people did. . .some people tried LSD and wanted to do it again. A lot of the people—people who had taken LSD would normally sit out about 6 a.m. on the beach watching the sunrise. The younger females that are English are taking Ecstasy and speed, not so much acid, but there was some of that going on as well. Yeah, normally it is the younger males."*

(Male raver, Age 20)

This is supported by findings from the U.S. study of spring breakers (Apostolopoulos et al., 2002; Sönmez et al., 2006) that young travelers experiment with drugs, binge drink, and take health risks in the pursuit of thrills and pleasure.

Not surprisingly, risk taking is not without serious ramifications. Information from one medical centre in Chalkidiki indicated that vaginal fungal infection was common amongst young holidaymakers and particularly among young British tourists engaging in sexual activities with multiple partners:

*"Young adults are exposed to high levels of sexual contact and unless using condoms, they are likely to contract some form of infection. Repetitive sexual intercourse with multiple partners can certainly lead to severe injuries and ailments. While they are aware of AIDS, they seem to have limited information and advice on safe sex."*

(Doctor, Local Medical Center, Kalimerya)

Although AIDS is known to be fatal, that knowledge does not appear to deter people from taking risks, because the effects of risk taking are not visible

(Giddens, 1991). It is clear that tourists take voluntary risks by 'bracketing out' the health dangers associated with their risky sexual behaviours—and "what could go wrong can be pushed to one side on the grounds that it is so unlikely that it can be put out of mind" (Giddens, 1991, p. 29).

A local pharmacist reported that she often prescribed medication to young English girls who complain of pain associated with 'cystitis'—the most common ailment experienced by female ravers—but also frequently sold condoms to young female tourists aged 20 and under (also supported by study respondents who reported packing 'an adequate supply of condoms'). The paradox associated with condom availability and access and the spread of STIs can be explained only by the fact that ravers ignore the use of protection while under the influence of alcohol. A finding that is clearly consistent with work reported by other researchers (e.g., Ryan & Robertson, 1997; Sönmez et al., 2006).

The Chalkidiki case study reinforces observations made by commentators that young travelers experiment with both sex and drugs and place themselves at great risks not only for a variety of STIs but also HIV/AIDS. Unfortunately, the significance of this type of research is underscored by growing numbers of HIV/AIDS cases among young people (15-24 years old) who account for half of all new HIV infections worldwide and more than 6,000 new infections daily.

## Conclusions

This chapter has discussed the health risk-taking activities of young people as revealed from evidence from Australia, Canada, New Zealand, and the U.S. Past and current research clearly shows that young adult travelers aged 25 and under indulge in unprotected sex, particularly when they are under the influence of alcohol and drugs, thus placing themselves at high risk for acquiring and transmitting STIs/HIV. Results of these studies were supported by the case study of young British travelers to Chalkidiki, in Northern Greece who commonly expose themselves to various STIs, including HIV.

Young travelers' risk taking behaviors are facilitated by a number of factors, including excessive alcohol consumption, the cloak of anonymity that being a tourist affords, substantial levels of social interaction, and an environment of permissiveness (from both peers and the destination community) and are further exacerbated by a complex biochemical relationship between alcohol consumption and sexual behavior. Considering the foregoing, youth travel has the potential to become an incubator for extreme risk taking by young adults through the convergence of drinking, drug use, casual sex, and irregular condom use. Therefore, a central conclusion from the foregoing discussion is that travel away from home for young tourists who are unaware of the ramifications of their risk behaviors is an important risk factor in the spread of STIs. Further, young travelers have the potential to bridge their home communities with the communities they visit and thus infect not only their own sexual partners but new partners they have sexual contact with; therefore, the implications for STI (including HIV) acquisition and transmission are serious and widespread.

A clear focus on situational and social contexts, rather than just behavior, has the potential to contribute more to the puzzle of the etiology of young adults' health risk behaviors, which in turn can assist in developing more effective interventions—especially considering the challenges involved. Developing successful and timely education and prevention messages for high risk behaviors relevant for youth travelers is particularly challenging. The evidence suggests that there is indeed an urgent need to adequately educate young travelers about the health risks they face and safe sex, including the use of condoms. While various creative ideas can be put forth in order to educate them about the potential health risks of careless behaviors and sway them away from reckless activities, it would be naïve to think that young travelers can be easily influenced. Preventive interventions need to be multipronged and to be rooted in multiple sources including the travelers themselves and their social networks, the tourism sector specializing in youth travel, destinations catering to this market segment, and the popular media.

## References

Abdullah, A., Fielding, R., & Hedley, A. (1998). Travel, sexual behavior, and the risk of contracting sexually transmitted diseases, *Hong Kong Medical Journal*, 4(2), 137-144.

Apostolopoulos, Y., Sönmez, S. & Yu C.H. (2002). HIV-risk behaviors of American spring break vacationers: A case of situational disinhibition? *International Journal of STD & AIDS*, 13(11), 733-743.

Balint, M. (1967). Cited In: Goffman, E. (1967). *Interaction Ritual*, London, UK: Penguin Books (pp. 196-197).

Beddoe, C. (1998). Beachboys and tourists: links in the chain of child prostitution in Sri Lanka. In (M. Oppermann, Ed.), *Sex Tourism and Prostitution: Aspects of Leisure Recreation, and Work*, (pp. 45-59). New York, NY: Cognizant Communication Corporation.

Bellis, M.A., Hughes, K., Thomson, R., & Bennett, A. (2004). Sexual behavior of young people in international tourist resorts, *British Medical Journal of Sexually Transmitted Infections*, 80(1), 43-47.

Black, P. (1997). Sexual Behavior and Travel: Quantitative and Qualitative Perspectives on the Behavior of Genitor-urinary Medicine Clinic Attendees. In S. Clift & P. Grabowski (Eds.), *Tourism and Health: Risks, Research and Responses*, (pp. 165-183). London, UK: Pinter.

Brown, J. & Minichello, V. (1994). The Condom: Why more people don't put it on, *Sociology of Health and Illness* 16, 229–51.

Boorstin, D. (1964). *The Image: A Guide to Pseudo-Events in America*, London, UK: Harper and Row.

Bruner, E. (1991). Transformation of Self in Tourism, *Annals of Tourism Research*, 18(1), 238-250.

Bryant, H.E., Csokonay, W.M., Love, M., & Love, E.J. (1991). Self-reported Illness and Risk Behaviors amongst Canadian Travelers While Abroad, *Canadian Journal of Public Health*, 82, 316-319.

Burns, P. & Holden, A. (1995). *Tourism: A New Perspective*, London, UK: Prentice Hall International.

Carter, S., Horn, K., Hart, G., Dunbar, M., Scoular, A., & MacIntyre, S. (1997). The Sexual behavior of international travelers at two Glasgow GUM clinics, *International Journal of STD & AIDS*, 8(5), 336-338.

Clift, S. & Grabowski, P. (1997). *Tourism and Health: Risks, Research and Responses*, London, UK: Pinter.

Cohen, E. (1971). Arab boys and Tourist Girls in a Mixed Jewish-Arab Community, *International Journal of Comparative Sociology*, 12(1), 217-233.

Cossar, J.H., Reid, D., Falcon, R.J., Bell, E.J., Riding, M.H., Follet, E.A.C., Dow, B.C., Mitchell, S., & Grist, N.R. (1990). A Cumulative Review of Studies on Travelers, Their Experience of Illness and the Implication of their Findings, *Journal of Infection*, 21(1), 27-42.

Daniels, D.G., Kelly, P., Nelson, M.R., & Barton, S. (1992). Sexual Behavior amongst Travelers: A Study of Genitourinary Medicine Clinic Attendees, *International Journal of STD & AIDS*, 3(1), 437-438.

Fenton, K. (2002). cited In J. Meikle, (Health correspondent) HIV Infections Head for Record Rise, London, *The Guardian*, November 30, pp. 2.

Ford, N. & Eiser, J.R. (1996). Risk and liminality: The HIV-related socio-sexual interaction of young tourists. In (S. Clift & S.J. Page, Eds.), *Health and the International Tourist* (pp. 152-178), London, UK: Routledge.

Giddens, A. (1991). *Modernity and Self-identity*, Cambridge, UK: Polity Press.

Giddens, A. (1992). *The Transformation of Intimacy, Sexuality, Love & Eroticism in Modern Societies*. Cambridge, UK: Polity Press.

Goffman, E. (1967). *Interaction Ritual*, London, UK: Penguin.

Herold, E.S., Maticka-Tyndale, E., & D. Mewhinney (1998). Predicting Intentions to Engage in Casual Sex, *Journal of Social and Personal Relationships*, 15(1), 502-510.

Josiam, B.M., Hobson, J.S.P., Dietrich, U.C., & B. Smeaton (1998). An Analysis of the Sexual, Alcohol, and Drug Related Behavioral Patterns of Students on Spring Break. *Tourism Management*, 19, 501-513.

Krippendorf, J. (1987). *The Holiday Makers: Understanding the Impact of Leisure and Travel*, Oxford, UK: Butterworth-Heinemann.

Lett, J. (1983). Ludic and Liminoid Aspects of Charter Yacht Tourism in the Caribbean, *Annals of Tourism Research*, 10(1), 35-56.

Lewontin, R. (1995). Sex, Lies and Social Science, *The New York Review*, (April 20, 1995), pp. 24-29.

MacCannell, D. (1976). *The Tourist: A New Theory of the Leisure Class*, Basingstoke, UK: MacMillan.

Maticka-Tyndale, E. & S. Herold (1997). The Scripting of Sexual Behavior: Canadian University Students on Spring Break in Florida. *The Canadian Journal of Human Sexuality*, 6(4), 317-328.

Maticka-Tyndale, E. & S. Herold (1999). Predicting Condom Use on Spring-break Vacation: The Influence of Intentions, Prior use, and Context. *Journal of Applied Social Psychology*, 29, 1011-1027.

Maticka-Tyndale, E., Herold, S., & M. Mewhinney (1998). Casual Sex on Spring Break: Intentions and Behaviors of Canadian students. *The Journal of Sex Research*, 35, 254-264.

Maticka-Tyndale, E., Herold, S., & M. Opperman (2003). Casual Sex among Australian Schoolies. *The Journal of Sex Research*, 40(2), 158-169.

Meikle, J. (2002). HIV Infections Head for Record Rise. *The Guardian*, London, (November 30, 2002) pp. 2.

Mewhinney, D., Herold, E.S., & E. Maticka-Tyndale (1995). Sexual scripts and risk-taking of Canadian university students on spring break in Daytona Beach, Florida, *The Canadian Journal of Human Sexuality*, 4(4), 273-288.

Oppermann, M. (1998) (Ed.). *Sex Tourism and Prostitution: Aspects of Leisure, Recreation and Work,* New York, NY: Cognizant Communication Corporation.

Pizam, A., Reichel, A., & Uriely, N. (2002). Sensation Seeking and Tourist Behavior. *Journal of Hospitality and Leisure Marketing,* 9(2), 17-33.

Pizam, A. (2002). The Relationship between Risk-taking, Sensation Seeking and the Tourist Behavior of Young Adults: A Cross–cultural Study. In *Reinventing A Tourism Destination Abstracts, International Tourism Research Conference.* Dubrovnik, Croatia (October, 2002), pp. 113.

Richards, G. & Wilson, J. (2003). (eds.), *Today's Youth Travellers: Tomorrow's Global Nomads*, International Student Travel Confederation (ISTC), Netherlands.

Ryan, C. (1997). Memories of the Beach. In C. Ryan (Ed.), *The Tourist Experience: A New Introduction* (pp. 155-170). London, UK: Cassell.

Ryan, C. & Kinder, R. (1996). Sex, Tourism and Sex Tourism: Fulfilling Similar Needs? *Tourism Management,* 17(1), 507-518.

Ryan, C. & Robertson, E. (1997). New Zealand student-tourists: Risk behavior and health. In (S. Clift & P. Grabowski, Eds.), *Tourism and Health: Risks, Research and Responses* (pp. 119-138), London, UK: Pinter.

Ryan, C. & Hall, M. (2001). *Sex Tourism, Marginal People and Liminalities,* London, UK: Routledge

Ryan, C. & Martin, A. (2001). Tourist and strippers: Liminal theatre. *Annals of Tourism Research,* 28 (1), 140-163.

Shields, R. (1992). *Places on the Margin: Alternative Geographies of Modernity.* London, UK: Routledge.

Smith, A.M.A. & Rosenthal, D. (1997). Sex, alcohol and drags? Young People's experience of schoolies week. *Australian and New Zealand Journal of Public Health,* 21(1), 175-180.

Sönmez, S., Apostolopoulos, Y., Yu, C.H., Yang, S., Mattila, A.S. & L.C. Yu (2006). Binge drinking and casual sex on spring break. *Annals of Tourism Research,* 33(4), 895-917.

Turner, V. (1973). The centre out there: Pilgrim's goal, *History of Religions,* 12, 191-230.

Urry, J. (1991). *The Tourist Gaze: Leisure and Travel in Contemporary Societies,* London, UK: Sage.

Vorakitphokatorn, S., Pulerwitz, J., & Cash, R.A. (1998). HIV/AIDS risk to women travelers in Thailand: Comparison of Japanese and western populations, *International Quarterly of Community Health Education,* 18, 69-87.

Wagner, U. (1977). Out of Time and Place: Mass Tourism and Charter Trips, *Ethnos,* 42(1), 38-52.

Wickens, E. (1994). Consumption of the Authentic: The Hedonistic Tourist in Greece. In (A. Seaton, C. Jenkins, R. Wood, P. Dieke, M. Bennett, L. MacLellan, & R. Smith, Eds.), *Tourism: The State of the Art*, (pp. 818-825). London, UK: John Wiley

Wickens, E. (1997). Licensed for Thrills: Risk-taking and Tourism. In S. Clift & P. Grabowski, (Eds.), *Tourism and Health: Risks, Research and Responses* (pp. 151-164). London, UK: Pinter.

Wickens, E. (2002). The Sacred and the Profane: A Tourist Typology. *Annals of Tourism Research*, 29 (1), 834-851.

WTO (2003). *Youth outbound travel from three major European generating markets*, News Release. Madrid: World Tourism Organization. www.world-tourism.org/ newsroom/Releases/ 2003/feb/youth_study.htm-6k (accessed 2/18/2005).

# Chapter 12

## In Search of the Exotic: Sex Tourism and Disease Risks

SEVIL SÖNMEZ, PH.D., EUGENIA WICKENS, PH.D., AND YORGHOS APOSTOLOPOULOS, PH.D.

*"Being mobile in and of itself is not a risk factor for HIV infection. It is the situations encountered and the behaviors possibly engaged in during mobility or migration that increase vulnerability and risk regarding HIV/AIDS"*

(UNAIDS 2001)

## Introduction

Although the link between human mobility and infectious disease spread is well established (Wilson, 1995), scholarly interest in the possible correlation between tourism and HIV/AIDS dissemination is fairly recent (Apostolopoulos & Sönmez, 2001a, 2001b, 2002; Apostolopoulos, Sönmez, & Yu 2002; Clift & Grabowski, 1997; Mulhall, 1996; Sönmez, Apostolopoulos, Yu, Yang, Matilla, & Yu, 2006; Wright, 2003). Sexual interactions that carry STI/HIV risks occur between travellers and locals or other travellers; however, "sex tourism" in particular is an important vector for STI/HIV transmission and has potentially explosive ramifications for public health (Wright, 2003). Sex tourism is specifically motivated by persons interested in finding sexual adventure at destinations where the social norms and restrictions of their home environments are suspended. By virtue of their behavioral interactions with sex workers (a "core group" of efficient transmitters of STIs/HIV) and sex partners back in their home environments, sex tourists have a high risk of both acquiring and transmitting STIs/HIV. Consequently, sex tourists themselves become an STI/HIV core group, along with sex workers, seafarers, and truckers—a concept based on the observation that an infection is endemic among a small sub-population of highly sexually active individuals, from whom it spreads in mini-epidemics to the population at large (Mulhall, 1996). The combination of sex tourists' financial resources, the inherently risky nature of their behaviors, and acute poverty at sex tourism destinations is alarming—particularly when viewed in light of the increasing globalization of both sectors of tourism and sex. This chapter will examine sex tourism in terms of social and economic factors that fuel the activity, discuss types of locations around the world where sex tourism flourishes, and provide case studies of sex tourism destinations where STIs/HIV have become problematic.

## Globalization of Tourism and Sex

The public health impacts of travelers' sexual risk taking need to be examined within the context of global tourism's expanding scope. The phenomenal growth of post-WWII tourism is demonstrated by increases of travelers from about 25 million in the 1950s to over 800 million in 2005—predicted to reach 1 billion by 2010 and 1.6 billion by 2020 (WTO, 2006). Revenues from international tourism have paralleled this extraordinary growth with global earnings of over US$2 billion per day in 2005 (WTO, 2006). Tourism is a major source of employment throughout the world and provides jobs directly or indirectly to over 260 million persons (or 1 out of every 9 jobs in the world), which is expected to increase by over 100 million jobs by 2010 with 70% just in the Asia-Pacific region. As the largest sector of business in the world, tourism is inextricably linked to increasing globalization and is viewed as *the* solution by countries anxious to market their resources in return for foreign currency. It is not coincidental that in economically troubled countries, the growth of the sex trade mirrors that of the tourism sector due to demand created by tourist influxes.

The globalization of sex tourism—as a growing segment of the tourism sector and a significant form of economic activity—has been linked to two parallel forces: the increase in migration and tourism and the increase in consumption (Wonders & Michalowski, 2001). While regular (legal) or irregular (illegal) migration involves the movement of people over borders from less to more developed or stable countries in search for work opportunities that often leave them vulnerable to exploitation (e.g., survival sex), tourism involves pretty much the opposite with more affluent people traveling from industrialized countries to less developed countries in search for exotic pleasures. As a result, increases in tourism and migration create more opportunities for sex work by increasing potential sex workers as well as consumers—creating both mobile sex workers and mobile sex consumers. The second force (of consumption) represents the continual development of new commodities or services. Therefore, it is argued that sex tourism both fosters and is fostered by the global commodification of desire and bodies (Wonders & Michalowski, 2001).

The globalization of sexual exploitation due to the growing profitability of the international sex trade is very much linked to the tourism sector. It is difficult to estimate annual earnings of the global sex industry, but trafficking (its illegal dimension) alone are believed to generate thousands of billions of dollars (Leidholdt, 2005). Prostitution has become industrialized and internationalized as big businesses have moved into various sectors of the sex trade and have entered the tourism sector via legalized brothel prostitution. This industrialization and internationalization have been linked to the growth of "prostitution tourism"[1] and increased demand by large numbers of travelers. The sale of sex is highly profitable not only for individuals and networks but also for governments that depend on sex tourism revenues. Profits from sex tourism in countries where significant portions of the population live below the poverty line have even led to government promotion of the activity, such as in Thailand and the Philippines. In both countries, where significant portions of the population are crippled by poverty and unemployment, monies earned from sex tourism are highly desirable and sometimes one of the few ways to survive. Thailand's billion-dollar tourism sector has been referred to as the "Thai economic miracle" and the linchpin of the country's economy at the same time sex was considered to be the linchpin of the tourist industry (*Economy*, 1997).

## *Femmigration,* Trafficking, and Prostitution

The interlinked problems of *femmigration* (increasing migration of women), trafficking, and prostitution contribute to the growth of sex tourism. The destabilization of economies since the 1980s has left fewer economic alternatives to large numbers of women, often already vulnerable due to their subordinate positions in society and the labor market. Development policies and political restructuring of the 1990s and in some cases, wars and state violence have further dislocated local economies and forced more women to migrate in search of jobs. A plethora of cases from various nations corroborate that women's economic position is first to be undermined in unregulated/illicit markets, especially when power and control are increasingly concentrated in male hands (Hughes, 2003). Over 70% of the world's poor are women with fewer economic options, who are far more vulnerable to coercive or forced sex or engaging in survival or transactional sex (GHC, 2005). *Femmigration* has also become a driving force behind sexual multipartnering and networking for women in transit and destination countries. As such, migrant settings oftentimes operate as sexual marketplaces rendering women vulnerable to exploitation and abuse, including trafficking for sexual exploitation (Van Liemt, 2004). Given that traffickers target regions and social groups where patriarchy is strongest and where women can be more easily manipulated (UN, 2004), gender inequality underpins and sustains trafficking—especially

---

[1] Preferred term by some to "sex tourism" as it stresses the seriousness of the exploitation and abuse of women and children and sets it apart from tourism that involves sexual activity by consenting adults (Jeffreys, 2002). In this paper, they are used interchangeably.

since supply (victims) and demand (sexual exploiters) of trafficking are firmly located within many countries (IOM, 2002). Under the cover of migration (whether regular or irregular), "human trafficking activities are rapidly becoming one of the most widespread forms of human rights abuses, affecting an ever wider range of countries of both origin and destination involving increasing numbers of women, adolescents, and children" (Erder & Kaska, 2003, p. 9).

Trafficking in women and children into the sex industry has evolved into a highly lucrative industry as well as a global problem (Hynes & Raymond, 2002). According to the U.S. Department of State (2005), nearly all countries around the world are one of source, transit, or destination for trafficking. Source countries have severe problems with poverty, either due to their level of development or economic collapse (e.g., Afghanistan, Albania, Angola, Bangladesh, Belarus, Cuba, Ethiopia, Jamaica, Moldova, North Korea, Russia, Rwanda, Sri Lanka, Sudan, Ukraine). Typically, destination countries are industrialized or have strong economies for other reasons, such as oil resources (e.g., Australia, Belgium, Canada, Denmark, France, Israel, Japan, Kuwait, Malaysia, New Zealand, Norway, Singapore, Sweden, Switzerland, Taiwan, U.A.E., U.K.). Transit countries often provide geographic convenience as persons are moved from one place to the other and often serve as temporary destinations as well, where trafficked persons are sold before moving to their final destinations (e.g., Greece, Germany, Hong Kong, Italy, Libya, Netherlands, Spain, Turkey). Some countries (e.g., Cambodia, Costa Rica, Dominican Republic, Haiti, Hungary, India, Kenya, Mexico, Philippines, South Korea, South Africa, Thailand, Venezuela, Vietnam) serve as source, destination, and transit countries when internal trafficking is involved.

Most nations have commercial sex industries into which trafficked women and children are integrated. Not surprisingly, foreign women are the lowest and most vulnerable within the hierarchy of sex work.[2] Their illegal status, social and cultural isolation, poverty, inability to speak the local language, and lack of familiarity with local customs and laws force them to work in a state of debt bondage, and in the worst, most unsanitary conditions, often without condoms while leaving them vulnerable to rapes, torture, and even murder. Most women in sex work do not work in their own towns or villages but instead move from rural areas to larger towns or cities or are moved either regionally or outside their own nations. For example, an estimated 20,000-30,000 Burmese women work in Thailand's sex sector (nearly all of who are illegal immigrants and 50% are HIV-positive); over 100,000 Nepalese

---

[2] While sex workers in developed countries have more power to insist on condom use, there is evidence of migrant sex workers with uncertain or illegal immigrant status being used in brothels to cater to clients that refuse to wear condoms (Pettman, 1997).

women work in India's sex industry with an additional 5,000 trafficked into the country annually; over the past decade an estimated 200,000 Bangladeshi women have been trafficked into Pakistan and thousands more into India while demand for Nepali women with fair skin and Mongolian features has increased; from the 80% of Asian female migrant workers who entered Japan in the 1990s as "entertainers" most were from the Philippines and Thailand; and Thai women work as sex workers throughout Asia and Australia, Europe, and the U.S. (Jeffreys, 1999).

## Sex: The "Dark Side" of Tourism

Tourism's dark side emerges when travel-related activities exploit vulnerable individuals and enter the realm of prostitution tourism. Too many people travel halfway around the world to pursue sexual experiences ranging from pedophilia to multiple anonymous sexual encounters with teens, women, and men or for unlimited access to Asian, Black, Latin women, men, and children. The sale of women and children in order to fulfill the desires of tourists fits into this model as they become a part of a country's tourist attractions.

### Who is the Sex Tourist?

Despite the establishment of the existence of both male and female sex tourists and serious disagreements among researchers about terms, definitions, and differences between them (e.g., De Albuquerque, 1998a, 1998b; Dahles & Bras, 1999; Jeffreys, 2003; Kempadoo, 1999a, 1999b, 2001; Opperman, 1998, 1999; Pruitt & Lafont, 1995; Sánchez Taylor, 2001; Wickens, 2002), men are more often linked than women to prostitution tourism. Male sex tourists are typically white men from affluent Western[3] or Asian countries ranging in age from their 20s to their 70s. Particularly men from Western countries who seek out women in Third World destinations are often described by researchers as believing that their masculinity and racialized power are affirmed away from home where women and girls are at their command and where Blacks, Latinas, and Asians serve them (O'Connell-Davidson, 2001). Online exchanges that male sex tourists engage in on websites dedicated to sex tourism illustrate exploitative views and behaviors. The World Sex Archives (http://www.worldsexarchives.com) describes its mission as "providing information about adult travel, prostitution, sex tourism" and posts messages

---

[3] Americans make up 25% of the world's sex tourists (about 3-5 million annually), 80% of sex tourists who travel to Costa Rica, and 38% of those who travel to Cambodia (ECPAT, 1996b).

and photos offered by its members (referred to as "fellow hobbyists") to share experiences or ask questions:

". . .will choose Madagascar because you have a nice mixture of Asian and Malgache girls at a very low price and less mosquitoes. . ."

"I joined a black dating website called afrointroductions.com. . .I hope to arrange some beautiful young women there. . .I know they want a meal ticket to the west but I can always string them along. . .this type of pussy is free not that I mind paying the going rate which I understand is $10-$15 a night."

". . .I'm constantly looking for women from Eastern Europe (18+ and free wheeling), both pro and non-pros, offering full sex WITHOUT A CONDOM. . ."

Another site, World Sex Guide (http://www.worldsexguide.org) offers advice about sex tourism destinations such as Thailand, Vietnam, Cuba, which clubs to go to and which to avoid, the best seasons to travel there, as well as advice on etiquette when dealing with sexworkers and other locals:

". . .you can get a 'dancing girl' for the equivalent of US$5 an hour. . ." (for Vietnam).

". . .they are, almost without exception, young, not terribly pretty, and fresh from the countryside. . .if your libido overcomes your empathy, select one (or more) and take them to your room. . .she'll probably do whatever you want. . ." (for Thailand)

". . .the girl. . .might become your girlfriend for 24 hours a day. . .you may not have to pay her any money, but you will have to feed her. . ." (for Cuba)

These casual exchanges between sex tourists are not only an indication of the extreme degradation that women are subjected to as sexual objects, but worse, it hints at the growing demand for consumption of sex tourism experiences as cheaply as possible—which then fuels the problem of human trafficking for sexual exploitation, which in turn carries risks for STI/HIV dissemination on a global scale.

## Hot Spots for Sex Tourism

Nearly all countries have a tourism sector and some form of prostitution, but some with serious economic problems have evolved into sex tourism destinations by providing travelers easy access to women and children in exchange for a boost to their earnings through prostitution. These destinations have developed into havens for sex tourists who can easily and cheaply find women, children, and other men for sex partners. Such locations are simultaneously targeted by internal or crossborder migrants in search of work, who often practice survival sex and by traffickers as source, transit, and destination countries. Ongoing human mobility and sexual mixing of individuals from areas of varying STI/HIV prevalences in the context of sex tourism may represent an overlooked at worst or underestimated at best epidemiologic phenomenon that could easily accelerate the global spread of STIs/HIV (Mulhall, 1996).

Southeast Asia

In the late 1990s, an International Labor Organization (ILO) report (Kaban, 1998) described Southeast Asia's (Indonesia, Malaysia, the Philippines, and Thailand) commercial sex sector as having become integrated into its economic, social, and political life. In the report, the ILO stated that the "economic and social forces driving the sex industry show no signs of slowing down, particularly in light of rising unemployment in the region." The sex industry of these four countries involves between .25% and 1.5% of the total female population and several million as pimps, managers, and owners of sex businesses in addition to sex workers while the industry accounts for 2-14% of the GDP. Government authorities benefit legally (licensing fees, hospitality industry taxes, gaming) and illegally (bribes). The growth of Southeast Asia's sex industry is attributed partly to the recent surge in migrant women who equal or outnumber migrant men. Overall, 20% of women engaged in sex work are enslaved, trafficked, or kept in prison in these countries (Kaban, 1998), therefore, the rapid, extensive, and uncontrolled spread of HIV in a number of countries in the region should come as no surprise—for example, Cambodia, India, Myanmar, Vietnam, and Malaysia continue to experience rapidly growing HIV epidemics.

*The Philippines*

A significant economic contributor to tourism earnings, sex tourism started around American military bases by providing sex to military personnel[4] (Jeffreys, 1999). Although military bases were abandoned in 1991, a new treaty was negotiated to permit American troops to return and have privileged access to 22 areas for "rest and relaxation" and potentially prostitution (Jeffreys, 1999). For example, Clark Air Force Base is the hub of Angeles City where prostitution is the only activity due to the absence of beach or tourist attractions and the presence of 152 nightclubs and many bars and hotels. Teen aged prostitutes are sold for as little as 0.50 cents to US$2.50 but there are also reports of people prostituting themselves in exchange for food or water (CATW, 2005). Although the country is experiencing a slower growth

---

[4] Engaging in prostitution is a violation of the U.S. Military Code of Conduct that is often ignored by many. In fact, the U.S. military has a "shameful history in Southeast Asia of fueling the growth of sex industries around military bases or at sites of R&R (rest and relaxation)" (Hughes, 2003, p. 4). In 2002, U.S. military police were filmed by a television reporter patrolling bars and brothels where trafficked women worked (Merriman, 2002 cited in Hughes, 2003). There are also documented cases of women from the Philippines, the Russian Federation, Bolivia, Peru, Mongolia, China, Bangladesh, Kyrgyzstan, and Uzbekistan being trafficked into bars and clubs around U.S. bases in South Korea (Lhagvasuren, 2001).

of its HIV epidemic compared with other countries in the regions[5] the Philippines continues to be a popular destination for sex tourists and one especially favored by pedophile sex tourists from the U.K., U.S., and Australia—in fact, it is known to be fourth among nine nations with the most children in prostitution.

*Thailand*

Although prostitution increased in Thailand when the country was opened to foreign laborers from China in the 1850s (Leheny, 1995), it grew into a major industry with help from the U.S. military and the World Bank. The U.S. Department of Defense entered into a contractual agreement with the Thai government during the Vietnam War to provide U.S. soldiers with "recreation and relaxation" (as in the Philippines) (Rogers, 1999). Prostitution became organized and expanded into a vibrant industry in Thailand and by the end of the Vietnam War the country had a reputation for a diverse and expanded sex market that attracted foreign tourists. The 1975 World Bank economic plan for Thailand further helped to develop the country's sex tourism sector, which grew into its leading export (Rogers, 1999) until prostitution yielded an annual income of US$22.5-$27 billion between 1993 and 1995 (Agnote, 1998). In the process, Thailand developed a reputation as the world's sex capital (Leheny, 1995) with sex slavery and child prostitution as its two main attractions (Hughes, 1996). There is also widespread male prostitution, also used by foreigners, which is numerically nearly as extensive as female prostitution. Another noteworthy pattern is that in addition to Thai women and those coming from Burma, China, and Laos, European women also work in brothels. Russian, Czech, and Romanian women trying to escape their own countries' harsh economic conditions and who are recruited by job placement agencies often wind up in Thai brothels servicing customers who think Europeans are less likely to be HIV infected. Sadly, the majority of brothel workers and women who work in the streets or by the railroad tracks earn shockingly little money while facing great disease risks. Although three quarters of a million people are estimated to be HIV-positive, Thailand's multi-sectoral prevention efforts have begun to take effect and are discussed later in the chapter.

*Cambodia*

Partially due to the publicized HIV/AIDS prevalence in Thailand, Cambodia has become an emerging travel destination for sex tourists and, in fact, has been placed on the map as "the new haunt of globe-trotting pedophiles" (Marks, 2003). The country's flourishing sex industry can be traced back to the early

---

[5] National behavioral studies conducted in the Philippines in the early 1990s attributed the slower growth of its HIV epidemic to lower numbers of clients and what is considered the indirect nature of sexwork.

1990s when tens of thousands of U.N. peacekeepers arrived for operation UNTAC (U.N. Transitional Authority in Cambodia) to end a long-running civil war (Richburg, 1998). By the mid-1990s, one quarter of the country's nearly half million annual visitors were sex tourists and shanty towns in Phnom Penh had become filled with Western men seeking children as young as four for sex (Bobak, 1996). The country's rampant corruption and extreme poverty have worked together to create a sex trade controlled by senior police and military officials[6] and even with the involvement of some cabinet ministers. The country's poverty has caused parents to sell their children into prostitution by exchanging them directly to brothel owners for a couple of hundred dollars. It has been reported that some children get paid US$2 for intercourse and have sex with an average of seven to eight men nightly (Bobak, 1996; Seper, 1998). Cambodia's HIV epidemic, which began in the late 1980s or early 1990s, is rooted in heterosexual multipartnering and shows no signs of slowing down.

*India*

Relaxed laws, abundant child prostitutes, and the false idea that one can not get infected with HIV by children has transformed India into an attractive sex tourist destination (Bedi, 1997). Men who believe that STIs and AIDS can be cured by having sex with a virgin are creating demand for increasingly younger girls (McGirk, 1997). The country has become the favored destination, particularly of pedophiles from Europe and the U.S. In Bombay's Falkland Road, tens of thousands of young women and children trafficked from Nepal and Bangladesh, known as "cage-prostitutes" are displayed for selection in zoo-like animal cages (CATW, 2005; Friedman, 1996). Eunuch Lane in Bombay has over 2,000 eunuchs in sex work—who are young boys abandoned or sold by their families to a sex ring and who have their genitals cut in a ceremony called *nirvana*. These child eunuchs are used more frequently than female sex workers in high-risk sex because many men believe they can not transmit HIV (Friedman, 1996). Many parts of India show evidence of uncontrolled and extensive spread of HIV, attributed to low condom use and high rates of STIs.

*Latin America and the Caribbean*

Latin American and Caribbean destinations are often associated with both "romance tourism" (involving men—often referred to as "beach boy," "beach bum," "gigolo," "hustler," "rent-a-dread," or "sanky panky"—as providers of sex to female tourists) and sex tourism (involving female sexworkers and male tourists) (Kempadoo, 2001). Since the 1960s, countries such as Barbados, Cuba, Jamaica, and the Dominican Republic, and more recently, Argentina and Brazil, have been receiving significant flows of sex tourists (Borland, Faas, Marshall, McLean, Schroen, Smit, & Valerio, 2004). This is partially due to

---

[6] A lieutenant in the Royal Cambodian Armed Forces became a brothel owner to supplement his salary (Bobak, 1996).

severe poverty at these countries that force locals to enter sex work in order to support themselves, partially due to demand shifts from Thailand, Sri Lanka, and other Asian countries, and partially to Western fantasies of Caribbean and Latin American women that can be traced back to colonial times when Black and Mulatto women were objectified as sexualized, racialized exotic "others" (O'Connell-Davidson, 1996). In fact, concern was expressed as far back as the 1960s specifically about the Caribbean becoming "the brothel of Europe" due to the neocolonial relationship established through the global tourism industry and the power and control exerted over Black women by European men (de Albuquerque, 1998; Kempadoo, 2001; Pruitt & LaFont, 1995; O'Connell-Davidson 1996). In recent years, Argentina, Brazil, Chile, Honduras, and Paraguay have become popular destinations for child sex tourists from Australia, Europe, and the U.S. as well as American and Australian human traffickers (Contreras, 2001). Although the spread of HIV/AIDS has been slower in the region than in others, the pandemic is considered to be well-established. In fact, rates of AIDS incidence in some countries (e.g., Haiti, Brazil) in the region are among the highest in the world. The current epidemiological profile of HIV/AIDS in the region is driven by high-risk situations favorable to the rapid spread of HIV infection. The growing sex tourism industry is identified as being among the sociocultural dynamics fueling the epidemic, along with sexual multipartnering, early initiation of sexual activity, and the involvement of young girls in sex work (CARICOM, 2005). Furthermore, the pandemic is believed to be dominating those countries facing the greatest socioeconomic hardships and where commercial sex ranges from informal networks to thriving and organized sex tourism businesses (World Bank, 2000). Nearly 2 million people were estimated to be living with HIV/AIDS in the region in 2002, including 1.5 million in Latin America and 440,000 in the Caribbean (Sullivan, 2003). Between 600 and 700 people are estimated to get infected with HIV in Latin America and the Caribbean each day—about one person every two minutes (UNAIDS, 2004).

*Cuba*

Flows of foreign travelers have been significantly affected over the years by U.S.-Cuba tensions. President Kennedy's 1963 Trading with the Enemy Act, which prohibited U.S. citizens and businesses from engaging in business with or visiting Cuba was further reinforced by the U.S. embargo in the 1970s. In the 1980s, following Cuba's new development plans that included tourism, steady increases were seen in visitors from Canada, Western Europe, Latin America, and the U.S. (Miller & Henthorne, 1997; Triana, 1995; Zúñiga, 2001). Despite tourism earnings, the Cuban economy crashed in the early 1990s leaving Cubans with an average monthly income of only about US$10. With the U.S. dollar as the only valued currency and the tourism sector as the primary source of money, tourists became the most accessible source of hard currency for Cubans. Visitors' offers of clothing and perfume in return for sex were followed by offers of cash. The loss of Soviet subsidies in the 1990s and growing economic desperation forced Cubans to agree to do virtually any-thing in return for a few dollars. Locals were exposed to luxuries afforded by tourists as jobs began to decline—and declining incomes and increasing material desires pushed many natives into prostitution (Faria, 2004). By the late-1990s, a sex worker in Havana could earn US$40 for a night of sex—which represented two months' salary for a Cuban university professor. *Jineteras (jockeys)* or professional prostitutes begin negotiations by requesting US$10 for oral sex or quick intercourse, but can agree to accept as little as US$2-4. On the other hand, inexperienced women and girls often get per-suaded into spending an entire night with a client in return for a meal, a few drinks, cooking oil, children's clothes, or even a bar of soap (O'Connell-Davidson, 1996). Some also earn money by procuring younger girls for Canadian and German tourists. One type of sex tourist to Cuba has been described as "macho men"—mostly Italians, Spaniards, Canadians, and Americans who pay about US$20-$40 plus meals for 12 to 24 hours of access and go by the motto: *"find them, feed them, fuck them, forget them"* (O'Connell-Davidson, 1996). Despite these worrisome behavioral patterns, until recently Cuba has maintained the lowest HIV prevalence rate in the Caribbean, largely due to the highly controversial AIDS program implemented in the early stages of the epidemic that required all HIV-positive individuals to be quarantined in government-run sanitariums (UNAIDS, 2004). Although this policy was even-tually abandoned, universal free access to antiretroviral therapy has kept the number of AIDS cases and deaths very low. It may be overly optimistic to believe, however, that low HIV prevalence rates will persist if the locals con-tinue to practice survival sex with sex tourists from around the world. In fact, Cuba's HIV epidemic is growing and an annual five-fold increase has been noted in newly reported HIV cases between 1995 and 2000 (UNAIDS, 2004).

*The Dominican Republic*

Years of colonialism, U.S. occupation, Trujillo's 32-year dictatorship, and international debt have weakened the economy. Too many Dominicans were living in poverty and one in five pre-school children was affected by chronic malnutrition. Beginning in the early 1980s, a debt crisis and negotiations with IMF and the World Bank led to efforts to stimulate tourism activity. By 1984, tourism replaced sugar as the country's leading export and turned the Dominican Republic into the fifth largest tourism earner in the Caribbean. Unfortunately, in addition to tourists looking for a tropical, romantic getaway, the destination drew increasing numbers of sex tourists. At Boca Chica, Puerto Plata, and Sosúa—main sex tourist sites—many businesses are owned and managed by North American and European sex tourists-turned-expatriates (referred to as *sexpatriates*) who have retired to permanently settle on the island and who are engaged in promoting sex tourism and organizing tourist-related prostitution to others interested in similar experiences (O'Connell-Davidson, 2001). Strong links have been established with U.S.-based travel clubs and the Internet is heavily used to market the Dominican Republic as a sex tourism destination. Many Dominican women migrate to the aforementioned towns in search of work and resources as well as hope of finding a boyfriend or husband to take them off the island to North America or Europe (Brennan, 2001)—but often find themselves servicing sex tourists instead. Despite prevention efforts aimed at encouraging safer sex practices, the Dominican Republic is faced with a serious HIV epidemic (UNAIDS, 2004). In fact, by sharing the island of Hispaniola with Haiti—which has 87% of all AIDS cases in the Caribbean—the Dominican Republic is at the epidemic's epicenter. Although Haiti represents only 24% of the Caribbean population, it has 61% of the region's AIDS cases, which has infected 5% of its population. In the Dominican Republic, over 140,000 people live with HIV/AIDS, which is about 46% among sex workers and 2% in the general population (Bryan, 2005).

Sex Tourism Destinations in the West

Increasing demand for sex tourism adds fuel to global human trafficking. The involvement of industrialized nations in global sex tourism is two-fold: they send the majority of tourists to destinations known for their sex industries and also have organized sex industries themselves. While Japanese men constitute the largest number of sex tourists originating in Asia, the majority of sex tourists originate in European and North American countries and Australia (Brennan, 2001). Sex tourism is also an attraction in industrialized countries in the form of upscale gentlemen's clubs, varied, specialized sexual services, and the availability of sex workers from all over the globe.

The Netherlands represents the main European destination for prostitution, where 30-40% (and in some cases 60%) of prostitutes are non-Europeans. Amsterdam's red light district with its sex clubs, sex shows, lingerie and S&M clothing stores, *condomories*, and porn shops, is described as the sex tourist's "mecca" (Wonders & Michalowski, 2001). Professional prostitutes are estimated at only 20,000-25,000 in the Netherlands; however, large numbers of non-professional sex workers representing at least 32 countries of origin as well as illegal immigrants and trafficked persons are likely to substantially increase this estimated number (Wonders & Michalowski, 2001). Although Amsterdam is known for its window brothels, other forms of sex work including private houses, clubs, escort services, and street prostitution also thrive. By deliberately attracting wealthy sex tourists and discouraging those interested in cheap labor Amsterdam's sex tourism sector differs very much—at least economically—from that of less developed destinations (Wonders & Michalowski, 2001).

## Child Sex Tourism

Child sex tourism—a multi-billion dollar industry—is defined as "tourism organized with the primary purpose of facilitating a commercial-sexual relationship with a child" (USDOJ, 1999, p. 32). The typical sex tourist who is a pedophile is a white, Western, heterosexual male in his 50s, 60s, and older. While there are also Black and Asian (primarily from Japan, Korea, and Taiwan tourists) who seek out children, the majority are from Western nations (e.g., Australia, Belgium, France, Germany, Italy, Spain, U.K., U.S.) (Contreras, 2001). They are often motivated by freedom from social constraints in environments where they enjoy anonymity and the absence of social taboos, by their views of Third World children as inferior, and by their misperceptions that children offer less risk for infectious diseases (Flowers, 2001). Child sex tourism destinations are expanding as poverty spreads[7] and while the activity was initially primarily located in Cambodia and Vietnam, it has expanded to include Indonesia, Taiwan, Thailand, the Philippines, Sri Lanka, South Korea, as well as various Central, Latin American (e.g., Argentina, Brazil, Costa Rica), and Eastern European countries.

Children are either lured away from poor homes with promises of employment or kidnapped and forced into sex work or are sold directly by their parents. In Thailand, the increase in the sale of children by their families to brothels has been correlated to the increase in consumerism fueled by the arrival of electricity and television in rural areas and the lure of cash paid for children. In Latin America, an estimated 40 million children work and live in the streets, often entering the street as early as the age of nine and many often engage in survival sex with adults for food, clothing, and shelter (Stillwaggon, 2000). The worldwide number of children prostituted is estimated to be as high as 100 million (Gorden, 1991) with one million children entering the sex trade annually.[8] It is not surprising that there are conflicting reports on the number of children being prostituted around the world and in addition to developing countries, there are reports of 200,000 children in sex work in Canada and 2.4 million (including teenage sex workers) in the U.S. (ECPAT, 1996a, 1996b; Namen, 1994, cited in Joseph, 1995, p. 8). Sexually abused children are permanently physically and emotionally scarred by their harsh experiences—that is, if they survive the beatings, rapes, and torture. They often become drug dependent and contract various STIs/HIV; in fact, the average rate for HIV infected children rescued from sex work ranges between 50% and 90% (ECPAT, 1996a, 1996b). The solution to the tragic problem of child sex tourism is very difficult and involves the prosecution of not only those who sell children to tourists but sex tourists themselves who create the demand for prostituted children.

---

[7] Children (between 3 and 17 years) are sold to sex tourists for literally pennies ($1-$5 for oral sex) (Bosch, 2004; Marks, 2003).

[8] It is important to note that children are not prostituted only to tourists. In some countries (e.g., Philippines), it is believed that sex with children restore virility while in others (e.g., Zambia), it is believed that children are free from disease and therefore safer sex partners (Joseph, 1995).

## Selling Sex Tourism

Specialized or "adventure" tours and inclusive packages[9] with airfare, hotel accommodations, and directions to local brothels and other sex establishments (Rodriguez-Garcia, 2001) are marketed in a manner that exploits sex tourists' desire to have guilt-free, casual sex in beautiful settings. For example, Thailand is depicted as the "pleasure center of the world" (Bishop & Robinson, 1998) where "indiscriminate love-making goes on in every hotel in the land. . . and the Thais consider love-making an indoor sport" and Thai women are described as "little slaves who give real Thai warmth" (Truong 1990, p. 178-179). In some cases, marketing literature points out the socio-economic conditions that push young women into sex work in order to help support her family, implicitly encouraging sex tourists to see themselves as benefactors helping them to earn a living (Bishop & Robinson, 1998). One Dutch brochure even notes that it is as easy to get a girl as it is to buy a package of cigarettes (Truong, 1990).

More recently, the Internet has fueled sex tourism through the development of numerous sites that inform sex tourists of destinations with potential to fulfill a multitude of desires and sexual proclivities as well as "how-to" guides that not only guide sex tourists to their desires but ironically, help them to avoid being exploited in the process (Bishop & Robinson, 1998). Examples are provided in Table 12.1 below:

# Health Costs of Sex Tourism

## Global STI/HIV/AIDS Rates

From an estimated 10,000 cases in 1980, HIV reached pandemic proportions by 2004, having infected 39.4 million and killed 3.1 million adults and children just in that year. It is predicted that an additional 45 million people will become infected with HIV by 2010—mainly concentrated in low- and middle-income countries (UNAIDS, 2004). It is estimated that by 2010, AIDS deaths will rival the 93 million caused by the bubonic plague (GHC, 2005).

The epidemic has become a major developmental issue affecting every country worldwide, with problematic concentrations in Sub-Saharan Africa, the Far East, India, and more recently Latin America and the Caribbean. The Caribbean's epidemic, in particular, is the worst in the Western Hemisphere and second in magnitude only to that in Sub-Saharan Africa (CAREC, 2001;

---

[9] A Philippine Adventure Tour costs US$1,645 and includes round trip airfare, hotel accommodations, and guided tours to bars where men can purchase sex services for as little as US$24 and tourists are promised that they'll never sleep alone on their vacation and are encouraged to enjoy different and multiple sex workers daily (CATW, 2005).

TABLE 12.1. A small sample of Internet sites offering sex tours

- **The Hedonist**, the "sex travel bible for exotic sex vacations" with detailed reviews of "the hottest red light districts in Mexico, Costa Rica, Caribbean, Brazil..." as well as brothels and massage parlors where men will be "treated like a king for $25" (http://www.theprofessional-bachelor.com):
  - *Cebu City, Philippines: "stunning white beaches, Azure blue water, and 1000s of young nymphos. . . sweet little girls competing to fuck for $20"*
  - *Rio de Jeniero, Brazil: "unbelievable display of stunning nympho Latinas, dancing samba topless and pulling you into back rooms . . ."*
  - *Tijuana, Mexico: "in-house brothels packed with strippers and models turned whores...all available and will race upstairs to fuck in a flash."*
  - *The FKK Health Spas in Frankfurt, Germany: "over 100 girls from all corners of the world, any shape, color and size can be yours. . . who compete for a session"*
  - *Bangkok, Thailand: "every sexual fantasy available in minutes. . . 100,000 wild, seductive, insatiable teenagers. . . Thai girls are uninhibited, tiny sex machines who never say no. . . you drink in a bar stool watching porn while getting a $9 blow job!"*
  - *Ibiza, Spain: "a buffet of Latinas and 18 yr. old jungle sistas. . . a new rotation of girls every 2 weeks. . ."*
- **The World Sex Guide**, offers advice on different destinations such as Thailand, Vietnam, Cuba, which clubs to go to/which to avoid, best seasons to travel, advice on etiquette when dealing with sexworkers and locals (http://www.worldsexguide.org).
- **The World Sex Archives**, "an interactive discussion and archive database dedicated to providing information about adult travel prostitution sex tourism," offers links to archives by country, members post messages and photos, share their experiences or ask questions, and men (referred to as "fellow hobbyists") rate the women, their attitudes, and performance between 1 and 10 (http://www.worldsexarchives.com).
- **Women of the World**, "the #1 resource for adult travel *infotainment*," provides links to women from Brazil, Thailand, Philippines, China, and Cambodia for a monthly membership fee of US$19.97 along with downloadable itineraries to guide sex tourists to "the hottest women at all the bangin' hot spots" (http://join.4womenoftheworld.com).
- **Travel and the Single Male**, a U.S.-based travel club run by/for male sex tourists with 5,000 members, guidebook, newsletters, discounts on hotels/brothels, information on travel/prostitution in various countries, access to softcore pornographic photos of sexworkers (http://www.tsmtravel.com).
- **Age of Consent** informs travelers of the youngest age sex partners they can find in each country without getting into legal trouble (e.g., 12 in Argentina, Colombia, Chile, Mexico, Paraguay, 13 in South Korea, Nigeria, Spain) (http://www.ageofconsent.com).

CARICOM, 2002; World Bank, 2000b). With a regional HIV prevalence rate ranging from 1.4% to 4.1%, the Caribbean's HIV epidemic—predominantly fueled by heterosexual sex and concentrated among sex workers in most places—is heavily concentrated in countries and territories with tourism-dependent economies, including the Bahamas, Barbados, Bermuda, the Dominican Republic, Jamaica, and Trinidad and Tobago (UNAIDS, 2005). In Latin America, approximately 1.2 to 2.1 million adults and children were estimated to be living with HIV by 2003 (UNAIDS, 2005). Within the region, Brazil accounts for over one third of people living with HIV and is followed by concentrations of high numbers of HIV cases in urban centers of Argentina, Uruguay, and in the Andean sub-region (among sex workers), as well as urban areas of Central American countries. In South and Southeast Asia, between 4.1 and 9.6 million adults and children were believed to be living with HIV in 2003 along with approximately 430,000 to 2 million newly infected adults and children that year (UNAIDS, 2005). The region's epidemic is as diverse as its countries but remains largely concentrated among core groups such as sex workers, their clients and their sex partners, men who have sex with men, and injecting drug users. Although the epidemic first hit Thailand, Myanmar, and Cambodia, it has been expanding rapidly in Indonesia, Nepal, Vietnam, and India—particularly among sex workers (UNAIDS, 2005). In India, HIV/AIDS is largely concentrated in the highest-risk populations of sex workers, injecting drug users, and truck drivers, but is disseminating into the general population. In some states of India (e.g., Tamil Nadu), HIV prevalence among sex workers has reached 50% (UNAIDS, 2005). Condom use among Indonesia's brothel workers is somewhere around 4% and in some parts of the country, HIV prevalence among sex workers was estimated at 17% in 2003. Increasing injecting drug use among sex workers fuels the epidemic even more, in fact in Vietnam's Ho Chi Minh City, 38% of 1,000 sexworkers surveyed reported injecting drugs— 49% of who were HIV positive.

Developing countries are disproportionately affected by the HIV/AIDS pandemic, which has become increasingly more complicated. Experts indicate that the pandemic has become fragmented and splintered into multiple epidemics distinguishable by transmission modes, geographic focus, HIV sub-types, sociodemographic and behavioral characteristics of affected populations, rapidity of or potential for HIV spread, maturity stage, and declining HIV incidence in some locations (IAS, 2004). AIDS has become a pandemic quickly and with extensive consequences for humankind, which has been fueled by human population movement (Davis-Lewis & Bailey, 1992/1993). As a result, a central link emerges between AIDS and international travel and, particularly tourism.

## Tourism, Prostitution, and Disease

Although the contribution of human mobility to the spread of infectious disease has long been established—irregular migration, human trafficking, prostitution, and sex tourism are inextricably linked with the common thread of STIs/HIV/AIDS (CATW, 2005). In the case of HIV, it is difficult to measure the level of contribution that travel may have due to the infection's clinically latent period, which may span years and because it may be diagnosed some time after initial exposure (NATHNAC, 2005). Nevertheless, sexual encounters—common among both leisure and business travelers—have the potential to be a major cause of morbidity with the risk being greatest for young travelers and sex tourists (Rogstad, 2004). The subgroup of sex tourists requires particular attention as it creates a growing demand for sexual services from vulnerable populations. The nature and types of sex work involved in sex tourism vary across locations and present different risk levels to those involved (Wright, 2003). Street-walkers and brothel workers who have less control over their work environment than sex workers in more organized venues (e.g., Amsterdam's window-based sex workers) are not only at greater risk of acquiring HIV/AIDS but also of transmitting it to sex tourists who function as bridges of transmission—simply because the chain of disease dissemination from the sex sector to the general population involves clients who have unprotected sex with their regular partners (Forsyth, 2000). In most places, foreign women are at the lowest end in the hierarchy of women working in prostitution and are subjected to unsanitary work conditions, are socially and culturally isolated, often remain illegal and have no freedom to move, they are usually unreachable by health services, and frequently work without condoms out of financial desperation. Table 12.2 illustrates possible correlations between prostitution and HIV/AIDS in the aforementioned countries.

Critical public health issues are linked to the relationship of transactional sex between those involved in the commercial sex industry and sex tourists. While sexual mixing, concurrency, and bridging among these populations have been anecdotally documented, empirical works have only touched upon them (Clift & Grabowski, 1997; Clift, Luongo, & Callister, 2002; Dahles & Bras, 1999; Herold, Garcia, & Demoya, 2001; Wickens, 2002). In fact, sexual mixing of sex tourists in the context of brothels, urban prostitution, and pedophilia and child prostitution have been linked to serious health repercussions (Clift & Forrest, 2000; Kempadoo & Ghuma, 1999; Luongo, 2000; O'Connell-Davidson & Sanchez-Taylor, 1999). Given the spatial and temporal dimensions of travel milieux along with the fact that travelers comprise a critical bridge population between different risk prevalence settings, leisure migration in general but sex tourism in particular, threatens extraordinary public health repercussions for tourist-generating and -receiving locales.

Travel may be difficult to isolate as a clear epidemiological component in understanding STI/HIV spread. Particularly because HIV has a clinically latent period that may span years and may be diagnosed much after initial exposure, the contribution of travel is difficult to measure. If co-infection with HIV prolongs or augments the infectiousness of individuals with STIs and if the same STIs facilitate HIV transmission—they may amplify one another in "epidemiological synergy" (Mulhall, 1996, p. 456), which in turn may lead to an explosive growth of the HIV pandemic in some populations.

## Strategies for Change

Many recommendations are offered by international organizations to combat the problems of trafficking and sexual exploitation of vulnerable populations. Although some activities appear to be successful, they are offset by the financial and political power of traffickers and organized crime groups in various countries that control the sex industry, which continues to thrive—particularly

TABLE 12.2. Population, poverty, prostitution, and HIV/AIDS prevalence[10]

| Country | Population (2005) | Population Living Under US$2 a Day (1990-2003) | Estimated Numbers of Persons in Prostitution | Estimated Numbers of Children in Prostitution | HIV/AIDS Cases (Adults/Children) (2003-2004) | HIV/AIDS Cases (% Sex Workers) |
|---|---|---|---|---|---|---|
| *World* | 6,377,643,000 | N/A | N/A | N/A | 39,400,000 | N/A |
| ***East and South Asia*** | | | | | | |
| Cambodia | 14,070,000 | 77.7% | ~10,000,000 | 400,000-500,000 | 170,000 | 45% (1998), 21% (2003) |
| India | 1,103,370,000 | 79.9% | 1,300,000 | 40,000-150,000 | 5,100,000 | 50%-70% |
| Indonesia | 222,780,000 | 52.4% | 43,000-142,000 | N/A | 110,000 | 5%-25% |
| Malaysia | 25,350,000 | 36.8% | 400,000-600,000 | 60,000-100,000 | 52,000 | 10% |
| Philippines | 83,050,000 | 46.4% | ~500,000 | 40,000-300,000 | 9,000 | 33% |
| Singapore | 4,330,000 | 13.1% | 1,000,000-2,000,000 | 800,000 (<15) | 4,100 | 50%-70% |
| Thailand | 64,230,000 | 32.5% | ~500,000 | ~3,500 | 570,000 | 50% (1991), 20% (2001) |
| Vietnam | 84,240,000 | 50.9% | ~200,000 | ~20,000 | 220,000 | 20% |
| ***Latin America and the Caribbean*** | | | | | | |
| Argentina | 38,750,000 | 14.3% | N/A | N/A | 130,000 | 15% |
| Brazil | 186,400,000 | 22.4% | ~1,000,000 | 100,000-500,000 | 660,000 | 60% |
| Cuba | 11,270,000 | 28.6% | ~100,000 | ~30,000 | 4,070 | N/A |
| Dominican Republic | 8,890,000 | 25% | ~200,000 | 25,000-30,000 | 140,000 | 46% |

[10] Figures in Table 12.2 come from a variety of sources (i.e., CARICOM, CATW, ECPAT, Global Health Council, ILO, IOM, UNAIDS, United Nations, World Bank) and vary as a result.

in countries ravished by poverty. Nevertheless, recommended solutions include the eradication of child sex tourism, the recognition of the abusive circumstances in which sex workers live and work, a more concentrated focus on broader structural issues that cause poverty and that facilitate and support the sex industry, and the examination of the health effects of sex work in terms of both sexworkers and clients (Lim, 1998). Some ongoing international efforts to end trafficking and sexual exploitation of women and children are noted below.

## Human Rights and Protection of Women and Children

Among the most distressing aspects of sex tourism is the exploitation of vulnerable persons, especially children. It has been argued that "prostitution tourism needs to be dealt with through human rights mechanisms that challenge all forms of men's prostitution behavior toward women and children as sexual violence" (Jeffreys, 1999, p. 180). Along these lines, a number of efforts have been undertaken to control or stop the sexual exploitation of individuals. While some focus on the problem of global trafficking, others try to stop sexual abuse of children by targeting child sex tourists for prosecution (examples are listed in Table 12.3 below).

## Education and Social Responsibility

A great deal of useful information is available to assist travelers in preventing potential health problems. The CDC, other governmental bodies, and the tourism sector offer health advice for travelers by addressing various health concerns. However, the potential health problems of behavioral risk-taking, particularly within the context of sex tourism remain an uncharted area for public-health practitioners. The thought of educating sex tourists only in terms of health risks to themselves and others is nothing more than naïve, particularly in light of the fact that sex tourism is considered by many to be the ultimate risk holiday (Rogstad, 2004). It is imperative to not only inform them of risks for STIs/HIV/AIDS but also in terms of the harm they inflict upon others through sexual exploitation. Particularly in the case of child sex tourists, efforts to educate must be combined with legal action to prevent individuals from continuing their exploitative activities for their own gratification. Along with multilateral efforts that have extra-territorial applications to find, prosecute, and punish child sex tourists, efforts need to focus on more socially responsible marketing of tourist destinations, rather than marketing certain places specifically as sex tourism locales.

Some Asian countries have addressed sexual transmission of HIV through large-scale prevention programs. In Bangladesh, Cambodia, Thailand, and the Philippines, fewer men visit sex workers—which unfortunately explains why sex tourist destinations in other regions of the world are flourishing—and condoms are used more frequently by commercial sex workers. Albeit, few,

TABLE 12.3. Efforts to combat trafficking in persons and child sexual exploitation

| | |
|---|---|
| 1989 | **U.N. Convention on the Rights of the Child (CRC)** ratified by 191 countries. |
| 1991 | **End Child Prostitution, Child Pornography, and the Trafficking of Children for Sexual Exploitation (ECPAT)** formed to combat the international child sex trade industry. |
| 1992 | **Program for Action for the Prevention of the Sale of Children, Child Prostitution; and Child Pornography** adopted by the U.N. Commission on Human Rights. |
| 1993 | **Declaration on the Elimination of Violence against Women** adopted following the passage of a resolution by the U.N. General Assembly for the purpose of ending trafficking. |
| 1996 | **First World Congress Against Commercial Sexual Exploitation of Children** met in Sweden with delegates from over 120 countries. |
| 1997 | **Task Force to Protect Children from Sexual Exploitation in Tourism** is a global action platform of tourism-related key players from government and industry established by the WTO. |
| 1998 | **Task Force to End Sexual Exploitation in Thailand** representing 24 government and private agencies. |
| 1999 | 24 countries have legislation with extra-territorial application to make child sex tourism a criminal offense (even when carried out overseas)[11] (David, 2000). |
| 2000 | **Trafficking Victims Protection Act** passed by the U.S. Congress, which created new laws to fight traffickers and new services to help victims and also authorized creation of the **Office to Monitor and Combat Trafficking in Persons**. |
| 2001 | Campaign by the **Coalition Against Trafficking in Women (CATW)** and the **U.N. Economic and Social Council** to ratify the **1949 Convention for the Suppression of the Traffic in Persons and of the Exploitation of the Prostitution of Others**, in order to define prostitution as a human rights violation and include the penalization of clients of sex workers. |
| 2003 | **Anti-Trafficking Strategy** announced by the U.S. Agency for International Development stating that *"organizations advocating prostitution as an employment choice or which advocate or support the legalization of prostitution are not appropriate partners for USAID anti-trafficking grants or contracts"* |
| 2003 | **National Security Presidential Directive** signed by President George Bush to combat the problem of trafficking in persons. |
| 2003 | **U.S. Protect Act** signed into law by President Bush (carries up to 30 year prison sentence). **Operation Predator**, a U.S. Immigration and Customs Enforcement (ICE) initiative to identify, investigate, and arrest child sex predators. |
| 2004 | **Code of Conduct for the Protection of Children from Sexual Commercial Exploitation in Travel and Tourism** launched as joint effort by UNICEF, ECPAT-USA, and the WTO—designed to create a more responsible tourism sector that is vigilant against child exploitation (50 companies signed on). |
| 2004 | U.S.-funded (US$500,000) advertising campaign created by World Vision and U.S. ICE targets American child sex tourists (25% of the world's total) with warnings of prosecution upon returning home to the States. Billboards with slogans such as: "Abuse a child in this country, go to jail in yours" have appeared in Cambodia, Costa Rica, Thailand, Mexico, Brazil, and the Dominican Republic. |

---

[11] Illegal prostitution often means that it is criminal to provide sexual services but not to pay for them—punishing sex workers instead of helping them to escape their situation while giving men the opportunity to find others to exploit. Therefore, sexual exploitation of persons may be prevented by changing the illegality of prostitution to assure that buyers of sexual services are arrested instead (Haney, 2000).

there are examples to show that solutions are possible, such as Thailand. In 1991, Prime Minister Panyaruchun made AIDS prevention and control a national priority. The following year, the Thai government legalized prostitution in order to control and monitor HIV infection rates and AIDS cases (*Economy*, 1997 cited in Neff-Smith, Spencer, & Tavai, 2001). The AIDS Control Program was moved from the Ministry of Public Health to the Office of the Prime Minister and its budget was increased from US$180,000 to US$44 million and later to US$80 million. A massive public information campaign was launched and anti-AIDS messages aired hourly on 488 state-owned radio and television stations. These and other efforts have been effective in controlling HIV spread, by reducing visits to sex workers by 50%, raising condom use, decreasing STIs, and in turn achieving substantial reductions in new HIV infections from 140,000 in 1991 to 21,000 in 2003 (World Bank, 2000). Thailand's three phase high profile campaign (1991-1995; 1996-2001; 2002-2006) with anti-AIDS messages, at first unpopular with the influential tourism sector, caused tourism to decline but opposition faded and support increased as AIDS took an increasingly popular place on the national agenda (World Bank, 1997).

To be realistic at the risk of sounding pessimistic, a few examples of success are insufficient to overcome the serious risks to public health that are associated with large volumes of sex tourism activity around the world. Travel health information is made available to anyone who seeks it in order to create awareness of health risks and offer suggestions to deal effectively with them. At the same time, many organizations around the world are working hard to curb the growth of the HIV/AIDS epidemic through a variety of education programs. But behavioral risk taking of travelers and the widespread use of women, children, and men in the international sex trade is a massive problem that requires creative, effective, and multi-pronged action by virtually everyone—governments, NGOs, various international organizations, including the IMF, the World Bank, the World Health Organization, and the World Tourism Organization. The problem reaches far beyond individual or public health and involves the need for broader structural improvements to eradicate the kind of poverty that forces people to sell themselves and their children in order to survive. As for individuals from developed countries who exploit the desperation of sex workers at sex tourist destinations, it is important for the governments of developed countries to become and remain involved in order to create and maintain a higher level of awareness and sense of responsibility. A problem as widespread as global exploitation, which carries explosive public health ramifications requires a global response.

## References

Age of Consent. http://www.ageofconsent.com (accessed 5/15/2005).

Agnote, D. (1998). Sex trade key part of S.E. Asian economies, study says. *Kyodo News*, August 18.

Apostolopoulos, Y. & S. Sönmez (2002). Sociocultural epidemiology of Caribbean tourism and development. *ReVista, Harvard Review on Latin America.* Winter: 79-80 (invited paper) (http://www.fas.harvard.edu/~drclas/publications/revista/Tourism/tcontent.html).

Apostolopoulos, Y. & S. Sönmez (2001a). Disease mapping and risk assessment for public health and sustainable tourism development in insular regions. In (Y. Apostolopoulos & D.J. Gayle, Eds.), *Island Tourism and Sustainable Development: Caribbean, Pacific, and Mediterranean Experiences* (pp. 225-248). Westport, CT: Praeger.

Apostolopoulos, Y. & S. Sönmez (2001b). Tourist migration, public health and sustainable development in the insular mediterranean. In (D. Ioannides, Y. Apostolopoulos, & S. Sönmez, Eds.), *Mediterranean Islands and Sustainable Tourism Development: Practices, Management, and Policies* (pp. 261-281). London, UK: Continuum.

Apostolopoulos, Y., Sönmez, S., & Yu C.H. (2002). HIV-risk behaviors of American spring break vacationers: A case of situational disinhibition? *International Journal of STD & AIDS,* 13(11), 733-743.

Bedi, R. (1997). *Bid to Protect Children As Sex Tourism Spreads.* News-Scan International Ltd. 3/19/1996. http://www.geocities.com/CapitolHill/Senate/8931/dbt-gem2.html?200614 (accessed 6/14/2005).

Bishop, R. & L.S. Robinson (1998). *Night Market: Sexual Cultures and the Thai Economic Miracle.* New York, NY and London, UK: Routledge.

Bobak, L. (1996). For sale: The innocence of Cambodia, *Ottawa Sun,* October 24.

Borland, R., Faas, L., Marshall, D., McLean, R., Schroen, M., Smit, M., & T. Valerio (2004). *HIV/AIDS and Mobile Populations in the Caribbean: A Baseline Assessment.* International Organization for Migration (IOM), Santo Domingo, Dominican Republic.

Bosch, X. (2004). Spain makes plans to combat sex tourism. *The Lancet.* 363, p. 542.

Brennan, D. (2001). Tourism in transnational places: Dominican sex workers and German sex Tourists imagine one another. *Identities.* 7(4), 621-663.

Bryan, A.T. (2005). The Caribbean's worst plague: HIV/AIDS. *Revista Inter-Forum.* Florida, US: Dante B. Fascell North-South Center, University of Miami. http://www.revistainterforum.com/english/articles/040802artprin_040802artprin_en2.html (accessed 4/10/2006).

CARICOM (Caribbean Community) Secretariat (2002). The Caribbean Regional Strategic Framework for HIV/AIDS: 2002-2006. Pan-Caribbean Partnership on HIV/AIDS.

CARICOM (Caribbean Community) Secretariat (2005). *Model CARICOM Youth Summit: HIV/AIDS in the Caribbean.* http://www.caricom.org/jsp/community_organs/aids.jsp?menu=cob (accessed 5/10/2006).

CAREC (Caribbean Epidemiology Centre) (2001). The HIV/AIDS Epidemic in the Caribbean. *CAFRA News,* June 26, 2001. http://www.cafra.org/article.php3?id_article=188 (accessed 2/10/2006).

CATW (Coalition Against Trafficking in Women) (2005). *The Economies of Sex Slavery: Follow the Money Trail.* June 22, 2005 Hearing Before the Subcommittee on Domestic and International Monetary Policy, Trade, and Technology. House of Representatives. 109th Congress: Combating Trafficking in Persons: An International Perspective. http://www.catwinternational.org/factbook (accessed 3/22/2006).

Clift, S. & P. Grabowski (Eds.) (1997). *Tourism and Health: Risks, Research, and Responses.* London, UK: Pinter.

Clift, S. & S. Forrest (2000). Factors associated with gay men's sexual behaviors and risk on holiday. *AIDS Care,* 11, 281-295.

Clift, S., Luongo, M., & C. Callister (Eds.) (2002). *Gay Tourism: Culture, Identity, and Sex.* London, UK: Continuum.

Contreras, J. (2001). The Dark Tourists. *Newsweek.* April 30, 2001. http://www. keepmedia.com/pubs/Newsweek/2001/04/30/313609 (accessed 5/1/2006).

Dahles, H. & K. Bras (1999). Entrepreneurs in romance: Tourism in Indonesia. *Annals of Tourism Research.* 26(2), 267-293.

David, F. (2000). Child Sex Tourism. Trends and Issues in Crime and Criminal Justice. No. 156. Canberra, Australia: Australian Institute of Criminology. http://www.aic. gov.au (accessed 5/3/2006).

Davis-Lewis, N. & J. Bailey (1992/1993). HIV, International Travel and Tourism: Global Issues and Pacific Perspectives. *Asia-Pacific Journal of Public Health*, 6(3), 159-167.

de Albuquerque, K. (1998a). Sex, beach boys, and female tourists in the Caribbean. *Sexuality and Culture.* 2, 87-111.

de Albuquerque, K. (1998b). In search of the big bamboo. *Transition.* 77, 48-57.

*Economy* (1997). The Economic Impact of AIDS in Thailand: A Comparison to Tanzania.

ECPAT (End Child Prostitution, Child Pornography, and the Trafficking of Children for Sexual Exploitation) (1996a). *The Paedo File.* Presented at the End Child Prostitution, Child Pornography, and the Trafficking of Children for Sexual Exploitation (ECPAT) International Conference, August 1996, Bangkok, Thailand.

ECPAT (End Child Prostitution, Child Pornography, and the Trafficking of Children for Sexual Exploitation) (1996b). *Child Sex Tourism.* http://www.missingkids.com/ html/ncmec_default_ec_tourism.html (accessed 5/16/2006).

Erder, S. & S. Kaska (2003). *Irregular Migration and Trafficking in Women: The Case of Turkey.* Geneva: International Organization for Migration (IOM).

Faria, Jr., M.A. (2004). Socialized medicine in Cuba part II: 'Doctor diplomacy,' sex tourism, and medical apartheid. *Surgical Neurology.* 62, 275-277.

Flowers, R.B. (2001). The sex trade industry's worldwide exploitation of children. *Annals, AAPSS,* 575, 147-157.

Forsythe, S. (2000). AIDS Brief for Sectoral Planners and Managers. *Tourism Sector.* Durban, South Africa: University of Natal.

Friedman, R.I. (1996). India's shame: Sexual slavery and political corruption are leading to an AIDS catastrophe. *The Nation,* April 8.

GHC (Global Health Council) (2005). Global Estimates of HIV and AIDS as of End 2003. http://globalhealth.org (accessed 11/17/05).

GBGM (General Board of Global Ministries) (2000). Global Deaths from HIV/AIDS 2000. http://gbgm-umc.org/health/wad01/2000global.stm (accessed 12/15/2005).

Global Health Reporting (2004). Facts at a Glance. http://globalhealthreporting. org/diseaseinfo.asp?id=23 (accessed 11/17/05).

*The Indian Express* (1997). Global law to punish sex tourists sought by Britain and EU, November 21, 1997.

Gorden, T. (1991). *Enslaved.* New York, NY: Pharos Books.

Haney, D. (2000). Third World Women's Health: Prostitution and Sex Tourism. http://www.arches.uga.edu/~haneydaw/twwh/traf.html (accessed 5/6/2005).

Herold, E., Garcia. R., & T. DeMoya (2001). Female tourists and beach boys: Romance or sex tourism? *Annals of Tourism Research.* 28(4), 978-997.

HIV and AIDS in Thailand (2005). AVERT. http://www.avert.org/aidsthai.htm (accessed 6/12/2006).

Hughes, D. (1996). Sex Tours Via the Internet. Coalition Against Trafficking in Women. 28, 71-76 (also on http://www.feminista.com/archives/v1n7/hughes.html)

Hughes, D. (2003). Trafficking of Women and Children in East Asia and Beyond: A Review of U.S. Policy. April 9 testimony before the Subcommittee of East Asian and Pacific Affairs, Senate Foreign Relations Committee.

Hynes, H.P. & J.G. Raymond (2002). Put in harm's way: The neglected health consequences of sex trafficking in the United States. In (J. Silliman & A. Bhattacharjee, Eds.) *Policing the National Body* (pp. 197-229). Cambridge, MA: South End Press.

IAS (International AIDS Society) (2004). Report on the XV International AIDS Conference. Bangkok, Thailand, July 11-16, 2004. http://www.iasociety.org/pdf/BangkokReport.pdf.

ILO (International Labor Organization) (1998). *Sex as a Sector: Economic Incentives and Hardships Fuel Growth.* World of Work, No. 26, September, 1998. International Labor Organization. http://www.ilo.org/public/english/bureau/inf/magazine/26/sex.htm (accessed 5/3/2006).

IOM (International Organization for Migration) (2002). *Journeys of Jeopardy: A Review of Research on Trafficking in Women and Children in Europe.* http://www.iom.int/documents/publication/en/mrs%5F11%5F2002.pdf (accessed 5/5/2006).

Jeffreys, S. (1999). Globalizing sexual exploitation: Sex tourism and the traffic in women. *Leisure Studies*, 18, 179-196.

Jeffreys, S. (2002). No hiding place: Child sex tourism and the role of extraterritorial legislation. *Contemporary Sociology*, 31(6), 687-689.

Jeffreys, S. (2003). Sex tourism: Do women do it too? *Leisure Studies*, 22, 223-238.

Joseph, C. (1995). Scarlet wounding: Issues of child prostitution. *The Journal of Psychohistory*, 23(1), 2-17.

Kaban, E. (1998). *UN Labor Body Urges Recognition of Sex Industry.* International Labor Office. August 18, Reuters.

Kempadoo, K. (1999a). *Sun, Sex, and Gold. Tourism and Sex Work in the Caribbean.* Lanham, MD: Rowman & Littlefield.

Kempadoo, K. (1999b). Continuities and change, In (K. Kempadoo, Ed.) *Sun, Sex, and Gold. Tourism and Sex Work in the Caribbean* (pp. 3-36). Lanham, MD: Rowman & Littlefield.

Kempadoo, K. (2001). Freelancers, temporary wives, and beach boys: Researching sex work in the caribbean. *Feminist Review.* 67, 39-62.

Kempadoo, K. & R. Ghuma (1999). For the children: Trends in international policies and law on sex tourism. In (K. Kempadoo, Ed.) *Sun, Sex, and Gold. Tourism and Sex Work in the Caribbean.* Lanham, MD: Rowman & Littlefield.

Lim, L. (Ed.) (1998). *The Sex Sector: The Economic and Social Bases of Prostitution in Southeast Asia.* Geneva: International Labor Organization (ILO).

Leheny, D. (1995). A political economy of Asian sex tourism. *Annals of Tourism Research.* 22(2), 367-384.

Leidholdt, D.A. (2005). Combatting Trafficking in Persons: An International Perspective. Hearing Before the Subcommittee on Dom6estic and International Monetary Policy, Trade, and Technology, House of Representatives. 109th Congress. The Economies of Sex Slavery: Follow the Money Trail. June 22, 2005.

Lhagvasuren, N. (2001). Waking up to a new reality. *Transitions Online.* August 21, 2001.

Luongo, M. (2000). The use of commercial sex venues and male escorts by gay tourists in New York City. In (S. Clift & S. Carter, Eds.) *Tourism and Sex: Culture, Commerce, and Coercion*, London, UK: Pinter.

Marks, K. (2003). British sex tourists turn killing fields of Cambodia into paedophiles' playground. *The Independent*. January 5, 2003. http://www.vachss.com/help_text/a2/british_sex.html (accessed 5/3/2006).

McGirk, T. (1997). Nepal's lost daughters, India's soiled goods. *Nepal/India News*, January 27.

Merriman, T. (2002). *Fox on the Record*. June 11, 2002.

Miller, M.M. & T.L. Henthorne (1997). *Investment in the New Cuban Tourist Industry: A Guide to Entrepreneurial Opportunities*. Westport, CT: Quorum Books.

Mulhall, B.P. (1996). Sex and travel: Studies of sexual behavior, disease and health promotion in international travellers—a global review. *International Journal of STD & AIDS*, 7(7), 455-465.

Namen, C. (1994). Telephone conversation. Rockville: National Victims Research Center, cited in C. Joseph (1995) Scarlet wounding: Issues of child prostitution. *The Journal of Psychohistory*. 23(1), 2-17.

NATHNAC (National Travel Health Network and Centre) (2005). Blood Borne and Sexually Transmitted Infections. *Foreign Travel-Associated Illness*, pp. 55-60. (http://www.hpa.org.uk/hpa/publications/travel_2005/travel.pdf).

Neff-Smith, M., Spencer, G., & V.R. Tavai (2001). AIDS in Asia: Linking tragedy in Thailand and Myanmar. *The Journal of Multicultural Nursing & Health*, 7(1), 17-20.

O'Connell-Davidson, J. (2001). The sex tourist, the expatriate, his ex-wife and her "other:" The policits of loss, difference, and desire. *Sexualities*, 4(1), 5-24.

O'Connell-Davidson, J. (1996). Sex tourism in Cuba. *Race & Class*, 37(3), 39-48.

O'Connell-Davidson, J. & J. Sanchez-Taylor (1999). Fantasy islands: Exploring the demand for sex tourism. In (K. Kempadoo, Ed.) *Sun, Sex, and Gold: Tourism and Sex Work in the Caribbean*. Lanham, MD: Rowman & Littlefield.

Opperman, M. (1998). *Sex Tourism and Prostitution: Aspects of Leisure, Recreation, and Work*. New York, NY: Cognizant Communications.

Opperman, M. (1999). Sex tourism. *Annals of Tourism Research*, 26(2), 251-266

Pettman, J.J. (1997). Body politics: International sex tourism. *Third World Quarterly*, 18(1), 93-108.

Pruitt, D. & S. Lafont (1995). For love and money: Romance tourism in Jamaica. *Annals of Tourism Research*, 22, 422-440.

Richburg, K.B. (1998). Spreading HIV threatens Cambodia government hard pressed to respond. *Washington Post Foreign Services*, August 9.

Rodriguez-Garcia, R. (2001). The health-development link: Travel as a public health issue. *Journal of Community Health*, 26(2), 93-112.

Rogers, B. (1999). Bitter harvest. *Ms. Magazine*, 9. New York: Liberty Media for Women.

Rogstad, K.E. (2004). Sex, sun, sea, and STIs: Sexually transmitted infections acquired on holiday. *British Medical Journal*, 329, 214-217.

Sánchez Taylor, J. (2001). Dollars are a girl's best friend? Female tourists' sexual behavior in the Caribbean. *Sociology*, 35(3), 749-764.

Seper, C. (1998). Police sweeps help clean up child prostitution. *Christian Science Monitor*, 8 January.

Sönmez, S., Y. Apostolopoulos, C.H. Yu, S. Yang, A.S. Mattila, & L.C. Yu (2006). Binge drinking and casual sex on spring-break. *Annals of Tourism Research*, 33(4), 895-917.

Stillwaggon, E. (2000). *Determinants of HIV Transmission in Africa and Latin America*. Unpublished manuscript.

Sullivan, M.P. (2003). *AIDS in the Caribbean and Central America*. Congressional Research Service (CRS) Report for Congress, November 17, 2003. The Library of Congress.

*The Economist* (1998). The sex industry: Giving the customer what he wants. February. 14, 23-25.

The Hedonist: World Sex Tours Guide for Single Male Travel. http://www. theprofessionalbachelor.com/webrigns/index.htm (accessed 11/10/2005).

Travel and the Single Male. http://www.tsmtravel.com (accessed 5/2/2006).

Triana, J.C. (1995). Consolidation of the economic reanimation. *Cuban Foreign Trade*. 1, 17-24.

Truong, T.D. (1990). *Sex, Money, and Morality: Prostitution and Tourism in Southeast Asia*. London, UK: Zed Books.

USDOJ (1999). Prostitution of Children and Child Sex Tourism: An Analysis of Domestic and International Responses. Alexandria, VA: U.S. Department of Justice, National Center for Missing and Exploited Children.

UNAIDS (2001). Population Mobility and AIDS. Joint United Nations Programme on HIV/AIDS, Technical Update. February, p. 5

UNAIDS & WHO (2003). *AIDS Epidemic Update: December 2004*. Geneva: Joint United Nations Programme on HIV/AIDS, World Health Organization.

UNAIDS (2004). Caribbean: HIV and AIDS Statistics and Features, End of 2002 and 2004. Joint United Nations Programme on HIV/AIDS. http://www.unaids. org/wad2004/EPIupdate2004_html_en/Epi04_06_en.htm (accessed 2/5/2006).

UNAIDS (2005). *Regional HIV and AIDS Estimates*. Joint United Nations Programme on HIV/AIDS. http://www.unaids.org (accessed 2/5/2006).

UNDP (2004). *Human Development Report*. United Nations Development Programme. http://www.undp.org/hdro/indicators.html (accessed 5/2/2006).

UN (1996). *The United Nations and the Advancement of Women 1945-96*. New York: United Nations Department of Public Information.

UN (2004). Economic Causes of Trafficking in Women in the UNECE Region. U.N. Economic and Social Council. October 5, 2004. http://www.unece.org/oes/gender/ documents/Secretariat%20Notes/ECE_AC.28_2004_10.pdf (accessed 4/4/2006).

USDOS (2005). *Trafficking in Persons Report*. U.S. Department of State. http://www.state.gov/g/tip (accessed 3/2/2006).

Van Liemt, G. (2004). *Human Trafficking in Europe: An Economic Perspective*. Geneva: IOL.

Wickens, E. (2002) Sacred and the profane: A tourist typology. *Annals of Tourism Research*, 29(3), 834-851.

Wilson, M.E. (1995). Infectious diseases: An ecological perspective. *British Medical Journal*, 311(7021), 1681-1685.

Wonders, N.A. & R. Michalowski (2001). Bodies, borders, and sex tourism in a globalized world: A tale of two cities—Amsterdam and Havana. *Social Problems*, 48(4), 545-571.

World Bank (1997). *Confronting AIDS: Public Priorities in a Global Epidemic*. New York, NY: Oxford University Press.

World Bank (1999). *World Development Report, 1998-1999*. New York, NY: Oxford University Press.

World Bank (2000a). Thailand's Response to AIDS: Building in Success, Confronting the Future. *Thailand Social Monitor*. http://siteresources.worldbank.org/INTTHAILAND/Resources/Social-Monitor/2000jan.pdf (accessed 2/10/2006).

World Bank (2000b). *HIV/AIDS in the Caribbean: Issues and Options, A Background Report*. No. 20491-LAO-2000. http://wbln0018.worldbank.org/LAC/lacinfoclient.nsf/145d45c4b49a8bb88525673600695e5f/0191899ca02a3f6885256905007be3d0/$FILE/HIVAIDSCaribbean.pdf (accessed 08/06/2005).

World Sex Archives. http://www.worldsexarchives.com (accessed 6/12/2005).

World Sex Guide. http://www.worldsexguide.com (accessed 6/12/2005).

Women of the World. http://join.4womenoftheworld.com (accessed 5/11/2005).

Wright, E.R. (2003). Travel, tourism, and HIV risk among older adults. *Journal of Acquired Immune Deficiency Syndrome*, 33, S233-S237.

WTO (2006). *Tourism Highlights, 2006 Edition*. Madrid, Spain: World Tourism Organization. http://www.world-tourism.org (accessed 12/5/2006).

Zúñiga, J. (2001). Cuba: The Thailand of the Caribbean. *The New West Indian*. http://www.awigp.com/default.asp?numcat=sextour2 (accessed 5/6/2006).

# Epilogue
## New Directions in Migration Health and Medicine

# Chapter 13

# Mapping and Modeling Disease Risk Among Mobile Populations

HENRY G. MWAMBI, PH.D. AND KHANGELANI ZUMA, PH.D.

## Human Mobility and Epidemiology

Human mobility patterns play an important role in the spread of many infectious diseases and in designing control strategies for them. Given that epidemiology is the study of the occurrence of disease in a person and at a time and place, this implies that mobility patterns and their distribution within and between countries or regions are important in explaining the dissemination of existing, emerging, or re-emerging diseases. Mobility patterns have been responsible for the introduction of infectious agents into areas where they never before existed. A well-known example is the spread of Human Immunodeficiency Virus/Acquired Immunodeficiency Syndrome (HIV/AIDS), which first emerged in the early 1980s. With the passage of time, HIV began to occur nearly on the entire face of the earth with varying proportions. A more recent example is the Severe Acute Respiratory Syndrome (SARS) an atypical pneumonia and part-time sexually transmitted infection (STI) spread through both sexual and casual contact that first appeared in November 2002 in China. First reported in Asia in February 2003, SARS was spread via international travelers in a few months to more than two dozen countries in Asia, North America, South America, and Europe before the global outbreak of 2003 was contained—but by the last case was recorded, there were a total of 8,437 known cases of the disease, with 813 deaths.

Mathematical and statistical models have been put to good use in understanding the spread of infectious pathogens and how best to contain them (Anderson, Fraser, Ghani, Donnelly, Riley, Ferguson, Leung, Lam, & Hedley, 2004; Donnely, 2004; Donnelly, Ghani, Leung, Hedley, Fraser, Riley, Abu-Raddad, Ho, Thach, Chau, Chan, Lam, Tse, Tsang, Liu, Kong, Lau, Ferguson, & Anderson 2003). The spread and persistence of highly pathogenic diseases, such as SARS, pose challenges to present day epidemiologists because their transmission is aided by key factors such as human mobility patterns including air travel, and the continued growth and overcrowding in big cities, as seen in many parts of the world, particularly in developing countries, as well as other risk factors. Considering the foregoing, epidemic outbreaks of new infectious agents are likely to become more common than ever, therefore, epidemiologists need to be equipped with quantitative tools and skills in order to counter such challenges. Data-oriented mathematical and statistical methods are crucial for the success of these efforts. It has been argued that international collaboration in the analysis of epidemiological and contact-network databases can provide further insight into the spread of emerging or re-emerging infections such as SARS and avian influenza (Donnelly et al., 2003).

Models incorporating geographic mobility among regions in the diffusion of infectious diseases are not new. Sattenspiel and Dietz (1995) developed a model for the spread of infectious diseases among discrete geographic regions that incorporated a mobility process describing how contact occurs between individuals from different regions. Their general mobility formulation included a range of mobility patterns from complete isolation of all regions to permanent migration between them. In addition, the authors showed how to incorporate mobility processes into the basic Susceptible-Infective-Recovered (SIR) epidemic model, which was applied to describe the 1984 measles epidemic on the Caribbean island of Dominica. For STIs including HIV/AIDS, a number of socioeconomic factors are definitely responsible for the recent rise in their incidence and prevalence but clearly most of the facilitating factors are linked to human mobility and migration (Lurie, Williams, Zuma, Mkaya-Mwamburi, Garnett, Sturm, Sweat, Gittelsohn, & Abdool Karim, 2003a; Lurie, Williams, Zuma, Mkaya-Mwamburi, Garnett, Sturm, Sweat, Gittelsohn, & Abdool Karim, 2003b; Zuma, Gouws, Williams, & Lurie 2005). Examples include increasing urbanization, migrant worker effect, expansion of the tourist travel sector, and new attitudes towards sexual behavior in modern societies. Generally, human mobility patterns and social networks in relation to the spread of infectious diseases are multilevel in nature. By design, it is expected that there will be more movements of humans within cities, towns and regions in the same country than movements between two or more countries. As one goes down to a finer geographic resolution, social networks and contacts become tighter. However, in developed countries where transport systems are highly efficient, communication between areas within a country and between countries in a modeling sense is more probable. This means that the transportation of an infectious agent between countries with such highly connected systems will be more efficient.

## Mathematical Modeling and Infectious Diseases

The earliest known mathematical model for infectious diseases is attributed to Daniel Bernoulli (1760) for the transmission of smallpox. After the work by Bernoulli there was a period of no further development in the area, possibly due to the lack of understanding of the mechanisms driving the infectious processes of diseases. Advances in biology and bacteriology reversed this situation and a major development followed with the first model for malaria, an indirectly transmitted disease, developed by Sir Ronald Ross (1909, 1911). In his model, Ross described the process whereby a human host acquires malaria from an infectious mosquito bite or conversely, a disease-free mosquito gets infected by biting an infected human host. Ross introduced a very important concept in disease control by suggesting that the eradication of malaria could be possible if the mosquito population could be reduced to a certain finite threshold number, say $N^{crit}$, suggesting that the complete eradication of mosquitoes is not necessary. This observation led to the threshold phenomenon in epidemiology. Following this, Kermack and McKendrick (1927) developed an epidemic model in which the infectivity of an individual depends on the time when the individual becomes infective or what essentially could be interpreted as an age of infection model. In this case, an epidemic is defined as a sudden outbreak of a disease, which infects a sizeable portion of the population in a region before it disappears. The Kermack-McKendrick SIR epidemic model is formulated as a two-dimensional system of ordinary differential equations representing transitions (in continuous time) from the Susceptible class (S) to the Infective class (I) and then from the Infective to the Recovered class (R). Since this period in history, there has been an increasingly rapid transition of biology and medicine from qualitative (descriptive) to quantitative (predictive) sciences in the form of mathematical and statistical models to explain the growth of human (and animal) populations and the spread of infectious diseases as well as the design of control strategies. A significant contribution in this field is the work of Anderson and May (1991) as well as a number of other model variants including contact rates, quarantine, and isolation which followed the recent SARS epidemic, and which can be grouped as infection models and analyzed using the Kermack and McKenderick approach.

## The Basic SIR Model

In this model the assumption is made that an individual can only occupy one of three possible disease states or classes. Firstly, an individual is uninfected and susceptible to the disease; secondly, if the individual comes into contact with the infectious agent and becomes infected then his/her state will change from that of susceptible to infected; and finally, the individual may develop some immunity to the disease and change from infective to the recovered or removed class. It should be noted, however, that this structure is in most cases a major simplification because in reality the disease stages may be more detailed. In order to briefly explain the formulation of the SIR epidemic model, the enticing approach developed by Daley and Ghani (1999) is followed. Let $x(t)$, $y(t)$ and $z(t)$ respectively denote the number of individuals in the susceptible, infected, and recovered classes of the disease at time $t$ respectively. The total number of individuals is $N = x(t) + y(t) + z(t)$ and assumed to be constant as in its original formulation (Kermack & McKendrick, 1927). The variables $x(t)$, $y(t)$ and $z(t)$ are taken as continuous deterministic variables, hence they can be modeled using a system of differential equations given by:

$$\frac{dx}{dt} = -\beta xy \tag{13.1}$$

$$\frac{dy}{dt} = \beta xy - \gamma y \tag{13.2}$$

$$\frac{dz}{dt} = \gamma y \tag{13.3}$$

The initial state of the system is $(x(0), y(0), z(0)) = (x_0 > 0, y_0 > 0, 0)$ assuming there is at least one infected person in the population otherwise the population will remain uninfected. In its basic form, the model assumes a closed population with no migration in or out of that population. The parameter $\beta$ denotes the rate of infection per individual per unit time or what may be called the hazard of infection. Note that susceptibles get infected at a rate that is proportional to the product of susceptible and infected individuals. This concept is known as "the law of mass action" governing the spread of infectious diseases assuming homogeneous mixing between those susceptible to and infected with the disease. The parameter $\gamma$ is the recovery or the removal rate of an infected individual. Written in this form the model assumes that the duration of infection follows an exponential distribution with a mean given by $1/\gamma$. An equation relating $x(t)$ and $z(t)$ can be obtained (Daley & Ghani, 1999) by first dividing the equation for $x(t)$ by the equation for $z(t)$ to yield:

$$\frac{dx}{dz} = -\frac{\beta}{\gamma} x = -\frac{x}{\rho} \text{ where } \rho = \frac{\gamma}{\beta} \tag{13.4}$$

Then the solution to equation (13.4) is easily obtained as

$$x = x_0 e^{-\frac{z}{\rho}} \tag{13.5}$$

where $\rho$ can be defined as a measure of the relative removal rate. This therefore means that

$$y = N - x_0 e^{-\frac{z}{\rho}} - z \tag{13.6}$$

hence

$$\frac{dz}{dt} = \gamma (N - x_0 e^{-\frac{z}{\rho}} - z) \tag{13.7}$$

The above equation has a parametric solution given by

$$\gamma t = \int_0^z \frac{dv}{N - v - x_0 e^{-\frac{v}{\rho}}}, \quad 0 \leq t \leq \infty \tag{13.8}$$

There are two main results which can be inferred from system (13.1)-(13.3). The first one is the criticality condition which comes from equation (13.2). Since at the start of the epidemic, this equation can be re-expressed as

$$\frac{dy}{dt} = \beta y (x_0 - \rho) \tag{13.9}$$

it follows that if the epidemic is ever to grow, then we require that

$$\frac{dy}{dt}\bigg|_{t=0} > 0 \; or \; x_0 > \rho$$

(i.e., the initial number of susceptibles must exceed a threshold value equal to $\rho$). The second important result from the work of Kermack and McKendrick (1927) is derived as follows. From equation (13.8), as $t \to \infty$, $z(t)$ approaches its limiting value $z_\infty < N$. Thus in the limit

$$N - z_\infty - x_0 e^{-\frac{z_\infty}{\rho}} = 0$$

Now suppose that $x_0$ is close to $N$; then $z_\infty$ is the approximate solution of

$$0 = N - N e^{-z_\infty/\rho} \approx N - z_\infty - N(1 - z_\infty/\rho + z_\infty^2/2\rho^2)$$

Thus if say $N = \rho + \upsilon$ with $\upsilon << \rho$ then

$$z_\infty \approx \frac{2\upsilon}{1 + \frac{\upsilon}{\rho}} \approx 2\upsilon$$

Thus if $x_0 \approx N = \rho + \upsilon$ with $\upsilon > 0$, then since $y_\infty = 0$, $x_\infty \approx \rho - \upsilon$ since $x_\infty + z_\infty = N$. According to this result, some susceptibles will ultimately survive the epidemic free from infection. An important fundamental property related to the first result noted above is that there is a basic reproductive number $R_0$ of the disease, determining whether the disease will die out without spreading or whether there will be an epidemic. $R_0$ is defined as the number of expected secondary infections caused by a single infective introduced into a wholly susceptible population of size $N$ over its entire infectious duration. In this case, since the mean infective period is $1/\gamma$, then $R_0 = \beta N/\gamma$, from the final size equation it is possible to calculate the fraction $x_\infty/N$ of the population that escapes the epidemic.

A more realistic model is one that includes a latent or exposed (incubating) class whose members progress to the infectious class at a rate of say $\sigma$ to which could also be included a disease-induced mortality at rate $\alpha$. If the time-scales of the disease process are much faster than the demographic processes, then the basic reproductive number of the disease becomes $R_0 = \beta N/(\gamma + \alpha)$. For a complete analysis of an age of infection model closely related to the original Kermack-McKendrick model, of which system (13.1)-(13.3) is a special case, the reader is referred to the work of Brauer (2005) in which general contact rates are allowed.

## Extensions to Incorporate Reactions to an Epidemic

An actual epidemic model differs considerably from the idealized model system (13.1)-(13.3) and its extension to the Susceptible-Exposed-Infected and Infectious-Recovered (SEIR) model with the SARS epidemic as a notable recent example follows. Some key differences are:

1. Various vaccination strategies are possible, such as the vaccination of health care workers and other first-line responders to the epidemic, vaccination of individuals who have been in contact with diagnosed infectious individuals, or vaccination of members of the population who are in close proximity to the diagnosed infectious individuals.
2. Those diagnosed as infected can be hospitalized, both for treatment and as a means of isolation from the rest of the population.
3. Contact tracing (Mueller, Kretzschmar, & Dietz, 2000) may be used to identify people at risk of becoming infective, and consequently so that they may be quarantined (or instructed to remain at home and to avoid contacts) and monitored so that they may be isolated immediately if and when they become infective.
4. Sometimes isolation may be imperfect, as in the case of in-hospital transmission of infection, which can be a major problem.

In hospitals, transmission can account for many new cases as was the case with SARS. This is an important heterogeneity in disease transmission which must be accounted for whenever there is any risk of transmission. Such details were accounted for in models for SARS (Anderson et al., 2004; Donnely et al., 2003) and approaches used for the SARS epidemic can also be relevant to other epidemics. The SARS outbreak attracted renewed effort to epidemic modeling, which is of great value in coping with future disease outbreaks. Thus if a vaccine is available for a disease that threatens to be an epidemic outbreak such as avian influenza, a vaccinated class that is protected at least partially ought to be included in the model development. But for an epidemic outbreak, where no vaccine protection is available, isolation and quarantine are the two main control measures available. Thus one can formulate a model for an epidemic once such control measures are in place, as in the work of Brauer (2005), who assumes that the epidemic has just started and so the number of infectious individuals is still small and almost all members of the population are still susceptible. In this approach, a class of quarantined individuals ($Q$) and another class of isolated ($J$) members are introduced. A general model with six compartments called the Susceptible-Exposed-Quarantined-Infected-Isolated-Recovered (SEQIJR) model is formulated in order to capture the course of the epidemic with no vaccine but with some control measures in place. The control reproductive number $R_C$ is then defined as the number of secondary infections caused by a single infective in a population consisting essentially only of susceptible individuals with control measures in place. In order to derive the expression for $R_C$ the following assumptions are necessary:

1. Exposed members may be infective with infectivity reduced by a factor $\theta_E$, where $0 \le \theta_E < 1$.
2. Exposed members who are not quarantined become infectious at rate $\sigma_1$.
3. Exposed members are quarantined at rate $\alpha_1$ per unit time. Although quarantine is not perfect, it should be assumed that it reduces the contact rate by, say $\theta_Q$.
4. Infective individuals are diagnosed at rate $\alpha_2$ per unit time and isolated. Quarantined members are monitored and isolated immediately on showing disease symptoms at rate $\sigma_2$.
5. There is a possibility of transmission of disease by isolated members, with an infectivity factor of $\theta_J$.
6. Infectious individuals who are not isolated leave the infective class at rate $\gamma_1$ with a fraction $f_1$ recovering, while isolated members leave the isolated class at rate $\gamma_2$ with a fraction $f_2$ recovering.

Without going into further details, an expression for $R_C$ is readily constructed (see full paper by Brauer, 2005):

$$R_c = \frac{\theta_E N\beta}{\Lambda_1} + \frac{N\beta\sigma_1}{\Lambda_1\Lambda_2} + \frac{\theta_Q N\beta\alpha_1}{\Lambda_1\sigma_2} + \frac{\theta_J N\beta\sigma_1\alpha_2}{\gamma_2\Lambda_1\Lambda_2} + \frac{\theta_J N\beta\alpha_1}{\gamma_2\Lambda_1} \quad (13.10)$$

where $\Lambda_1 = \alpha_1 + \sigma_1$ and $\Lambda_2 = \alpha_1 + \gamma_1$ giving the overall rate of leaving the exposed and infectious classes respectively. The epidemiological interpretation of each term in $R_C$ is as follows. The mean duration in the Exposed class is $1/\Lambda_1$ with contact rate modified to $\theta_E\beta$, giving a contribution of $\theta_E N\beta/\Lambda_1$. A fraction $\sigma_1/\Lambda_1$ goes from the Exposed class to the Infectious class, with contact rate $\beta$ and mean duration of $1/\Lambda_2$, giving a contribution of $N\beta\sigma_1/\Lambda_1\Lambda_2$. Next, a fraction $\alpha_1/\Lambda_1$ goes from the Exposed class to the Quarantined class, with contact rate $\theta_Q\beta$ and mean duration $1/\sigma_2$, giving a contribution to $R_c$ of $\theta_Q N\beta\alpha_1/\Lambda_1\sigma_2$. A fraction $\sigma_1\alpha_2/\Lambda_1\Lambda_2$ move from the Exposed to the Infectious class then to the Isolated class (J), with contact rate $\theta_J\beta$ and a mean duration of $1/\gamma_2$, giving a contribution of $\theta_J N\beta\sigma_1\alpha_2/\gamma_2\Lambda_1\Lambda_2$. Lastly a fraction $\alpha_1/\Lambda_1$ move from E to Q to J with contact rate $\theta_J\beta$ and a mean duration of $1/\gamma_2$ giving a contribution of $\theta_J N\beta\alpha_1/\Lambda_1\gamma_2$. Adding all these contributions together leads to the expression of $R_C$.

## Modeling Epidemics on Social Networks

Localized spread of infectious diseases has been successfully captured through various spatial models such as those developed by Mollison (1977), Durrett and Levin (1994), and Grenfell and associates (2001), among others. Such approaches recognize that the predominantly local nature of disease transmission leads to high degree of spatial heterogeneity and hence the population is not well mixed. As an alternative, the use of social network analysis has increasingly become an important tool to further our understanding of the spread of epidemics, particularly when proximity in space is no longer the determining risk factor for transmission. The approach is most useful in the development of more effective targeted control and treatment strategies. A wide range of communicable human diseases can be considered as spreading through a network of possible transmission routes. The implied network structure of a particular disease is vital in determining its dynamics, mixing pattern, and spread. The structure becomes particularly crucial when the average number of connections per individual is small as is the case for many STIs including HIV/AIDS. The use of social network models in epidemics is ideally an extension of the traditional population-level, pathogen-focused analysis of epidemics to one that is focused more closely on the host. Attention is no longer only on an individual's risk behavior, but focused on that individual's risk environment—which can accordingly increase or decrease an individual's risk behavior depending on the infectious status and behaviors of the people with whom s/he typically interacts. Thus, routinely collected contact tracing data is a critical source of information in the construction of disease networks for specific areas of occurrence; however in many parts of the world such data are either partially available or non-existent. This problem is further magnified in developing countries whose health budgets are highly constrained. Nonetheless it is recommended that centralized computer-based data systems be kept at all cost to cumulatively capture the contact tracing information gathered by public-health workers and physicians.

Social network models have already been applied to study infectious diseases in the study of STI transmission patterns (e.g., Wylie & Jolly, 2001). A mathematical model to address the question of heterogeneity in the rates of partner change and sexual mixing patterns was developed to investigate ethnic inequalities in the incidence of STIs in south-east London (Turner, Garnett, Ghani, Sterne, & Low, 2004). A more general analysis of (sexual) network models is found in a paper by Eames and Keeling (2002), who developed an intuitive mathematical framework to deal with the heterogeneities implicit within contact networks and those that arise because of the infection process. The researchers demonstrated how such models can be used to estimate parameters of epidemiological importance, and how they can be extended to examine the effectiveness of various control strategies, particularly screening and contact tracing.

In general, a network model for an infectious disease focuses on one of the fundamental issues of epidemiology—such as, who can acquire infection from whom (Lurie et al., 2003b). Such networks represent an individual within a population as a *node*, with connecting *edges* denoting relationships that could lead to the transmission of the disease. For many of the common airborne diseases it may be difficult to define which contacts form an edge, but for STIs, edges are more precisely defined as and correspond to sexual partnerships, thus networks are disease dependent. The initial spread and long-term behavior of any infectious disease are determined by both its epidemiological characteristics and the graph theoretical properties of the network. Some of these properties include an average number of neighbors, degree of clustering and the path length between nodes (Ghani & Garnett, 1998; Kretzschmar & Morris, 1996; Morris & Kretzscmar, 1995). One of the key features of an infection occurring within the constraints of a network is the rapid build-up of correlations in the infectious status of connected individuals. This aggregation will have the net effect of reducing the average number of susceptible partners per infected individual and consequently slow the spread of an epidemic. Note that standard epidemiological models such as the SIR model ignore this important correlation structure. In practice, however, the chains of transmission detected are seldom more than a few individuals long. This necessitates the need for modeling approaches that are capable of utilizing the available detailed information about the network, but does not require the complete network to be reconstructed. This goal was achieved by modeling partnerships as dynamic variables, developing a set of differential equations for the various types of connected pairs within the network in the study of STIs (Eames & Keeling, 2002). The beauty of this approach is that the models can easily be parameterized through the use of readily attainable contact tracing data, yet retain a high degree of generality.

Standard models for the dynamics of diseases or the mean-field models (Anderson & May, 1991) classify individuals according to their infection history by keeping track of the densities of susceptible, infected, and immune hosts. In general, these models consider the proportion of individuals in each class and ignore the underlying network or spatial structure. For STIs and childhood respiratory diseases (e.g., the respiratory synctial virus [RSV]) there is generally little or no immunity, so individuals return to the susceptible state upon recovery hence a suitable model for such infections is the SIS. The simplest correlation dynamics equations keep track of states of neighboring pairs of hosts on the lattice (Van Baalen, 2005). The general pair-wise network model for the Susceptible-Infective-Susceptible (SIS) model dynamics, following Keeling (1997), is outlined as follows. First label individuals as $S$ or $I$ and superscripts to denote their number of partners. Thus $[I^n]$ denotes the number of infected individuals with $n$ partners and $[S^n I^m]$ the number of partnerships between a susceptible with $n$ partners and an infected with $m$ partners. It is through such partnerships between susceptible and infected individuals that infection can be transmitted. Considering the dynamics of infectious individuals, two basic events can occur: either the infectious individual recovers, assumed to occur at rate $\upsilon$ or a susceptible individual gets infected by an infectious individual assumed to occur at rate $\gamma$. This leads to the following equation for the number of infected individuals with $n$ partners:

$$\frac{d[I^n]}{dt} = -\nu[I^n] + \gamma \sum_m [S^n I^m]$$  (13.11)

The second term on the right hand side gives the total number of infected partners of all $S^n$, each of whom transmits infection at rate $\gamma$. By making the standard assumption of ignoring partnerships but using contact data to estimate mixing between classes, this number can be estimated by:

$$[S^n I^m] \approx \frac{[S^n]}{[n]} \times \frac{[I^n]}{[m]} \times [nm]$$  (13.12)

where [n] denotes the number of individuals with n partners (with a similar meaning for [m]) and [nm] the number of partnerships with n and m partners. Although this mean-field approximation includes risk-structured hetero-geneities, it ignores the correlations in infection status that emerges between connected individuals. To model the dynamics of pairs, such as the $[S^n I^m]$ pair, equations of the form given below can be constructed.

$$\frac{d[S^n I^m]}{dt} = \gamma \sum_p ([S^n S^m I^p] - [I^p S^n I^m]) - \gamma [S^n I^m]$$
$$- \nu [S^n I^m] + \nu [I^n I^m] \tag{13.13}$$

The terms in the above equation refer to the creation of the $[S^n I^m]$ pair caused by infection of an $S^m$ within an $[S^n S^m]$ pair, loss of the pair caused by infection of the $S^n$ from outside or within the partnership, loss of the pair because of the recovery of the infected individual, and the last term which is specific to an SIS process represents the creation of the pair due to an $[I^n]$ recovery (which will be absent from the SIR model). In a similar manner, one can construct equations for all types of pairs by considering all possible events that can lead to that pair. This process could in theory be extended to model triplets, such as $[S^n S^m I^p]$, in terms of quadruples and so on, but the system rapidly becomes more compli-cated and in addition, the amount of data available to characterize the triplets is limited. This problem can be alleviated by making use of the *moment closure approximation* (Dushoff, 1999; Van Baalen, 2005), which allows the estimation of the number of triplets in terms of pairs, which closes the system, enabling one to calculate the behavior of individuals and pairs.

The impact of network models can be explained when important epidemio-logical quantities are considered, such as the basic reproduction ratio, $R_0$, already defined as the average number of secondary cases produced by an aver-age infectious individual in a wholly susceptible population. It is calculated as a measure of initial growth of an infinitesimal infection in an otherwise sus-ceptible population. For a structured population, however, the growth rate may depend on which class of individuals is infected. It might therefore be necessary to allow the level of infection to equilibrate between classes (so that high-risk individuals are more likely to be infected) before calculating $R_0$. For network models, $R_0$ should be calculated only once early spatial correlations (which develop within a couple of generations) have formed (for a detailed analysis, refer to Eames and Keeling, 2002 and Keeling, 1999). For an SIR version of the pair-wise network model, the basic reproduction ratio is given by

$$R_0 = \frac{\gamma (\lambda - 1)}{\nu} \tag{13.14}$$

where $\lambda$ is the dominant eigenvalue of the matrix $M$ given by:

$$M_{mn} = \frac{[nm](m - 1)}{m \times [m]} \tag{13.15}$$

The matrix $M$ is therefore a useful means of quantifying the connectedness of contact networks. Thus the strong correlations between the infection statuses of neighboring individuals play two roles. First, the negative correlation between susceptible and infectious individuals acts to dampen the epidemic spread and therefore reduces $R_0$. Second, in standard mean-field models, which ignore partnerships and correlations, $R_0$ is the same for both the SIS and SIR models. However in a pair-wise SIR structure, infectious individuals have a high proportion of recovered individuals as their neighbors, which will limit further spread of the disease. This limitation does not exist in the SIS formulation, and hence epidemic growth is more rapid. Thus equation (13.14) above offers only a lower bound for the SIS disease process. The importance of taking partnerships into account was demonstrated by using simulation studies where the mean-field model consistently overestimated initial spread of an infection over a range of values of the dimensionless infection parameter here given by $\gamma/\upsilon$ (Eames & Keeling, 2003). The key aim of modeling epidemics and analysis is to help in the design of control and treatment strategies. Clearly a control strategy focused on high-risk individuals (those with high numbers of contacts), taking advantage of the heterogeneities present in the network of partnerships, is likely to be more successful than that applied homogeneously across the population. More importantly at the verge of eradicating the disease, the high-risk classes can act as both reservoir and possible invasion routes for new infections. Hence when an intervention is about to achieve success it becomes increasingly important to target those individuals most central to disease spread.

## Migrant Worker Effect: A Real Application

### Introduction

HIV was identified as the cause of AIDS two years after its identification as a disease. Today, HIV affects all countries of the globe, making it and its disease consequences the most significant emerging infection of the late 20th century (Nicoll & Gill, 1999). To date, epidemiological factors determining the geographical spread of STIs/HIV are still not completely understood.

The geographical spread of STIs/HIV is determined by an interaction of factors related to demography, socioeconomics, and sexual behavior. HIV, like other infections that spread from person to person, follows the movement of people (Decosas & Adrien, 1997; Decosas, Kane, Anarfi, Sodji, & Wagner, 1995; Mabey & Mayaud, 1997; Quinn, 1994). The predominant socioeconomic factor (particularly in developing regions) is the rural-urban *labor migration* of young sexually active men leaving their sexual partners behind (Decosas, et al., 1995; Pison, Le Guenno, Lagarde, Enel, & Seck, 1993). Mobile people are at higher risk of STIs/HIV than those in stable living arrangements (Lagarde, Pison, & Enel, 1996; Pison, et al., 1993), primarily because the conditions of migration bring, for instance men into heterosexual contact with commercial sex workers and other women at high risk of STIs/HIV (Jochelson, Mothibeli, & Leger, 1991). The consequent sexual networking between urban and rural areas determines the diffusion rate of STIs/HIV into local societies (Fleming & Wasserheit, 1999). Furthermore, the women left behind sometimes have to exchange sex for favors as a survival strategy (Evian, 1993). The stark reality of the impact of STIs/HIV on society requires deeper understanding of factors determining the spread of STIs/HIV and further understanding of the relationship between STIs and HIV.

## Migration and HIV Diffusion Risks

In a study of the effects of migration in the transmission dynamics of HIV, migrant men from two adjacent health districts in South Africa's northern province of Kwa-Zulu/Natal were recruited at two primary migration destinations, Richards Bay (an industrial area) and Carletonville (a mining town). Migrant men were eligible to participate in the study if they were from Hlabisa or Nongoma districts, if they had at least one regular partner living in at least one of the two districts, and if they had been a migrant for at least the last six months (study methodology and results have been reported elsewhere, see Lurie et al., 2003a, Lurie et al., 2003b; Zuma et al., 2005; Zuma & Lurie, 2005). Migrant men gave information to locate their rural partners who were then invited to participate in the study. Non-migrant men and their partners living within a one kilometre radius from a migrant couple's home were asked to participate in the study. A detailed questionnaire was administered and urine and blood were collected for STI/HIV testing respectively.

A total of 168 couples were recruited into the study, of whom 98 (58.3%) were couples in which the male partner was a migrant, and 70 (41.7%) in which the male partner was not a migrant. The overall prevalence of HIV was 19.9% with 24.4% of men and 15.5% of women infected and among 69.6% of the couples, none of the partners was infected with HIV. Migrant couples were as likely as non-migrant couples to have neither partner infected with HIV (65.3% versus 75.7%) that is, to be HIV-concordant[1]. In 9.5% of the couples, both partners were infected with HIV, but this did not differ significantly by the migration status of the male partner (Lurie et al., 2003b). In 20.8% of the couples, one of the partners was infected with HIV. Migrant couples were 2.5 times more likely than non-migrant couples to be HIV-discordant[2] (26.5% versus 12.8%). Of the 35 discordant couples, the man was HIV-positive in 25 (71%) of the cases and the woman in the remaining 10 (29%) cases. The proportion of men who were infected in the migrant discordant couples was essentially the same as in non-migrant HIV discordant couples (Lurie et al., 2003b).

---

[1] Both sexual partners have the same HIV status
[2] Only one sexual partner is infected with HIV in a couple

## The Mathematical Model

In order to estimate the relative risk (RR) of infection for migrant and non-migrant men and women from their spouses and from partners outside the relationship, a set of parameters need to be defined (for greater detail of the model and results, see Lurie et al., 2003b). For a man and a woman in a sexual partnership, the man may be infected from outside the relationship with probability $\alpha$, the woman may be infected from outside the relationship with probability $\beta$. The man may also be infected by his wife with probability $\gamma$ (if she is already infected) and the woman may be infected by her husband with probability $\delta$ (if he is already infected). If the probabilities of infection are known, then the probabilities of each of the four concordance possibilities can be calculated. Combining probabilities gives:

$$P_{nn} = (1 - \alpha)(1 - \beta)$$
$$P_{pn} = \alpha(1 - \beta)(1 - \delta)$$
$$P_{np} = \beta(1 - \alpha)(1 - \gamma)$$
$$P_{pp} = \alpha\beta + \alpha\gamma + \beta\gamma - \alpha\beta(\gamma + \delta)$$

where the first subscript indicates the HIV status of the man (positive or negative) and the second indicates that of the woman. The parameters are varied in order to maximize the likelihood of the fit of the estimated probabilities to the observed probabilities assuming binomial errors. Since there are four parameters and only three independent observations, an appropriate value for the ratio of the likelihood that an infected man infects his wife to the likelihood that an infected woman infects her husband, is assumed to be $\delta/\gamma$.

Fitting this mathematical model to the above described data shows that both men and women are more likely to be infected by partners outside the relationship than to be infected by their spouses, irrespective of the migration status of the man. Migrant men are 26 times more likely to be infected by partners outside the relationship than from inside the relationship, whereas, women whose partners are migrants are 2.1 times more likely to be infected from outside the relationship than from inside. The same is true for non-migrant couples but with smaller RR of 10.5 for non-migrant men and 0.8 for their partners.

The impact of migration on the transmission dynamics of HIV can be better understood by comparing the RRs of infection for migrants as against non-migrants from outside versus inside their primary relationship for both men and women. Both men and women are likely to be infected from outside the primary relationship 1.44 and 1.53 respectively; however, they are less likely to be infected by their spouse if they are part of the migrant couple (Lurie et al., 2003b). The model assumes that within a spousal relationship, male-to-female HIV transmission is twice as likely as female-to-male transmission. Changing the relative transmissibility from men to women in either direction changes the RR estimates by less than 1.5% in all cases.

Discussion

It has long been assumed that the primary direction of spread of HIV has been from returning migrant men, who become infected while away at work, to their rural partners upon their return home. If this were the case, the male would be the HIV infected partner in most of the discordant couples; however, in nearly one-third of the discordant couples the female was the infected partner. Although this confirms the importance of migration as a risk factor for infection in both men and women, it changes the understanding of the way in which migration enhances risk.

The analysis in this chapter has focused on the man as a migrant and a woman as a non-migrant. In recent years, female circular migration has increased in South Africa as well as other places. The impact that migration has on the health of female migrants has not been investigated as extensively as it has been for men and most studies have concentrated on the migration of men and the risk that this entails for them and their non-migrant female partners (Decosas et al., 1995; Jochelson et al., 1991; Pison et al., 1993). Fewer have explored explore HIV infection risk factors among migrant women (Brewer et al., 1998; Zuma, Gouws, Williams, & Lurie, 2003) but have demonstrated that migrant women are also at high risk of HIV infection during their migration periods. There is a need to take drastic steps to address the social and economic pressures that migrant men, migrant women, and partners of migrant men face in the process of migration—such as the encouragement of industrial decentralization and regional developments to reduce the need for migration as well as to improve the conditions of migration.

# Mapping Disease Risk

## GIS, Mapping, and Clustering

Disease mapping and geographical information systems (GIS)[3] are becoming necessary as new technologies to improve decision-making processes in disease surveillance and control activities. These tools provide health professionals the ability to quickly analyze spatial relationships and disease risk factors in order to facilitate policy planning and implementation. The technique is used to visualize spatial patterns in the geographical distribution of disease, usually for explorative and descriptive purposes, to gain important clues about the etiology of a disease, and to provide information for further studies. As a result, disease mapping has become a valuable approach to hypothesis generation in explorative epidemiology.

Because of its growing usefulness, the development of methods for disease mapping has received great attention. The mapping and GIS program

---

[3]GIS is a surveillance system that uses remote sensing to predict disease spread.

of the World Health Organization (WHO) has spearheaded a global partnership in the promotion and implementation of GIS to support decision-making for a wide range of infectious diseases and as early as 1997, the WHO held a workshop in Rome on "Disease Mapping and Risk Assessment for Public Health Decision-Making." The workshop concluded with the general belief that geographical analysis of the distribution of risk factors can be useful in prioritizing preventive measures. Disease mapping was identified as useful for health service provision and targeting interventions if avoidable risk factors are known. It was however agreed that, no methodology of choice can be recommended in general and that analytical methods should be selected on the basis of the structure of the data to be analyzed and of the hypotheses to be investigated. In most circumstances, it might be helpful to envisage a first level of descriptive analysis, to be followed by more specific and problem-dependent analyses involving parameter estimation and hypothesis testing (Lawson, Biggeri, Boehning, Lesaffre, Viel, & Bertollini, 1997).

Numerous disease-mapping methods exist from the simple to the complicated (Lawson et al., 1997). While many of the earlier methods adopted a frequentist approach, Bayesian approaches based on Markov Chain Monte-Carlo (MCMC) methods have been gaining importance. In one of the earliest applications of the latter method, an empirical Bayes approach was used to shrink the Standardized Mortality Ratio (SMR) towards a local or global mean (Besag, York, & Mollié, 1991; Clayton & Bernardinelli, 1992). In the paper by Besag and associates (1991) the method was generalized to allow for different spatial heterogeneity. In their model Clayton and Bernadinelli (1992) discuss a Markov Random Field (MRF) approach as representing spatially structured heterogeneity. A nonparametric Bayesian approach was later proposed for the detection of clusters of elevated (or lowered) risk for the identification of unknown risk factors regarding the disease (Knorr-Held & Raer, 2000).

## Mapping Mobile Populations

The first two case studies illustrate the use of GIS techniques in disease mapping and control. The third case study is on modeling disease risk in space and time, where data are both longitudinal in time and spatial in nature.

(1) Using Remote Sensing and GIS to Identify Villages in Uganda at High Risk for Sleeping Sickness

GIS and remote sensing were used to identify villages at high risk for sleeping sickness (also known as human Africa trypanosomiasis, caused by *Trypanosoma brucei rhodesiense* and *Trypanosoma brucei gambiense*), as defined by reported incidence (Odiit, Bessel, Fevre, Robinson, Kinoti, Coleman, Welburn, McDermott, & Woolhouse, 2006). Sleeping sickness is a vector disease spread by the riverine tsetse fly species *Glossina fuscipes fuscipes*; therefore, tsetse fly densities and infection rates are major entomological determinants of sleeping sickness which is regarded as a re-emerging disease (WHO, 1986).

Landsat Enhanced Thematic Mapper (ETM) satellite[4] data were classified to obtain a map of land cover, and Normalized Difference Vegetation Index (NDVI) and Landsat band-5[5] were derived as unclassified measures of vegetation density and soil moisture, respectively. GIS functions were used to determine the areas of land cover types and mean NDVI and band-5 values within 1.5 km radii of 389 villages where sleeping sickness incidence had been estimated. Analysis was carried out using backward logistic regression, and proximity to swampland and low population density were found to be predictive factors of reported sleeping sickness presence, with distance to a sleeping sickness hospital as an important confounding variable. The study area comprised the Tororo district in eastern Uganda (Odiit et al., 2006). A sample of 389 villages out of a total of 884 census villages was selected with each village covering an area of approximately 0.5 to 5km², in an area that has two distinct wet (September-November and March-May) and dry (June-August and December-February) seasons. Increasing land pressure has forced people to encroach on marginal habitats to expand the area under cultivation. In eastern and southern Africa, where sleeping sickness occurs, reservoir hosts are a major contributing factor to its persistence. The human population in the area is split between rural mixed farmers, growing subsistence crops and rearing small holdings of cattle, and those living in the region's urban centers. The movement of infected cattle from endemic areas has been implicated in the re-emergence of sleeping sickness in areas where it was not known to be endemic (Fevre et al., 2001) but where tsetse flies are prevalent. Such movements of cattle bring the sleeping sickness agent into contact with the causal vector, which in turn transmits it to humans.

In this study logistic regression was used to first asses the statistical significance of satellite-derived variables, distance to a sleeping sickness hospital and population densities. For logistic regression, a binary response was defined as taking a value of 1 if sleeping sickness was present in a village and 0 otherwise, then using the presence and absence of disease as a predictor variable, backward logistics regression analysis of variables with associations of significance was carried out. After this, backward-stepwise logistic regression was performed to find the most parsimonious model of sleeping sickness risk (Greenland & Maldonado, 1994). This is a typical example in which human and animal mobility critically affects the spread of an infectious disease.

---

[4] A series of satellites by the USGS and NASA.
[5] Band designated to discriminate moisture content of the soil and vegetation and also able to penetrate thin clouds.

## (2) Bayesian and GIS Mapping of Childhood Mortality in Burkina Faso

Investigators used GIS ArcView and an empirical Bayes smooting technique to map the annual childhood mortality rates for each of 39 villages in the Nouna Demographic Surveillance Area (DSA) in Burkina Faso, West Africa (Sankoh, Berke, Simboro, & Becher, 2002). The study was restricted to children under the age of five years and was carried out between 1993 and 1998. The annual population of children younger than five years per village ranged from 15 to 454, showing a wide range of village size. In summary, annual mortality rates for each village in the study area was calculated using mid-year populations of children under five as the denominator. Two mapping techniques were implemented: first, the GIS software ArcView was used to map the crude mortality rates, and then the data were smoothed by the method of empirical Bayes (shrinkage) estimation[6]. The geostatistical method of Krigging was then administered to spatially interpolate the data for successive years. As an output of the above analysis, a semivariogram (the spatial dependence structure) of the mortality rates was estimated. The method of Krigging was used to produce isopleth maps showing the risk of children living in a certain place in the study region to die in a given year (Sankoh, et al., 2002). The maps showed no clear spatial trend pattern but the authors found that there was a tendency of villages in the northeastern region to produce higher incidence or risk values, which confirmed clustering of disease reported earlier by Sankoh and associates (2001). It is important to note that disease mapping was used primarily as an explorative tool to provide a general insight as opposed to precise estimates of incidence or spatial trends (Kafadar, 1999).

In general, the Bayesian smoothing technique is used to address the issue of heterogeneity in the population at risk and it is therefore a useful tool to use in explorative mapping of disease and mortality. In this study the method was helpful for visual identification of clustering in the northeastern side of the study region.

## (3) Modeling Risk from a Disease in Time and Space

Both models for longitudinal and spatial data were combined in a hierarchical Bayesian framework, with particular emphasis on the role of time- and space-varying covariate effects (Knorr-Held & Besag, 1997). Data analysis was implemented via Markov chain Monte Carlo methods and the methodology was applied to the Ohio lung cancer data covering the period of 1968 to 1988. The state of Ohio is located in northeastern United States and is divided into 88 counties. The database consisted of the population size and the number of deaths from lung cancer, stratified by age, gender, and race (white or non-white), for each year between 1968 and 1988 and for each

---

[6]Other smoothing techniques include the loess, kernel smoothing, or head-banging to name a few (Elliot et al., 2000).

county. Two approaches that adjust for unmeasured spatial covariates, particularly tobacco consumption, were used; the first included the use of random effects model to account for unobserved heterogeneity and the second involved the addition of a simple urbanization measure as a surrogate for smoking behavior. The Ohio data set has been of particular interest because of the suggestion that a nuclear plant located in the southwest of the state may have caused increased levels of lung cancer. The authors, however, concluded that Bayesian smoothing may not be the most appropriate tool for a focused analysis of this nature, and that the Ohio dataset does not provide enough information for any proper conclusion to be drawn. Thus the authors' main interest in the data was to illustrate the use of Bayesian mapping in time and space.

It is important to note that disease occurrence data in time and space is in the form of counts that nominally follow binomial or Poisson distributions. The key property with data of this type is that the outcomes are naturally correlated in time and space. The challenge is then to incorporate this correlation structure in any model one adopts to model the process. The generalized linear model (GLM) therefore is the starting point in an attempt to model such data statistically because the GLM neatly synthesizes likelihood-based approaches to regression analysis for a variety of outcome measures (McCullagh & Nelder, 1989). Extensions of the GLM involve models with random terms in the linear predictor giving rise to generalized linear mixed models (GLMMs). These models are useful for modeling the dependence among outcome variables inherent in longitudinal or repeated measures designs and for producing shrinkage estimates in multi-parameter problems, such as the construction of maps of small area disease rates (Clayton & Kaldor, 1987). For more details about these models including inference methods in GLMMs the reader is referred to the work of Breslow (1993).

## Conclusions and Future Research

This chapter has presented the SIR model as the basic mean-field epidemic model (Anderson & May, 1991; Daley & Gani, 1999) upon which further extensions and modifications can be implemented to capture more complex disease processes, in order to introduce basic concepts associated with disease modeling in order to enhance understanding and analysis of such processes. The extension of the above basic model has been particularly directed towards the understanding of the recent SARS epidemic and other general properties which have been described more elegantly by Brauer (2005). Further, the chapter has emphasized the need to develop statistical methods to enable the estimation of key parameters of a disease process and to enable the evaluation of the significance of some key factors driving epidemics such as HIV. As an example of the effect of population mobility on disease transmission, migrant worker effects and the spread of HIV/AIDS in Africa have been discussed.

The chapter has highlighted the concept of social networks as a means of enhancing present understanding of the local dynamics of infectious diseases, particularly when proximity of individuals in space is no longer the determinant factor of whether or not and individual infects or gets infected. Spatial explicit models have been used (e.g., Durett & Levin, 1994) when spatial heterogeneity plays a significant role in the spread of a disease. The discussion has been focused on sexual network models because partnerships are more easily defined with these infections. The spread of STIs, especially HIV/AIDS depends very much on patterns of sexual contact prevalent in a given population. In some societies serial monogamy may be the norm such that having more than one partner at the same time is an exception, while in other societies polygamy is the norm or at least widely accepted. Understanding of such differences is therefore important to understanding the spread of such infections and to help in designing control and intervention strategies. This chapter has also presented GIS and disease mapping techniques, which are becoming increasingly more applicable by improving decision-making process in disease surveillance control activities. The technique is useful as a tool to visualize spatial patterns in the geographic distribution of disease, for explorative and descriptive purposes as well as to provide information for further studies. Many earlier methods for disease mapping methods adopted the frequentist approaches, but currently Bayesian inference methods (parametric and nonparametric) are gaining popularity because of the advent of powerful computational methods such as the MCMC methods of parameter estimation and inference generation. The combination of standard statistical and Bayesian modeling approaches in order to understand the spread of the highly pathogenic diseases such as HIV/AIDS, Malaria, TB, and childhood diseases in Africa are among the future research interests of the authors of this chapter. Finally, it is our goal to enhance capacity in the continent in the field of disease modeling and mapping to inform policy on the most optimal control strategies that have high efficiency and of minimal cost relative to some existing methods.

## References

Anderson, R.M. & May, R.M. (1991). *Infectious Diseases of Humans*. Oxford, UK: Oxford University Press.

Anderson, R.M., Fraser, C., Ghani, A.C., Donnelly, C.A., Riley, S., Ferguson, N.M., Leung, G.M., Lam, T.H., & Hedley, A.J. (2004). Epidemiology, transmission dynamics and control of SARS: The 2002-2003 epidemic. *Philosophical Transactions of the Royal Society, London B*, 359, 1091-1105.

Besag, J., York, J., & Mollié, A. (1991). Bayesian image restoration with two applications in spatial statistics (with discussion). *Annals of the Institute of Statistical Mathematics*, 43, 1-59.

Brauer, F. (2005). The Kermack-Mackendrick epidemic model revisited. *Mathematical Biosciences*, 198, 119-131.

Breslow, N.E. & Clayton, D.G. (1993). Approximate inference in generalized linear mixed models. *Journal of American Statistical Association*, 88(421), 9-25.

Brewer, T.H., Hasbun, J., Ryan, C.A., Hawes, S.E., Martinez, S., Sanchez, J., Butler de Lister, M., Constanzo, J., Lopez, J., & Holmes, K.K. (1998). Migration, ethnicity and environment: HIV risk factors for women on the sugar cane plantations of the Dominican Republic. *AIDS*, 12(14), 1879-1887.

Clayton, D.G. & Bernardinelli, L. (1992). Bayesian methods for mapping disease risks. In (J. Cuzick & P. Elliot, Eds.) *Small Area Studies in Geographical and Environmental Epidemiology*, pp. 205–220, Oxford, UK: Oxford University Press.

Clayton, D.G. & Kaldor, J. (1987). Empirical Bayes estimates of age-standardized relative risks for use in disease mapping. *Biometrics*, 43, 671-681.

Daley, D.J. & Gani, J. (1999). *Epidemic Modelling. An Introduction.* Cambridge Studies in mathematical Biology. Cambridge, UK: Cambridge University Press.

Decosas, J., Kane, F., Anarfi, J.K., Sodji, K.D., & Wagner, H.U. (1995). Migration and AIDS. *Lancet*, 346(8978), 826-828.

Decosas, J. & Adrien, A. (1997). Migration and HIV. *AIDS*, 11(Suppl A), S77-S84.

Donnelly, C.A., Ghani, A.C., Leung, G.M., Hedley, A.J., Fraser, C., Riley, S., Abu-Raddad, L.J., Ho, L.M., Thach, T.Q., Chau, P., Chan, K.P., Lam, T.H., Tse, L.Y., Tsang, T., Liu, S.H., Kong, J.H., Lau, E.M., Ferguson, N.M., & Anderson, R.M. (2003). Epidemiological determinants of causal agents of severe acute respiratory syndrome in Hong Kong. *Lancet*, 361, 1761-1766.

Donnelly, C.A. (2004). Infectious Disease Epidemiology and Surveillance. Workshop on the epidemiological Methods and Clinical Trials for Preventive Health, 7-9 July 2004, Sydney, Australia.

Durret, R. & Levin, S.A. (1994). Stochastic spatial models: a user's guide to ecological applications. *Philosophical Transactions of the Royal Society, London B*, 343, 329-350.

Dushoff, J. (1999). Host heterogeneity and disease endemicity. A moment-based approach. *Theoretical Population Biology*, 56, 325-335.

Eames, K.T. & Keeling, M.J. (2002). Modelling dynamic and network heterogeneities in the spread of sexually transmitted diseases. *Proceedings of the National Academy of Sciences*, 99(20), 13330-13335.

Elliot, P., Wakefield, J.C., Best, N.G., & Briggs, D.J. (2000). *Spatial Epidemiology: Methods and Applications*. Oxford, UK: Oxford University Press.

Evian, C. (1993). The socio-economic determinants of the AIDS epidemic in South Africa—a cycle of poverty. *South Africa Medical Journal*, 83, 653-656.

Fevre, E.M., Coleman, P.G., Odiit, M., Magona, J.W., Weburn, S.C., & Woolhouse, M.E.J. (2001). The origins of a new *Trypanosoma brucei rhodensiense* sleeping sickness outbreak in eastern Uganda. *Lancet*, 358, 625-628.

Fleming, D.T. & Wasserheit, J.N. (1999). From epidemiological synergy to public health policy and practice: the contribution of other sexually transmitted diseases to sexual transmission of HIV infection. *Sexually Transmitted Infections*, 75(1), 3-17.

Ghani, A.C. & Garnett, G.P. (1998). Measuring sexual partner networks for transmission of sexually transmitted diseases. *Journal of the Royal Statistics, A*161, 227-238.

Greeland, S. & Maldonado, G. (1994). The interpretation of multiplicative-model parameters as standardized parameters. *Statistics in Medicine*, 13, 989-999.

Jochelson, K., Mothibeli, M., & Leger, J.P. (1991). Human immunodeficiency virus and migrant labor in South Africa. *International Journal of Health Services*, 21(1), 157-173.

Kafadar, K. (1999). Simultaneous smoothing and adjusting mortality rates in U.S. counties: Melanoma in white females and white males. *Statistics in Medicine*, 18, 3167-3188.

Keeling, M. (1999). The effects of local spatial struture on epidemiological invasions. *Proceedings of the Royal Society, London, B,* 266, 859-869.

Keeling, M. (1997). Modelling the persistence of measles. *Trends in Microbiology,* 5, 513-518.

Kermack, W.O. & McKendrick, A.G. (1927). A contribution to the mathematical theory of epidemics. *Proceedings of the Royal Society, A,* 115, 700-721.

Knorr-Held, L. & Besag, J. (1997). *Modeling risk from a disease in time and space.* Technical Report Series, NRCSE-TRS No. 005, University of Munich, Germany.

Knorr-Held, L. & Raer, G. (2000). Bayesian detection of clusters and discontinuities in disease maps. *Biometrics,* 56, 13-21.

Kretzschmar, M. & Morris, M. (1996). Measures of concurrency in networks and the spread of infectious disease. *Mathematical Biosciences,* 133, 165-195.

Lagarde E., Pison, G., & Enel, C. (1996). A study of sexual behavior change in rural Senegal. *Journal of Acquired Immune Deficiency Syndromes,* 11, 282-287.

Lawson, A., Biggeri, A., Boehning, D., Lesaffre, E., Viel, J.F., & Bertollini, R. (1999). *Disease Mapping and Risk Assessment for Public Health.* Chichester, UK: Wiley.

Lurie, M.N., Williams, B.G., Zuma, K., Mkaya-Mwamburi, D., Garnett, G.P., Sturm, A.W., Sweat, M.D., Gittelsohn, J., & Abdool Karim, S.S. (2003a). The impact of migration on HIV-1 transmission in South Africa: a study of migrant and nonmigrant men and their partners. *Sexually Transmitted Diseases,* 30(2), 149-156.

Lurie, M., Williams, B.G., Zuma, K, Mkaya-Mwamburi, D., Garnett, G.P., Sweat, M.D., Gittelsohn, J., & Abdool Karim, S.S. (2003b). Who infects whom? HIV-1 concordance and discordance among migrant and non-migrant couples in South Africa. *AIDS,* 17(15), 2245-2252.

Mabey, D. & Mayaud, P. (1997). Sexually transmitted diseases in mobile populations. *Genitourinary Medicine,* 73(1), 18-22.

McCullagh, P. & Nelder, J.A. (1989). *Generalized Linear Models* (2nd Ed.). London, UK: Chapman and Hall.

Mueller, J., Kretzschmar, M., & Dietz, K. (2000). Contact tracing in deterministic and stochastic models. *Mathematical Biosciences,* 164, 61-75.

Morris, M. & Kretzschmar, M. (1995). Concurrent partnerships and transmission dynamics in networks. *Social Networks,* 17, 299-318.

Mollison, D. (1977). Spatial contact models for ecological and epidemic spread. *Journal of the Royal Statistical Society, B,* 39, 283-326.

Nicoll, A. & Gill, O.N. (1999). The global impact of HIV infection and disease. *Communicable Disease and Public Health,* 2(2), 85-95.

Odiit, M., Bessel, P.R., Fevre, E.M., Robinson, T., Kinoti, J., Coleman, P.G., Welburn, S.C., McDermott, J., & Woolhouse, M.E.J. (2006). Using remote sensing and geographic information systems to identify villages at high risk *rhodesiense* sleeping sickness in Uganda. *Transactions of the Royal Society of Tropical Medicine and Hygiene,* 100, 354-362.

Pison, G., Le Guenno, B., Lagarde, E., Enel, C., & Seck, C. (1993). Seasonal migration: A risk factor for HIV infection in rural Senegal. *Journal of Acquired Immune Deficiency Syndromes,* 6, 196-200.

Quinn, T.C. (1994). Population migration and the spread of types 1 and 2 human immunodeficiency viruses. *Proceedings of the National Academy of Sciences,* 91, 2407-2414.

Ross, R. (1911). *The Prevention of Malaria,* (2nd Ed.). London, UK: Murray.

Sattenspiel, L. & Dietz, K. (1995). A structured epidemic model incorporating geographic mobility among regions. *Mathematical Biosciences*, 128, 71-91.

Sankoh, O.A., Ye, Y., Sauerborn, R., Mueller, O., & Becher, H. (2001). Clustering of childhood mortality in rural Burkina Faso. *International Journal of Epidemiology*, 20, 485-492.

Sankoh, O.A., Berke, O., Simboro, S., & Becher, H. (2002). Bayesian and GIS mapping of childhood mortality in rural Burkina Faso. SFB 544 *Control of Tropical Infectious Diseases*, Discussion Paper 03/2002, Uni-Heidelberg, Germany.

Turner, K.M.E., Garnett, G.P., Ghani, A.C., Sterne, J.A.C., & Low, N. (2004). Investigating ethnic inequalities in the incidence of sexually transmitted infections: mathematical modeling study. *Sexually Transmitted Infections*, 80, 379-385.

Van Baalen, M. (2005). Contact networks and the evolution of virulence. In: *Adaptive Dynamics of Infections Diseases: In Pursuit of Virulence Management*. Diekmann, U., Metz, J.A.J., Sabelis M.W. and Sigmund, K. (Eds), pp. 85-103. Cambridge, UK: Cambridge University Press.

WHO (1986). Epidemiology and control of human African trypanosomiasis. Report of WHO expert committee on sleeping sickness. Geneva: World Health Organization, Technical Report Series No. 739.

WHO (1997). Disease mapping and risk assessment for public health decision-making. Report on a WHO worksop, Rome, Italy, 2-4 October, 1997. EUR/ICP/EHRO 02 03 01 (In Lawson et al. 1999: pp. 453-468).

Wylie, J.L. & Jolly, A. (2001). Patterns of Chlamydia and Gonorrhea infection in sexual networks in Manitoba, Canada. *Sexually Transmitted Diseases*, 28(1), 14-24.

Zuma, K., Gouws, E., Williams, B.G., & Lurie, M. (2003). Risk factors for HIV infection among women in Carletonville, South Africa: Migration, demography and sexually transmitted diseases. *International Journal of STD & AIDS*, 14, 814-817.

Zuma, K., Lurie, M., Williams, B.G., Mkaya-Mwamburi, D., Garnet, G.P., & Sturm, A.W. (2005). Risk factors of sexually transmitted infections among migrant and non-migrant sexual partnerships from rural South Africa. *Epidemiology and Infections*, 133, 421-428.

Zuma, K. & Lurie, M. (2005). Application and comparison of methods for analyzing correlated interval censored data from sexual partnerships. *Journal of Data Science*, 3, 241-256.

# Chapter 14

## Ethical and Legal Issues Impacting Migrant Health

SANA LOUE, J.D., PH.D., M.P.H.

## Issues in the International Context

### *Migration and the Containment of Infectious Disease*

History documents the inadvertent facilitation of disease transmission by tourism, migration, and international trade networks to locations that are far flung from the discrete geographical regions of the globe from which the diseases were thought to originate (Cartwright & Biddis, 2000; Evans, 1992; Hays, 1998). As an example, during recent years, cases of "imported" and "airport" malaria have surfaced in Europe, North America, and other regions of the world (Gratz, Steffen, & Cocksedge, 2000; World Health Organization Regional Office for Europe, 1999). Of the 8,353 cases of imported malaria identified in the U.K. between 1987 and 1992, it was found that immigrants accounted for 11% of the cases, while the remainder were attributable to U.K. nationals who had visited friends and family members in malaria-endemic regions of the world (49% of the cases), visitors and tourists to the U.K. (35%), and expatriates (5%) (WHO, 1999). The 2002-2003 epidemic of severe acute respiratory syndrome (SARS) similarly demonstrated how quickly disease could spread from country to country as a result of the increased international mobility of individuals for a variety of purposes, including tourism, global investment and trade, and permanent migration (Catto, 2003; deLisle, 2004).

Because disease does not respect political boundaries, the international community has made efforts to address the risk of contagion that may be associated with migration between nations. The United Nations (UN) has as one of its primary objectives international health cooperation (UN Charter, 1945). The World Health Organization (WHO), one of the first specialized agencies created under the UN system, sought to develop international rules relating to the control of infectious disease (Sharp, 1947). Under Article 21 of its Constitution, the WHO has the authority to adopt regulations relating to "sanitary and quarantine requirements and other procedures designed to prevent the international spread of disease" (WHO Constitution, 1948).

Under this authority, the World Health Assembly (WHA) adopted in 1951 the International Sanitary Regulations, which were renamed the International Health Regulations (IHR) in 1969 and were last revised in 1981.

The IHR are intended to "ensure the maximum security against the international spread of diseases" while minimizing the impact of these efforts on international traffic and trade. In order to achieve this objective, the IHR provides for the establishment of a global surveillance system for yellow fever, plague, and cholera; requires specified health-related capabilities at ports and airports, such as safe drinking water and a mechanism for the disposal of excrement; and sets forth provisions relating to the enumerated diseases, such as the use of isolation against an individual arriving at an airport who is suspected of carrying cholera. Under these regulations, Member States may prevent the departure of an individual or carrier and may require health certificates relating to these diseases from individuals seeking entry into a State.

The past emphasis on the use of quarantine has diminished in favor of increasing reliance on epidemiological surveillance and the improvement of basic health services, in recognition of the inability of even rigid quarantine measures to provide security against disease. Unfortunately, however, the IHR-authorized and -suggested measures appear to have little effect on the global control of infectious disease due to countries' failure to report cases (DeLeon, 1975; Fidler, 1999). Accordingly, efforts are ongoing to revise the regulations (IHR, 2005).

Despite the IHR's increased emphasis on surveillance as a means of curtailing the globalization of disease, many countries have adopted exclusionary provisions that deny individuals the ability to cross legally through and into their borders. Disagreement exists among commentators regarding the legality of these measures under international law. Some have argued that such restrictions constitute a violation of human rights, while others emphasize the legal right of each nation to determine who may enter into its borders and the corollary right to define the class or classes of persons who may be excluded (Fidler, 1999; Gostin & Lazzarini, 1997).

## International Protections and Restrictions Related to Immigrants and Health

International law governs the relationships between the states, that is, nations that represent discrete entities that are responsible to themselves with respect to political, economic, and social matters. Treaties and customs provide the basis for these laws. The obligations that derive from the laws may be bilateral (between two nations), multilateral (between more than two states), or complex (linked to the creation of an international institution, such as the UN) (Goodwin-Gill, 1996). Two basic principles of international law are the sovereignty of each nation state and the equality between states (UN Charter, 1945).

International law has only relatively recently begun to address issues within the framework of human rights. Human rights are premised on the idea that individuals possess certain rights because of their humanity and governments must respect them; the existence of the rights does not depend on the beneficence of governments (Gostin & Gable, 2004).

It has been asserted that international law confers upon individuals the right to health. Table 14.1 provides a listing of the various international docu-

TABLE 14.1. International Documents and the Right to Health, and Limitations on Freedoms in Order to Protect Health

| International Document | Health-Related Rights and Limitations |
| --- | --- |
| WHO Constitution, 1946 | "The enjoyment of the highest attainable standard of health is one of the fundamental rights of every human being without distinction of race, religion, political belief, economic or social condition." |
| Universal Declaration of Human Rights, 1948 | Article 2: Everyone is entitled to all the rights and freedoms set forth in this Declaration, without distinction of any kind, such as race, colour, sex, language, religion, political or other opinion, national or social origin, property, birth or other status. |
| | Article 25: Everyone has the right to a standard of living adequate for the health and well-being of himself and of his family, including food, clothing, housing and medical care and necessary social services, and the right to security in the event of unemployment, sickness, disability, widowhood, old age or other lack of livelihood in circumstances beyond his control. |
| | The U.N. Sub-Commission on the Prevention of Discrimination and the Protection of Minorities has determined that "other status" in this context encompasses health status. |
| American Declaration of the Rights and Duties of Man | Article 11: "Every person has the right to the preservation of his health through sanitary and social measures relating to food, clothing, housing and medical care, to the extent permitted by public and community resources |
| International Covenant on Economic, Social and Cultural Rights (ICESCR), 1966 | Article 12(1): "States Parties to the present Covenant recognize the right of everyone to the enjoyment of the highest attainable standard of physical and mental health." |
| | Article 26: All persons are equal before the law and are entitled without any discrimination to the equal protection of the law. In this respect, the law shall prohibit any discrimination and guarantee to all persons equal and effective protection against discrimination on any ground such as race, colour, sex, language, religion, political or other opinion, national or social origin, property, birth or other status. |
| Protocol of San Salvador, negotiated 1988 | Article 10: "Everyone shall have the right to health." State Parties must agree to adopt various enumerated measures including the extension of health services to all individuals; the provision of preventive services and treatment for endemic, occupational, and other diseases; and the provision of primary health care to all individuals and families in the community |
| United Nations Convention on the Rights of the Child | Article 24(2): States are to take "appropriate measures" to implement "the right of the child to the enjoyment of the highest attainable standard of health and to facilities for the treatment of illness and rehabilitation of health" |

ments that contain references to a right to health and that provide the basis for this perspective. Commentators have noted that because the right to health as embodied in these documents is so broad, it essentially lacks coherent meaning and cannot be adequately monitored (Fidler, 1999). Consequently, it is difficult to identify the minimum level of responsibility that nations have. Gostin and Lazarrini have argued that "the state would have a responsibility, within the limits of its available resources, to intervene to prevent or reduce serious threats to the health of individuals or populations" (1997, p. 29). This would presumably apply to individuals within the territorial limits of each country, including immigrants.

Table 14.2 enumerates the source of governments' responsibility to protect the public health and the individual rights that may be impinged upon in this process. The government's right to infringe upon individuals' freedom of movement may provide justification for the imposition of quarantine measures and for limitations on the ability to travel. As can be seen, there exists a tension between, on the one hand, the State's sovereignty and its corollary right of self-preservation and duty to protect public health and, on the other hand, the rights of each individual.

Even refugees do not have the right to enter into another country. Although the expression the "right of asylum," suggests otherwise, the Refugee Convention does not obligate the state to permit refugees entry; rather, it obligates signatory states to conform to the principle of *nonrefoulement*, meaning that the state may not return a refugee to the territories where his life or freedom would be threatened due to his race, religion, nationality, membership in a particular social group, or political opinion (Convention Relating to the Status of Refugees, 1951; Protocol Relating to the Status of Refugees, 1967). Indeed, the "right of asylum is the right of the state to grant protection, which in turn is founded on the 'undisputed rule of international law' that every state has exclusive control over the individual within its territory" (Goodwin-Gill, 1996, p. 138).

TABLE 14.2. International Documents and Governmental Powers Associated with the Protection of Public Health

| International Document | Governmental Right |
|---|---|
| European Convention on Human Rights and Fundamental Freedoms (ECHR), 1950 | Persons may be deprived of the right to liberty "for the prevention of the spreading of infectious disease." Public authority may interfere with rights to privacy, freedom of religion, freedom of expression and freedom of assembly for the protection of health. |
| International Covenant on Civil and Political Rights (ICCPR), 1966 | Protection of public health is a legitimate reason for restricting the rights of freedom of movement, freedom of religion, freedom of expression, right of peaceful assembly, and right to freedom of association. |
| American Convention on Human Rights (ACHR), 1969 | Rights to freedom of expression, peaceful assembly, freedom of association, freedom of movement may be restricted for public health reasons. |

This conflict is reflected in the response of the U.S. to efforts by individuals infected with the human immunodeficiency virus (HIV) to enter its borders. U.S. law provides specifically for the exclusion of all HIV-infected individuals who are not citizens or lawfully permanent residents ("green card" holders or "mica" holders), absent a waiver of this provision. Waivers, discussed in greater detail below, are potentially available to refugees and several other classes of persons, but are relatively difficult to obtain. This policy is premised both on fears of contagion and fears that HIV-infected immigrants will drain available publicly-funded health care. In a scenario that raised widespread shock and claims of racism, the U.S. government attempted to deny HIV-infected Haitian refugees entry into the U.S. and subjected them to detention in a refugee camp without the provision of adequate medical care and sanitary precautions (*Haitian Centers Council v. Sale*, 1993). This move was widely criticized as a violation of international law and/or human rights because the consideration of refugees' HIV seropositivity nullified their ability to exercise their rights to the same degree as other refugees, thereby violating the principle of nondiscrimination. Additionally, it was argued, the *per se* exclusion of refugees due to health status could not be justified as related to public health or public expense because HIV is not a threat to either in the absence of specific individual behaviors, which were not in evidence (Goodwin-Gill, 1996).

Commentators have argued that the denial of entry by a country to individuals because of their HIV seropositivity constitutes a form of status discrimination that contravenes the internationally recognized principle of nondiscrimination and the right to privacy (Gostin, Cleary, Mayer, Brandt, & Chittenden, 1992). Others have countered these arguments by noting that it is the right of every country to decide who may enter (Fidler, 1999; Goodwin-Gill, 1996) and the infringement of the right to privacy arises from the improper use of information relating to an individual's seropositivity, rather than the denial of admission into the country (Fidler, 1999).

## Refugees and Access to Care

Data indicate that there may be upwards from 20 million refugees in the world; approximately half of who are children (Hakansson, 1999). As noted, although provisions in international documents appear to assure immigrants of a right to health care, that right is broad and subject to varying interpretations. A relatively recent analysis of international treaty provisions related to health care concluded that these protections afforded to refugees apply to only those who are lawfully resident within the territorial boundaries of a nation and not to those who may have entered illegally (Goodwin-Gill, 1996). It has been argued that nations' refusal and failure to make these same health services available to refugees and asylum seekers who have entered their borders illegally in search of a refuge constitutes constructive refoulement and a violation of the international principle of *nonrefoulement* (Cholewinski, 2000).

A recent survey of health care services provided to refugees and asylum seekers found vast differences among European nations. Germany restricts access to government-funded medical and dental treatment during the first 12 months of residence to cases involving "serious illness or acute pain" (Cholewinski, 2000: 741). Many countries have adopted similar policies and practices, although Italy and Sweden provide pregnant refugees with free access to their national health care systems for the duration of their pregnancies. Romania does not provide any state-funded medical services to refugees and asylum seekers (Cholewinski, 2000).

## Issues in the U.S. Context

Both permanent and temporary immigrants to the U.S. face significant issues in their attempts to maintain health and to access care. First, individuals suffering from conditions that impact their health may be denied admission to the U.S. Second, those who do enter, whether legally or illegally, may face significant challenges in accessing needed care due to a lack of health insurance coverage and barriers to qualifying for and obtaining publicly funded medical health insurance programs, such as Medicaid and Medicare. Even those immigrants who have sufficient resources to pay for the desired medical care, such as organ transplantation, may be denied that care due to policy concerns governing the allocation of scare resources. Immigrants who are detained may find that their ability to obtain care is further limited by policies specific to detention facilities. Each of these issues is explored in greater depth below.

### The Exclusion of Health-Impacted Immigrants

Despite the inscription at the base of the Statute of Liberty and its seeming welcome of the poor and downtrodden, the U.S. has a long history of excluding from its shores individuals who are believed to be burdened by disease. Historical accounts indicate that even in colonial America, individuals traveling to the colonies could be quarantined on ship and denied entry if cases of smallpox were detected aboard the ship or if the ship sailed from an area in which smallpox was endemic (Duffy, 1953). As an independent nation, the U.S. has provided for the exclusion of individuals for health-related reasons since 1882, with a prohibition against the landing of idiots or lunatics (Act of August 3, 1882). This provision was expanded further by the Act of March 3, 1891 to encompass "persons suffering from loathsome or contagious disease." The Act of February 5, 1917 enumerated additional classes of persons to be excluded as threats to the nation's well-being:

"... all idiots, imbeciles, feeble-minded persons, epileptics, insane persons; persons who have had one or more attacks of insanity at any time previously; persons of constitutional psychopathic inferiority; persons with chronic alcoholism; ... persons afflicted with *tuberculosis in any form or with a loathsome or dangerous contagious disease; [and] persons not comprehended within any of the foregoing excluded classes who are found to be and are certified by the examining surgeon as being mentally or physically defective, such physical defect being of a nature which may affect the ability of such alien to earn a living...”*

*(Act of February 5, 1917)*

This legislation provided the basis for the exclusion of individuals as mentally retarded persons, insane persons, and imbeciles (*Casimano v. Commissioner of Immigration*, 1926; *Patton v. Tod*, 1924; *Saclarides v. Shaughnessy*, 1950).

Subsequent legislation eliminated the bar against "persons of constitutional psychopathic inferiority" and replaced it with "aliens afflicted with psychopathic personality" in an attempt to provide for the exclusion of homosexuals (Act of June 27, 1952); provided for the exclusion of individuals suffering from mental defects or leprosy and those found to be "narcotic drug addicts" (Act of June 27, 1952); eliminated language relating to the "feeble-minded" and provided, instead, for the exclusion of those who were retarded (Immigration and Nationality Act Amendments of 1965); eliminated epilepsy as a ground of exclusion (Immigration and Nationality Act Amendments of 1965); added "sexual deviation" as a ground of exclusion to provide further for the exclusion of homosexuals (Immigration and Nationality Act Amendments of 1965); and authorized the exclusion of individuals infected with HIV (Act of July 11, 1987). The prohibition barring homosexuals from entering legally into the U.S. was not removed until 1990, 17 years after the American Psychiatric Association had determined that it is not a mental disorder (Foss, 1993; Minter, 1993).

Current immigration law provides for the exclusion of noncitizens who are determined "to have a communicable disease of public health significance" and those found

*(I)    to have a physical or mental disorder and behavior associated with the disorder that may pose, or has posed a threat to the property, safety, or welfare of the alien or others, or*

*(II)    to have had a physical or mental disorder and a history of behavior associated with the disorder, which behavior has posed a threat to the property, safety, or welfare of the alien or others and which behavior is likely to recur or to lead to other harmful behavior, or*

*(III)    who is determined . . . to be a drug abuser or addict*
(Illegal Immigration Reform and Immigration Responsibility Act of 1996; Immigration Act of 1990).

Regulations specify which diseases are to be considered "communicable disease of public health significance." At the time of this writing, these diseases are infectious syphilis, HIV, chancroid, gonorrhea, granuloma inguinale, lymphogranuloma venereum, active tuberculosis (TB), and infectious leprosy (Code of Federal Regulations, 2005). Individuals seeking admission as permanent residents are also subject to exclusion if they lack vaccinations against

mumps, measles, rubella, polio, tetanus, diphtheria, pertussis, hepatitis B, vari-
cella, haemophilus influenza type B, and pneumococcus unless medically
contraindicated or contrary to religious beliefs. Although it has been argued
that the health-related exclusion provisions and the corresponding medical
examinations are necessary to protect the public's health, history reveals that
efforts to bar the entry of disease and immigrants as their repositories were
and are often intertwined with tinges of homophobia, racism, anti-Semitism,
xenophobia, and generalized fear (Fairchild, 2003; Foss, 1993; cf. Gilmore &
Somerville, 1994; Markel, 1997; Somerville & Wilson, 1998).

A waiver of the exclusion bar for communicable diseases of public health
significance is potentially available to refugees, asylum applicants, and specified relatives of U.S. citizens and permanent residents. Such status or relationship is not a prerequisite for a waiver of a mental or physical disorder. No
waivers are available for the bars against admission of those determined to be
drug addicts or abusers.

The health-related reason for an individual's exclusion from the U.S. is
determined based upon a medical examination by a government-authorized
physician that is required of all who apply for permanent residence in
the U.S. as well as specified classes of individuals who may be coming
for temporary, but potentially long, periods of time. In addition, an
immigration officer conducting a legal inspection of the individual's
documents at the time of his or her entry into the U.S., such as at the airport,
may refer all non-U.S. citizens to an officer of the Public Health Service
(PHS) for a medical examination if the officer believes that an examination
might provide information that would indicate that a health-related reason
for exclusion exists (Code of Federal Regulations, 2005; USDHHS, 1992a,
1992b).

## Access to Health Care for Documented and Undocumented Persons

After entry into the U.S., access to health care for both documented and
undocumented immigrants is limited in the absence of health care insurance.
Data indicate many immigrants may lack such coverage. The 1989 and 1990
National Health Interview Surveys and the 1989 Insurance and 1990 Family
Resource Supplements indicate that, compared to native-born residents,
foreign-born residents of the U.S. were more likely to be uninsured, less likely
to have private insurance or Medicare, and somewhat more likely to have
Medicaid (Thamer & Rinehart, 1998).

Reliance on publicly-funded health insurance programs, such as Medicare
and Medicaid, is problematic for many immigrants and intending immigrants.
First, immigration law provides that individuals who are "likely to become a
public charge" may be excluded from entry into the U.S.. This provision has
been interpreted to mean that individuals applying for either temporary or
permanent residence into the U.S. may be denied admission if, based on

present circumstances, it is believed that they may rely on public funding for support. As an example, consider the situation of an individual seeking entry into the U.S. as a tourist. The immigration officer at the airport believes that he looks quite ill and refers him to the PHS officer for further examination. Upon questioning, it is determined that the individual is suffering from cancer that has metastasized. The PHS officer may indicate to the immigration official that the individual will likely require medical attention if he remains for any period of time in the U.S., but he does not have the resources to cover such medical expenses. The immigration officer may deny him admission into the U.S.and the individual will be forced to physically leave.

Individuals who have obtained permanent residence may also face penalties for reliance on publicly funded medical care. Immigration law provides that individuals who become a public charge within five years after having received status as permanent residents may, under certain circumstances, be deported (United States Code, 2005).

Subsequent legal reforms at both the state and federal levels have impacted even further immigrants' ability to obtain medical care due to a lack of health care coverage. As an example of state-level legal changes, the ballot initiative known as Proposition 187 was passed by California voters in 1994. If implemented, this initiative would have barred undocumented individuals from using public benefits, including Medicaid. (Palinkas & Arciniega, 1999; Ziv & Talo, 1995), and would have required that specified health care providers report their undocumented patients to law enforcement officers. Following the passage of Proposition 187, the California Department of Health Services developed a special program in collaboration with the then-Immigration and Naturalization Service (INS) to demand that foreign-born noncitizen women returning to the U.S. through California ports of entry and airports repay Medicaid for any benefits they had used. [The INS was disestablished and its functions incorporated into the Bureau of Immigration and Customs Enforcement (BICE) of the Department of Homeland Security (DHS). For ease of reference, this chapter will continue to refer to the agency as the INS.] The women were advised that failure to repay these sums could result in a denial of their re-entry into the country (California State Auditor, 1999; Wiles, Wright, Parks, & Clayton, 1997). However, no such requirement for repayment existed under either Medicaid law or immigration law (Schlosberg & Wiley, 1998). These efforts to garner payments from the women exacerbated fears among even legal immigrants that their legitimate reliance on Medicaid benefits could lead to their characterization by INS as "public charges" and result in their exclusion or expulsion from the U.S. (Berk, Schur, Chavez, & Frankel, 2000; Schlosberg & Wiley, 1998; Sun-Hee Park, Sarnoff, Bender, & Korenbrot, 2000).

The implementation of various provisions of Proposition 187, including the cessation of prenatal care to undocumented mothers, was ultimately enjoined by various California courts. However, subsequent to voter passage in California of Proposition 187, the U.S. Congress passed the Personal

Responsibility and Work Opportunity Reform Act (PRWORA) and the Illegal Immigration Reform and Immigrant Responsibility Act (IIRAIRA), which became effective on August 22, 1996. PRWORA created two classes of immigrants for the purpose of determining potential eligibility for specified publicly funded benefits, including nonemergency medical services, such as prenatal care. Immigrants who obtained their legal permanent resident status prior to August 22, 1996, the date of the law's enactment, were to be known as "qualified aliens." Individuals who obtained their legal permanent resident status after the date of enactment were to be classified as "nonqualified aliens." Pursuant to provisions in the legislation, most such individuals would be ineligible to receive publicly funded benefits, including Medicaid-funded services, for a period of five years following their receipt of their legal status.

Exceptions were created for certain classes of immigrants, including refugees, asylum seekers, immigrants with 40 quarters of qualifying work history, and noncitizens who had served in the U.S. military. Somewhat later, an exception was created for specified noncitizens whose need for publicly funded medical care was attributable to domestic violence. Nonqualified aliens would be subject to a deeming requirement, whereby the income of the U.S. citizen or permanent resident individual(s) who sponsored them for immigration would be considered in calculating eligibility for the benefit. In addition to the restrictions that were imposed on the receipt of benefits by certain legally immigrated individuals, the federal legislation provides that states may not provide nonemergency services to nonqualified aliens, including undocumented persons, without first passing new state legislation providing for the use of state funding for this coverage.

Findings relating to the effect of immigration and welfare reforms on immigrants' ability to access care have been inconsistent. Asch and colleagues reported that the passage of Proposition 187 in California may have discouraged immigrants in Los Angeles County from seeking screening and/or early treatment for TB infection (Asch, Leake, Abderson, & Gelberg, 1998). The passage of Proposition 187 was also found to be associated with a decrease in new walk-in patients at an ophthalmology clinic at a major public inner-city hospital in Los Angeles County (Marx, Thach, Grayson, Lowry, Lopez, & Lee, 1996) and a decrease in patients at an STD clinic (Hu, Donovan, Ford, Courtney, Rulnick, & Richwald, 1995). However, Loue and colleagues found no statistically significant difference in time between onset of gynecological illness and seeking of care, or length of time between seeking care and receipt of care among women of Mexican ethnicity of varying immigration statuses in San Diego County (Loue, Cooper, & Lloyd, 2005). Another study of immigrants of various nationalities, languages, and immigration statuses in Cuyahoga County, Ohio similarly found no effect of the reform laws on immigrants' ability to access care (Loue, Faust, & Bunce, 2000). A high proportion of respondents in this latter study, however, had entered the U.S. as refugees and, as such, were not subject to the restrictions on their receipt of publicly funded health care.

The denial of care to immigrants under both federal and state legislation and the reporting requirements that were mandated under Proposition 187 raise significant ethical, as well as legal, issues. Commentators have argued that immigrants, even those who are undocumented, have a moral claim to health care because they pay taxes and contribute more to the system than they utilize (Nickel, 1986). Additionally, it has been argued, all individuals have moral claims against others to obtain needed assistance. Counterarguments have been voiced, contending that (1) any response to a need for assistance is a matter of charity, rather than duty; (2) citizenship is a prerequisite to a valid moral claim to the state's services; and (3) at least some undocumented immigrants have forfeited any moral claim because they chose to enter into or remain in the U.S. illegally (Nickel, 1986).

## Health Care in the Context of Detention and Imprisonment

The U.S. Supreme Court has interpreted the prohibition of the Eighth Amendment to the U.S. Constitution against the imposition of cruel and unusual punishment of prisoners to encompass a prohibition against the deliberate indifference to an inmate's serious medical needs (*Estelle v. Gamble*, 1976). "Deliberate indifference" requires "a culpable state of mind" (*Farmer v. Brennan*, 1994). "Deliberate indifference" may be evidenced by prison physicians in the nature of their response to a prisoner's needs or by the intentional interference of prison guards in an inmate's access to medical care or to prescribed treatment (Pereira, 2004; Sylla & Thomas, 2000). This same standard applies to the states through the Fourteenth Amendment to the U.S. Constitution. The standard to be applied in the context of immigration detention, which is not considered criminal imprisonment, remains unclear, however. The lack of adequate medical care to immigrants in detention in the U.S. has been a continuing theme in human rights reports (Kerwin, 2001).

## Conclusion

Significant cooperation is needed across countries to interrupt the transmission of disease across political boundaries. Unfortunately, the efforts of individual countries to protect the public health may not accurately reflect the state of our knowledge and may unnecessarily target immigrants as the purveyors of disease. In addition, although international law seemingly assures immigrants and refugees access to health care, this ability to access care is broad and undefined and actual access and the nature of the care provided consequently vary across nations.

U.S. law reflects the tensions that exist between the principles of national sovereignty, self-protection, and nonrefoulement of refugee and asylum seekers. Consensus is lacking with respect to the appropriateness of the measures that the U.S. has implemented in an effort to reduce the likelihood of disease transmission by permanent and temporary immigrants and the consequent burden to public resources.

## *References*

Act of August 3, 1882, ch. 376, 22 Stat. 214.

Act of March 3, 1891, Ch. 551, 26 Stat. 1084.

Act of February 5, 1917, Ch. 29, 39 Stat. 874.

Act of June 27, 1952, Ch. 477, 66 Stat. 163.

Act of July 11, 1987, Pub. L. No. 100-71, 101 Stat. 391.

Asch, S., Leake, B., Abderson, R., & Gelberg, L. (1998). Why do symptomatic patients delay obtaining care for tuberculosis? *American Journal of Respiratory and Critical Care Medicine,* 157, 1244-1248.

Berk, M.L., Schur, C.L., Chavez, L.R., & Frankel, M. (2000). Health care use among undocumented Latino immigrants. *Health Affairs,* 19, 51-64.

California Department of Health Services. (1996). Adequacy of prenatal care utilization—California 1989-1994. *Morbidity and Mortality Weekly Report,* 45, 655.

California State Auditor. (1999). *Department of Health Services: Use of its Port of Entry Fraud Detection Program is no Longer Justified.* Sacramento, CA: California Bureau of State Audits.

Cartwright, F.F. & Biddess, M. (2000). *Disease & History.* Gloucestshire, UK: Sutton Publishing Limited.

*Casimano v. Commissioner of Immigration.* (1926). 15 F.2d 555 (2d Cir.).

Catto, S. (2003). Travel advisory: Toronto contends with SARS outbreak. *New York Times,* April 27, 152 (52466), 3.

Cholewinski, R. (2000). Economic and social rights of refugees and asylum seekers in Europe. *Georgetown Immigration Law Journal,* 14, 709-755.

Code of Federal Regulations. (2005).Title 42, § 34.2(b).

Convention Relating to the Status of Refugees, July 28, 1951, 189 U.N.T.S. 137.

Convention on the Rights of the Child. Adopted and opened for signature November 20, 1989, 1577 U.N.T.S. 3, entered into force September 2, 1990; http://www.un.org/documents/ga/res/44/a44r025.htm

DeLeon, P.J. (1975). *The International Health Regulations: A Practical Guide.* Geneva, Switzerland: World Health Organization.

deLisle, J. (2004). Atypical pneumonia and ambivalent law and politics: SARS and the response to SARS in China. *Temple Law Review,* 77, 193-245.

Duffy, J. (1953). *Epidemics in Colonial America.* Baton Rouge, LA: Louisiana State University Press.

*Estelle v. Gamble.* (1976). 429 U.S. 96.

Evans, R.J. (1992). Epidemics and revolutions: Cholera in nineteenth-century Europe. In (T. Ranger & P. Slack, Eds.), *Epidemics and Ideas: Essays on the Historical Perception of Pestilence* (pp. 149-173). Cambridge, UK: Cambridge University Press.

Fairchild, A.L. (2003). *Science at the Borders: Immigrant Medical Inspection and the Shaping of the Modern Industrial Labor Force.* Baltimore, MD: Johns Hopkins University Press.

*Farmer v. Brennan.* (1994). 511 U.S. 825.

Fidler, D.P. (1999). *International law and infectious disease.* Oxford, UK: Clarendon Press.

Foss, R.J. (1993). The demise of the homosexual exclusion: New possibilities for gay and lesbian immigration. *Harvard Civil Rights-Civil Liberties Law Review*, 29, 439-466.

Gilmore, N. & Somerville, M.A. (1994). Stigmatization, scapegoating and discrimination in sexually transmitted diseases: Overcoming them and us. *Social Science and Medicine*, 39, 1339-1358.

Goodwin-Gill, G.S. (1978). *International Law and the Movement of Persons between States*. Oxford, UK: Clarendon Press.

Goodwin-Gill, G.S. (1996). *The Refugee in International Law*. Oxford, UK: Clarendon Press.

Gostin, L.O. & Gable, L. (2004). The human rights of persons with mental disabilities: A global perspective on the application of human rights principles to mental health. *Maryland Law Review*, 63, 20-121.

Gostin, L.O., Cleary, P.D., Mayer, K.H., Brandt, A.M., & Chittenden, E.H. (1992). Screening and restrictions on international travelers for public health purposes: An evaluation of United States travel and immigration policy. In (L.O. Gostin & L. Porter, Eds.), *International law & AIDS: International response, current issues, and future directions*. Washington, DC: American Bar Association.

Gostin, L.O. & Lazarrini, Z. (1997). *Human Rights and Public Health in the AIDS Pandemic*. New York, NY: Oxford University Press.

Gratz, N.G., Steffen, R., & Cocksedge, W. (2000). Why aircraft disinfection? *Bulletin of the WHO*, 78, 995-1004.

*Haitian Centers Council v. Sale*. (1993). 823 F. Supp. 1028 (E.D.N.Y.).

Hakansson, G. (1999). International adoption and refugee children. *Whittier Law Review*, 21(1), 245-249.

Hays, J.N. (1998). *The Burdens of Disease: Epidemics and Human Response in Western History*. New Brunswick, NJ: Rutgers University Press.

Hu, Y., Donovan, S., Ford, W., Courtney, K., Rulnick, S., & Richwald, S. (1995). The impact of Proposition 187 on the use of public services by undocumented immigrants in Los Angeles County [abstract 1008]. 123rd Meeting of the American Public Health Association Meeting, 3.

Illegal Immigration Reform and Immigration Responsibility Act of 1996. Immigration and Nationality Act § 212(a)(1), 8 U.S.C. § 1182(a)(1).

Immigration Act of 1990. Immigration and Nationality Act § 212(a)(1), 8 U.S.C. § 1182(a)(1).

Immigration and Nationality Act Amendments of 1965, Pub. L. No. 89-236, 79 Stat. 911, 919.

International Covenant on Civil and Political Rights (ICCPR). Dec. 16, 1966, 999 U.N.T.S. 171, entered into force Mar. 23, 1976; ratified by 144 States as of 2000.

International Covenant on Economic, Social, and Cultural Rights (ICESCR). Dec. 16, 1966, 993 U.N.T.S. 3, entered into force Jan. 3, 1976; ratified by 141 States as of 2000.

International Health Regulations (2005). http://www.who.int/csr/ihr/en/

Kerwin, D. (2001). *Looking for asylum, suffering in detention*. American Bar Association, Human Rights Magazine, 28, 1. Washington, D.C: American Bar Association. http://www.abanet.org/irr/hr/winter01/kerwin.html

Loue, S., Cooper, M., & Lloyd, L.S. (2005). Welfare and immigration reform and use of prenatal care among women of Mexican ethnicity in San Diego, California. *Journal of Immigrant Health*, 7, 37-44.

Loue, S., Faust, M., & Bunce, A. (2000). The effect of immigration and welfare reform legislation on immigrants' access to care, Cuyahoga and Lorain Counties. *Journal of Immigrant Health,* 2, 23-30.

Markel, H. (1997). *Quarantine! East European Jewish immigrants and the New York City epidemics of 1892.* Baltimore, MD: Johns Hopkins University Press.

Marx, J.L., Thach, A.B., Grayson, G., Lowry, L.P., Lopez, P.F., & Lee, P.P. (1996). The effects of California Proposition 187 on an ophthalmology clinic utilization at an inner-city urban hospital. *Ophthalmology,* 103, 847-851.

Minter, S. (1993). Sodomy and public morality offenses under U.S. immigration law: Penalizing lesbian and gay identity. *Cornell International Law Journal,* 26, 771-818.

Nickel, J.W. (1986). Should undocumented aliens be entitled to health care? *Hastings Center Report,* Dec., 19-23.

*Patton v. Tod.* (1924). 297 F. 385 (2d Cir.)

Pereira, A. (2004). Live and let live: Healthcare is a fundamental human right. *Connecticut Public Interest Law Journal,* 3, 481-503.

Protocol Relating to the Status of Refugees, Jan. 31, 1967, 606 U.N.T.S. 267.

*Saclarides v. Shaughnessy.* (1950). 180 F.2d 687 (2d Cir.).

Schlosberg, C. & Wiley, D. (1998). *The impact of INS public charge determinations on immigrant access to care.* Washington, DC: National Health Law Program and National Immigration Law Center, May. Available at http://healthlaw.org/pubs/19980522publiccharge.html (accessed 4/25/2004).

Somerville, M.A. & Wilson, S. (1998). Crossing boundaries: Travel, immigration, human rights, and AIDS. *McGill Law Journal,* 43, 781-834.

Sun-Hee Park, L., Sarnoff, R., Bender, C., & Korenbrot, C. (2000). Impact of recent welfare and immigration reform on use of Medicaid for prenatal care by immigrants in California. *Journal of Immigrant Health,* 2, 5-22.

Sylla, M. & Thomas, D. (2000). The rules: Law and AIDS in corrections. *HIV Education Prison Project News, November.* http://www.aegis.com/pubs/hepp/2000/HEPP2000-1101.html

Thamer, M. & Rinehart, C. (1998). Public and private insurance of US foreign-born residents: Implications of the 1996 welfare reform law. *Ethnicity and Health,* 3 (1,2), 19-29.

United Nations (1945). Charter; http://www.un/org/aboutun/charter/

United Nations Sub-Commission on the Prevention of Discrimination and the Protection of Minorities. U.N. Doc. E/CN.4/Sub.2/1994/L.42.

United States Code. (2005). §§1227.

United States Department of Health and Human Services, Public Health Service. (1992a). *Technical instructions for the medical examination of aliens, July.* Washington, DC.

USDHHS-PHS (1992b). *Technical instructions for the medical examination of aliens in the United States, July.* Washington, DC: U.S. Department of Health and Human Services, Public Health Service.

Universal Declaration of Human Rights. (1948). G.A. Res. 217 A, U.N. GAOR, 3d Sess., U.N. Doc. A/311.

WHO (1948). Constitution. Geneva, Switzerland: World Health Organization. http://www.who.int/ about/en/

WHO (1999). *Report on infectious diseases: Removing obstacles to health development.* Geneva, Switzerland: World Health Organization.

World Health Organization Regional Office for Europe. (1999). *Strategy to Roll Back Malaria in the WHO European Region.* http://www.euro.who.int/document/e67133.pdf

Wiles, M.H., Wright, D.F., Parks, M., & Clayton, J. (1997). Abuse by official at the border. *Los Angeles Times, Dec.* 23, B6 (editorial).

Ziv, A. & Talo, B. (1995). Denial of care to illegal immigrants. *New England Journal of Medicine, 332,* 1095-1098.

# Chapter 15

## Migration in a Mobile World: Health, Population Mobility, and Emerging Disease

BRIAN D. GUSHULAK, M.D.
AND DOUGLAS W. MACPHERSON, M.D. M.SC (CTM), F.R.C.P.C

### The Historical Relationships Between Population Mobility and the Control of Emerging Diseases

Mobile populations[1] and outbreaks of disease are associated with some of the oldest recognized, institutionalized public health interventions. Disease epidemics that followed the arrival of travelers, merchants or trade goods stimulated the implementation of risk-mitigation and control responses in the Middle Ages. Unanticipated health threats that were often related to epidemics of infectious diseases continue to create national and international response activities that reflect those patterns of practice developed in the past (Levison, 2003). The factors that stimulate disease control responses are based on the management of both real and perceived risk. As we look at the history of the interaction between migration and emerging disease threats, it can be observed that the perception of threat can be more important than the real disease risk itself.

Public health interventions follow a recurrent pattern of stimulus and response. This pattern is the result of two main factors that influence the perception of threat and the subsequent conversion to a measurable and managed risk. Understanding those factors helps to explain some of the recurrent challenges in modern public health approaches directed at mobile, migrant populations. The two major factors that link migration and disease threat and risk are: 1) the uncertainty due to deficiencies in knowledge level, experience, and understanding of the disease, including the fear of inability to control the event, and 2) the real and perceived disease outcomes in terms of

---

[1] Due to the plurality of populations and groups that are encompassed by the term migrant or immigrant (immigrants, emigrants, refugees, asylum seekers, displaced populations, migrant workers, foreign workers, etc.) the term mobile population is used extensively in this chapter. In this context a mobile population is one which resides, works, travels, or lives outside of its nation of birth.

death, or morbidity, and other consequences including loss of livelihoods, population displacements, security considerations, and economic impacts.

## The Role of Disease Uncertainty in the Development of Response Strategies

Limited understanding, experience and knowledge of a disease or condition, in the context of migration and population mobility can result from two situations. The disease may be a new event for which there is no historical information to guide management, control and prevention activities (Zuckerman, 2004). Alternatively, the re-emergence of a previous prevalent disease threat that has been controlled or absent for an extended period of time may create health sector management challenges due to experience or knowledge limitations in health care workers unfamiliar with the condition. Both of these situations are important in the context of migration and both affect control and intervention strategies.

## The Role of Disease Outcome in the Development of Response Strategies

The perceived consequences posed by a disease threat influence the political and public communication of risk. This real or perceived level of risk in turn can affect the investment of public health efforts directed at mitigating the disease threat. Historically, fear of the disfiguring, disabling, or disgusting outcomes of disease drove public health responses. This was characterized by medieval interventions introduced to prevent the introduction of and control of leprosy, a disease much feared at the time. Fear has always been significant in measures to limit the introduction or spread of disease. Fear and uncertainty regarding the impact of new or novel infectious disease threats have influenced public health response for centuries. This historical linkage continues into today's context. Current health legislation and regulation often continues to make reference to "loathsome" diseases.

The two factors of fear and lack of knowledge, working together in the 14th century produced one of the most enduring public health interventions: quarantine. Faced with a new epidemic disease of unknown cause and high mortality, city states attempted to protect their inhabitants and their economic interests by restricting the entry of new arrivals. Some 500 years later, the expansion of quarantine practice in the 1800s occurred in the midst of three important events that today continue to influence the practice of public health interventions for mobile populations.

Those events were the great wave of European colonization in North America; the Irish Potato Famine causing forced population displacement, and the Asiatic cholera epidemics in Western Europe with subsequent spread to the Americas. The expansion of quarantine practice ("holding off for 40 days") included the regular medical screening examination of arriving immigrants. Concurrent with these events in 1851, 12 European nations began a series of international conferences to standardize and harmonize Port of Entry sanitation and health interventions for goods, conveyances, and travelers (Goodman, 1971). This process with revisions evolved into the International Health Regulations (IHR) and played a significant part in the formation of the World Health Organization's role in international disease control (WHO, 1951).

Dealing with disease control and the movement of people set the stage for the more organized approaches to medical management of migrants at the beginning of the 20th century (Birn, 1997). These activities became integral parts of the formal immigration process for those nations with active immigration programs. Public health and infectious disease control practices were expanded, and the basis of many current immigration health practices flow from pre-existing quarantine procedures. Those practices owe their own origin to fear and uncertainty related to disease threats, and the potential for imported disease-associated death and morbidity (Abel, 2004). Consideration of the use of quarantine as a method of infectious disease control is a recurring theme in situations involving new diseases. In late 2005, quarantine practices were included in national contingency plans to manage pandemic influenza (U.S. Homeland Security Council, 2005).

Modern migrants often originate in areas of the world were new or emerging infections generate concerns based on disease novelty, poor clinical outcomes, and lack of knowledge. As a consequence, migrants from these source regions are more likely to be the target of public health interventions or activities. Balancing the nature of the interventions against the real risks of disease importation in terms of cost benefit and global health and development goals represents a significant international health challenge as indicated in the differential public health responses to malaria, HIV/AIDS and severe acquired respiratory syndrome (SARS).

## Current Nature of Population Mobility and Interventions Directed at Controlling International Disease

The evolution of the migration processes since the mid-20th century makes the application and reference of traditional approaches to public health difficult and in some cases irrelevant. New approaches to the management of health and migration will be necessary as the world moves along the pathway to greater integration over shorter periods of time. The often confusing relationship and linkages between migration and attempts to control or limit the impact or outcome of emerging and re-emerging disease challenges can be effectively approached from an integrated perspective. Using this integrated model, called the five "Ps" of the Migration Health Paradigm, it is possible to consider, measure and balance several disparate but related factors that act together in national and international migration health policies and practices.

## The Five Ps of Migration Health

Population Mobility

The first aspect is the consideration of the individual, group or population involved in international movement from the perspective of mobility rather than from an administrative immigration perspective. This is important as it allows for the consideration of different risks between groups and populations that are included in broad classifications of immigration. As traditional patterns of immigration evolve, the changing patterns affect some of the health issues related to migration. Considering migrants in terms of more defined groups and communities moving across and between different health environments and systems, as opposed to a homogeneous group, allows for better assessment of the impact of those differences and provides an improved framework for dealing with health concerns.

Several of the major changes in migration and migrant demography that have occurred during the last 40 years are encompassed in this population mobility concept (Rodriguez-Garcia, 2001). They include:

- Post-colonial population flows;
- Major immigration source country evolution;
- Changes in refugee dynamics, including displaced persons, refugee claimants and asylum seekers;
- The collapse of the East-West Cold War Dynamic;
- Travel and globalization; and
- Persistent disparities in development indices.

In 1960, about 90% of regular immigration to western, developed nations originated in nations, in Europe and the Americas, that often shared similar demographic and biometric characteristics. By the end of the 20th century approximately 80% of that immigration movement had shifted to source nations that were tropical, sub-tropical or developing. This situation resulted in the movement of people across marked differences in the prevalence of certain health characteristics between source and destination locations. These dramatic shifts over significant prevalence gaps in communicable diseases in source countries to receiving regions are also associated with migration between different levels of socio-economic status, genetic/biological, cultural/behavioral, and environmental risk patterns. Each of those differences can significantly influence health outcomes. Additionally, while the offspring of foreign-born are usually considered in the same context as the host population, some of the differences in health indicators, as described above, continue to influence health outcomes in combination with those basic health determinants and through return travel and contact with ancestral migrant origins. Traditional approaches designed to control disease control at the border were not designed to deal with these issues.

The evolving patterns of migration that have occurred over the last 40 years have changed many of the characteristics of current migrants and mobile populations in comparison with those of previous migrant groups. Modern refugee and other displaced population movements occur rapidly and international assistance is provided more expediently than in refugee situations of 50 or 60 years ago. As a consequence, more vulnerable migrants, the young, the old, the ill, and females may be more frequently encountered in these populations. These forced, mass movement situations, which now occur more commonly with involvement of the international community, have personal, public, and population health implications (Zlotnik, 1995).

Together, the new facets of migration combine to make traditional migration health practices that were conceived as a single event, frontier-associated process, less relevant or applicable in the modern context of migration. The management of the migrant's individual health as well as aspects of national public health activities and international disease control efforts is not adequately served by traditional immigration practices.

Prevalence Gaps

The second component in this paradigm is the concept of movement across and between epidemiological and systematic disparities in health determinants. In spite of extensive efforts directed at health and development, the world remains marked by regional, national and geographic disparities in health determination, health service utilization, and health outcomes. While these differences, particularly those with a geographic or environmental origin have always existed; the impact of globalization as manifest through the ease and speed of current international travel has greatly increased their impact. Now more than at any time in recorded human history, individuals are moving rapidly between and across boundaries that separate regions of different disease incidence and prevalence (Boggild, Correia, Keystone, & Kain, 2004).

Tuberculosis (TB) provides an illustrative model of how international disease flow, development, and migration are integrally related. Many migration receiving nations in North America and Europe have long-standing established, TB control programs. Several of those programs are directed towards domestic elimination of the disease. Disease elimination programs, when followed to completion result in the expenditure of increasingly large amounts of public health and capital resources per case eliminated as the incidence of the disease falls.

Globalization requires that national disease control programs have an international focus that extends beyond the national boundaries. Those programs that do not include a global component will be continually challenged by population mobility (Harper, Ahmadu, Ogden, McAdam, & Lienhardt, 2003). Using TB as an example, in spite of efforts directed at the national, domestic level, TB control programs will be unable to eliminate or eradicate the disease as long as migrants originate in areas of higher endemicity. Population mobility demands that national disease control programs must contain a significant international focus that should be integrated with national and international development assistance programs and policies.

Failure to integrate development assistance programs with domestic public health program planning, in nations with existing immigration programs, will ensure that the domestic outcomes will always be challenged by international factors. The sustained disparity in disease prevalence between migrant source and destination regions will impair the future success of domestic public health control strategies in migrant receiving nations of lower disease prevalence.

## Process: The Phases of Population Mobility

Traditional approaches to migration and the health of migrants have been most commonly based on the uni-directional flow from a point of origin to a resettlement destination. Immigrants and refugees usually arrived at their new destination and remained there permanently. Through a process of assimilation, the new arrivals adopted and adapted to the characteristics and patterns of the host population, resulting in a shifting of baselines for both populations. Studies and evaluations that examined the health and health outcomes of migrants were often separated on the basis of foreign versus domestic birth and the foreign-born cohorts analytically aggregated into one homogeneous population.

While this was a relevant approach for the large immigrant waves of the early and mid 20th century, these aggregative approaches to the assessment of the health of migrants are not currently sensitive enough to the changing demography of migration. The end of the Cold War, for example, brought a liberalization of restricted travel in Eastern Europe and parts of East Asia that meant many refugees and other migrants could now return to their own or ancestral place of origin. As temporary asylum and return migrations have become more common, the associated migratory movements have become dynamic circular processes in the short-term that also spin across generations.

Other changes in the process and patterns of population mobility have been in the technical aspects of travel itself. Current air travel has become more easily available, accessible, and affordable for many migrants, and transit is much more rapid. Opportunities for return visits to migrants' places of origin are more common and within the reach of more people than they were even two decades ago. This facilitation of travel and continued journeys between source and destination locations affects the health aspects associated with migration and can extend the exposure to existing health and disease risks for the migrant and subsequent generations (Bacaner, Stauffer, Boulware, Walker, & Keystone, 2004). Additionally, the ease of travel is allowing for the expansion of the globally mobile cohort who divides their residence time between different locations. When these locations transit significant inter-regional prevalence gaps, these multinational residents may also experience an increase in their health risk exposures resulting in personal, public, and population-based health risks.

Public Health and Population Health

The fourth component is composed of the activities directed at what historically was broadly known as "public health." Traditionally, the approach to public health has been directed at the regulated activities of surveillance, detection, intervention and reporting of contagious infectious diseases of significance to the health of the public. The modern concept of public health is evolving to encompass more than those functions. Public health now involves the consideration of population-based health determinants; including maternal-child health, environmental health, trauma prevention, chronic diseases, substance abuse, socio-economics, emergency response, and security. This population-based approach to public health focuses on the health of both individuals and groups. It is a conceptual extension of traditional public health practice integrating demographics and biometrics with the broad determinants of health. This approach to public health includes the impacts of non-infectious diseases and health determination factors such as genetics and biology, socio-economics, behavioral activities, environmental factors, cultural and linguistic characteristics in determination of health impacts and outcomes systematically for the population.

Historically, interest in health and migration has centered on the challenges posed by virulent, communicable diseases. Recently, interest in the preventive and control of infectious disease has been growing at national and international level. Much of this renewed interest has been in response to the emerging infectious disease threats and situations, often originating outside of the regional health jurisdiction. This combined attention on infections of international importance, provides an obvious convergence point. To be most effective, modern approaches to public health will have to include the broader implications of population mobility. This convergence also means that greater international collaboration is and will be necessary to meet the challenges posed by diseases of multinational importance (CDC, 2004).

This primary interface between migration and public health is the major reason that the impact and consequences of emerging disease threats are intimately related to population mobility. Globalization requires and supports greater population mobility. The economic and demographic future of many nations is more closely tied and appreciated to be migration-dependent. At the same time, there is significant and growing awareness of the implications of emerging diseases and the renewed importance of communicable disease public health management as a major component of the health services and management sector (Patz, Daszak, Tabor, Aguirre, Pearl, Epstein, Wolfe, Kilpatrick, Foufopoulos, Molyneux, & Bradley, 2004).

Perception of Risk

The fifth component is related to one of the basic historical aspects that govern the sociological response to imported disease, which is the perception of risk. How nations and the public at large perceive the importance of a health threat even before it may be demonstrated to be a true risk—particularly in a world of virtual instant, world-wide communication, is a major factor in the health and population mobility paradigm. Global communication technology now allows for the worldwide reporting of actual events and situations as they happen, even before the quality of the information has been evaluated or processed. This has played a significant role in risk perception in many disease outbreaks (Grein, Kamara, Rodier, Plant, Bovier, Ryan, Ohyama, & Heymann, 2000). Fear of serious illness or death caused by a "loathsome contagion" can quickly exceed concerns about other risks of mortality and morbidity that may be of greater epidemiological importance.

Many of the factors that affect risk appreciation and risk acceptance are often compounded when the event is one of a new or re-emerging disease and also associated with uncertainty. When the public observes uncertainty in the scientific, medical or political arenas that are entrusted with protecting the public well being, high levels of concern are not surprising. In a migration-related context, the perception of risk and the sociological pressures for counter measures can generate significant reflex responses in both the immigration and public health sectors (Speakman, Gonzalez-Martin, & Perez, 2003). In many locations, particularly in the developed world where infectious disease mortality and morbidity are rare, there are often demands to manage what are, in global terms, very small risks.

Immigrant populations are often involved or associated in emerging disease situations (Fauci, 2001). Their status and legal requirements to interact with border, frontier or immigration officials present a controlled opportunity for intervention. As a group, they may be the recipients of public health control measures that are not applied to other travelers. It is important that when the risk perception is associated with the implementation of health or travel interventions, that the outcome, rationale and justification of those interventions be evaluated. It is also important to avoid the stigmatization and potential marginalization of migrant populations based on the fear of disease. Failure to manage or address these issues results in the risk of expending resources and efforts on activities of low or questionable return, at the expense of other more relevant and necessary needs.

# The Health of Mobile Populations—How the Five Ps Come Together

Having faded from its level of importance in the early part of the 20th century, activities directed at the health of migrants continued at a rudimentary administrative level following World War II. Traditionally an interest of border control officers and the medical sectors of nations with formal, long-standing immigration policies, the health of migrants had resurgence in association with large-scale refugee resettlement activities after the conflict in Viet Nam in the late 1970s.

The rapid movement of large numbers of individuals from a tropical, developing region was associated with imported infectious diseases not seen in previous movements. The prevalence of many diseases of national public health importance in the destination countries was in some cases significantly much higher in Southeast Asia. As a consequence, the risks associated with importing relatively large numbers of cases of TB, malaria, intestinal parasites and other infections were greater than had been observed during the previous 30 years when most immigration and refugee movements had been European in origin.

Flowing from the historical basis of quarantine and the desire to protect the host population from the direct risks and consequences of imported disease, the strengths and weakness of immigration medical screening became subjects of increased study and comment. In response to growing public and political interest, the historical use of the immigration medical screening process as a tool for denying or delaying admission to the country of destination often becomes a topic of discussion and debate. Each new emerging disease threat or challenge with a migration component is subject to this reflection on national domestic levels.

Migration health response patterns and practices tend to be based on responding to the threat at the time of international travel. This response is often done in an immediate and reactive manner to the perceived threat before risk assessment has been done. Migration-related health interventions have also tended to be individually focused, as opposed to population-based. They have usually been directed towards surveillance or treatment interventions as opposed to prevention, and have been of short duration in application. As such, they can be costly on an individual basis, are often of limited public health effectiveness in terms of community health, and do little in terms of health promotion and disease prevention. These approaches are not only limited to immigration screening situations. For examples in the past 15 years, cholera in Peru, plague in India, cyclosporiasis in Central America, and SARS in Asia have resulted in the wide spread, reactive application of traditional quarantine-based health interventions often with extensive, economic consequences locally and elsewhere.

Better science and improved understanding of outcomes related to population mobility and health are beginning to lead to changes in the philosophy and practice of migration health. These initiatives are recent and while they have not yet been in place sufficiently long enough to demonstrate their enduring effectiveness, they represent the beginning of a new approach to health and population mobility that is based on the available scientific evidence that best encompasses the components of health and population mobility, beyond the antiquated public health practices based on quarantine principles.

## Migration Health Challenges and Consequences Resulting from Globalization

Several of the factors and events that are associated with the perception of threat and risk and the current interest in migration and emerging disease threats are similar to those which have occurred earlier in human history. The movement of conveyances, individuals, and goods across and between areas and regions where gaps in disease prevalence and risk exist has been historically a recurrent theme. Sometimes the implications have been dramatic and serious as exemplified by plague, smallpox, and cholera introduction in the Americas, pandemic influenza in 1918, and *Plasmodium falciparum* malaria in South America in the 1930s.

At other times, the inevitable consequences of the global sharing of disease epidemiology have been less consequential, although public concern has been high. This has been most evident in the international public health approaches towards HIV/AIDS. In spite of significant comment and rhetoric, actual interventions have neither affected the globalization of the disease nor significantly affected global migration. Population mobility globalizes disease risk. The epidemiological consequences resulting from the fact that many migrants originate in areas of the world where development indices and health conditions are lower than those at destination countries, are that migrants will continue to be groups at greater risk of disease (MacLean et al., 2004).

As mobility continues to bridge regions of different disease prevalence, any organized, integrated public health endeavor or planning process designed to mitigate or manage the risks of emerging diseases must include a migration and population mobility component (Lee & Henderson, 2001). Failure to recognize and anticipate these situations is likely to create interventions and activities that may not effectively deal with the intricacies and complexities of migratory processes. The lack of effective programs that can explain and manage the health aspects of migration may actually increase fear, xenophobia, stigmatization and marginalization of migrant groups who may be blamed for what are the simple consequences of global developmental disparities (Siem, 1997).

Program weaknesses will also result from the differential appreciation and communication of risk factors that vary considerably among and between populations (Mayer, 2000). Migrant populations may have different valuations of risk than those of host populations and may require specific preventive and health promotional interventions in that context. Globalization and migration will require adjustments in the medical and health services sector in host nations for large numbers of migrant and mobile populations. Modern examples include the relatively recent creation of a global pharmacotherapeutic network that encompasses large numbers of mobile populations.

National pharmaceutical and drug regulatory programs and strategies are increasingly tested and stressed by the capacity of mobile populations to acquire, import, or otherwise obtain medications or therapeutic and diagnostic agents from areas beyond domestic pharmaceutical or vaccine regulatory control. While it may be possible to intercept and interdict commercial or high volume shipments, it is logistically difficult to control or even monitor personal use of pharmaceuticals acquired from international sources. At the same time, globalization factors such as the Internet allow for transborder drug shopping between nations. Those health care providers who work with migrants and international travelers are increasingly aware of the issue. Numerous postings on websites and automated listserves used by these practitioners are directed at the identification and intended use of these agents.

Similar activities take place with regard to food and other nutritional items. The globalization of food distribution poses its own challenges to the regulation and standard applications of food safety provisions (Keiser & Utzinger, 2004). It is increasingly recognized that the unofficial importation and international exchange of food and regional nutritional items is beyond the capacity of most regulatory and enforcement agencies. As a consequence, there will be a greater globalization of risk in terms of food-associated disease with the attendant public health implications. As the stimuli that produce and sustain the international exchanges of "local" or ethnic items cross major economic divides, migrants at their new destination may create increasing demand for the goods than may exist at the origin resulting in new market-demand forces.

Costs of drugs, vaccines, and other pharmaceuticals at the migrants' new destination may be higher than those for similar agents at the place of origin. Global communication technology and frequent travel between these two sites is now more accessible and available at affordable costs. These factors allow for unofficial markets in traditional and regulated medications and pharmaceutical agents that cross many national boundaries. While organized in more formal manners in Asian communities where traditional pharmacies are regular component of migrant societies from Asia, the practice includes many other migrant groups. The size and extent of these exchanges is difficult to estimate as many of the acquired agents are for personal or family use only and are imported with personal effects or baggage. Yet health care providers who work with migrant communities commonly encounter the use of imported agents from the migrants' home country.

## Future Directions and Policy Development

In terms of migration and development, planners and policy makers will need to become much more lateral and tangential in their thinking and consultative planning processes. Globalization of population mobility brings the consequences of distant events, situations, and health factors as close as the next international arrival by air, sea or land (McMichael, 2004). Until more robust systems are in place to allow for the better assessment and quantification of real risk with outcome based analysis and clarity in communication of risk, public and systematic perceptions of international threats and risk will continue to be an important component of mitigation and response activities. While potentially a significant paradigm shift, the recognition that health intervention needs to be multi-dimensional (e.g., five P's), broader and more widely applied, including being focused at migrant source areas, will be challenging to those who traditionally direct their resources at new arrivals at the time of arrival.

One of the most important aspects of a new and modern understanding of migration and health in the current global context will be the necessity to assess and approach the issue from a horizontal and systematically integrated perspective (Lee, 2000). Policies designed to deal with development and globalization will increasingly need a specific component to measure and describe the migration related impact and benefits of the proposal. Globalization will continue to support and require the facilitated movement of large numbers of migrants, workers, and travelers. Many of those individuals will originate in, or transit through, areas of the world where health conditions and epidemiological risk factors differ significantly from those at the travelers' destination (Sattar, Tetro, & Springthorpe, 1999). Real-time electronic media will continue to report world events of public health and population health interest as they occur, independent of their local or global context or veracity.

Policy and program initiatives will require greater and sustained collaboration at regional and international levels to ensure that procedures, protocols, and undertakings are balanced and harmonized. The management of the various aspects of the issue in general is complicated by the lack of centralized focus on the issues of health and mobile populations. The nature and requirement for immigration medical services is a function of the administrative and/or legal status of the individual or population. Migrant workers, foreign students, visiting family members, travelers, returning residents, or other mobile individuals who may be at equivalent or, in some cases, greater risk of an adverse health or disease outcome, are often excluded from routine national immigration medical interventions.

Further compounding the weaknesses of existing immigration medical interventions in those nations that maintain them is the fact that they are fundamentally related to the immediate entry or arrival process. They are for the most part concerned with a limited number of listed or scheduled diseases or conditions. Given the rapid development of real and perceived emerging disease threats, the historical and policy basis behind existing formal immigration screening processes makes them unwieldy tools for addressing issues of temporal or immediate relevance.

## Health Interventions

Historically, health interventions directed towards migrants and arriving mobile populations were based on the general application of risk as a function of immigration status. Investigations or screening were required for all members of certain migrant classes on arriving vessels, while citizens or nationals of the host country arriving at the same time from the same source country were exempted from the health processes. As the true epidemiological risks of disease importation became more defined for immigration processing nations, immigration medical screening became part of the immigration selection process and was directed off shore at the migrant in their place of origin.

As the world moves to a more integrated approach to the medical management of the risks of imported diseases, the full impact of globalization has yet to become apparent (DesMeules, Gold, Kazanjian, Manuel, Payne, Vissandee, McDermott, & Mao, 2004). Traditional immigrant-receiving nations have existing health programs and medical practices that can be modified to deal with newly arising disease threats. Recent examples include: 1) the introduction of immunization either actively or as an administrative review of existing records, as a component of immigration-related medical screening activity, 2) the population-based mass treatment of certain infections in migrants before departure to low endemic areas, and 3) the move away from disease screening for the purposes of denying admission on public health grounds to screening for diagnosis and treatment. These strategies and capacities are being successfully used to manage public concern regarding emerging and re-emerging diseases in migrants. However the same approaches are not often applied to non-immigrant travelers; including for example retuning citizens, foreign students, and business and tourist travelers.

When situations develop, where risk management and mitigation strategies are needed for all mobile populations, the systematic tendency is to return to the basic concepts and principles of isolation, exclusion, and inspection under quarantine practices, and denial of admission to the ill or potentially ill (Samaan, Patel, Spencer, & Roberts, 2004). The economic and social consequences of this rather blunt response will require the need to move away from a *one size fits all* approach to traditional public health to a more risk management-based approach that will strive to ensure that those at greater risk receive the attention required to manage the demand for effective but rational intervention. This population-based, risk assessment and mitigation strategy will require fundamental and paradigm shifts in the policy structure, rationale, and practice of immigration and migration health.

## Health System Implications

It has already been noted that traditional international and domestic public health sectors and programs within nations with significant migration programs will need increasing and regular attention to international public health activities. The effects of globalization and migration will also impact on other areas of the health sector (Collins, 2003). As migrant and mobile populations grow in both size and diversity, they will produce ever more substantial effects on domestic health policy, management, and care delivery services; in addition to health education, training, registration, certification,

and standards enforcement activities. This shift in focus is already evident in
areas of disease epidemiology in the developed world for maladies that have
primarily been controlled or eliminated in the host population. Mobile populations make up the majority or increasing components of those affected
with several chronic infections. Travel patterns and population mobility also
combine to create situations where these groups are at greater risk of other
acute infections not endemic in the source country. As many of these conditions may not have been encountered or have been rarely seen by health care
providers in host communities, diagnostic acumen and clinical indices of
suspicion can be low. This can lead to delayed clinical recognition, diagnosis,
and management. As migration and globalization continue to impact on
health care delivery sectors, education and training of service providers in
these areas will be increasingly required.

In addition to the clinical aspects of health care delivery that require attention in order to better meet the future health challenges related to migration,
population mobility generates other demands. The diversity in both culture
and language associated with many migrant populations can affect access to
and delivery of health care services. To improve the effectiveness and efficiency
of health care services, host nations will need to examine and increase their
health sector capacities in the areas of cultural and linguistic competencies.

## Implications for International Cooperation

A common thread that runs through the issues of immigration, population
mobility, emerging disease threats, globalization, and international development is the degree of interdependency that exists in today's world (Baretto,
2003). The factors that support and create many of the challenges that
emerging disease threats pose inter-regionally result from or are influenced by
globalization and global integration. These interacting and confounding risk
factors; both real and perceived, can extend well beyond national boundaries
and across domestic control programs through the effects of population
mobility. The solutions and responses necessary to meet these challenges will
originate and resonate through the same factors.

The global nature of threat is reflected in the progressive inability of
national activities to effectively deal in any long term or sustained manner
with those threats as they convert to both quantifiable and qualitative risk.
The great cost and effort placed in national and domestic programs designed
to detect threats and mitigate risks that arise beyond national boundaries
may be more effectively expended to manage the situation at the source rather
than at the destination.

Integrated and virtually simultaneous travel, communication and information exchange now more than ever, allow for rapid recognition and appreciation of developing disease threats. A more globalized and integrated health
sector component can, if properly supported and structured, effectively

harness knowledge and capacity that extends across and between disparate health systems (Loewenson, 2004). More integrated and empirical analysis and risk mitigation planning on a broad scale can both define the extent of threats and new disease challenges and propose effective international strategies to manage those events.

Some of these activities are already underway. The IHR have been revised by WHO (Hardiman, 2003) and have been accepted at the World Health Assembly in 2005 (WHO, 2005). Many of the factors that have generated the momentum for this revision have been the result of emerging disease threats and population mobility. When completed and promulgated, the IHR are intended to provide a standard reference source that governs and guides both local and international response systems faced with emerging disease threats (Fidler, 2003).

While the IHR will deal with the disease component of the equation, the population mobility and immigration aspects of the relationship remain somewhat more of an international policy challenge. Nations with formal immigration programs maintain and support health services designed to deliver and sustain those activities of medical screening predominately for exclusion directed at a limited scope of the global migrant population. For the most part, these immigration medical screening activities continue to be based on national and domestic frameworks and there is a lack of international, academic, scientific and analytical attention on the design, delivery and effectiveness of these programs in a global context.

Some international organizations and agencies, such as the United Nations Agencies, the International Labor Organization, and the International Organization for Migration, have interests in aspects of the relationships between population mobility, migration and health. Additionally, WHO has addressed specific migration health topics and there are some sections of the IHR that deal with a few defined migration issues. Other organizations, agencies, national immigration and health departments, municipal and metropolitan health departments and universities address health issues in mobile populations, often from a situational or local perspective.

In 2003, in response to the Secretary General of the United Nations, a Global Commission on International Migration was convened. The commission was directed to provide a framework for the formulation of a coherent, comprehensive and global response to the issue of international migration. During its tenure, the Commission prepared a detailed report on the aspects of migration that was delivered to the UN in October 2005 (Global Commission on International Migration, 2005). The Commission's work noted that health issues related to migration were important but their nature and scope exceeded the Commission's capacity and they were not addressed in the final report. As a consequence there remains a continuing lack of an integrated, globally focused undertaking that is actively engaged in the coordinated, collaborative study and investigation of the many aspects of health and population mobility.

The creation of an area of study of this scope and magnitude will not be an easy task; however, it is necessary and essential that it be done.

In the absence of such an integrated approach to the multifaceted relationships between health, international disease control and population mobility, responses and resource allocations will be less effective. They will tend to be situation specific as opposed to policy directed. They will more likely be reactive as opposed to anticipatory and they will continue to be directed at receiving locations as opposed to migrant origins. All of those factors will combine to make them less cost effective and more limited in scope than forward looking disease prevention and health promotion approaches that should more effectively be components of integrated, globally focused social and economic development programs.

## References

Abel, E.K. (2004). "Only the best class of immigration:" public health policy toward Mexicans and Filipinos in Los Angeles, 1910-1940. *American Journal of Public Health*, 94, 932-939.

Bacaner, N., Stauffer, B., Boulware, D.R., Walker, P.F., & Keystone, J.S. (2004). Travel medicine considerations for North American immigrants visiting friends and relatives. *Journal of the American Medical Association*, 291, 2856-2864.

Barreto, M.L. (2003). Science, policy, politics, a complex and unequal world and the emerging of a new infectious disease. *Journal of Epidemiology and Community Health*, 57, 644-645.

Birn, A.E. (1997). Six seconds per eyelid: The medical inspection of immigrants at Ellis Island 1892-1914. *Dynamis*, 7, 281-316.

Boggild, A.K., Correia, J.D., Keystone, J.S., & Kain, K.C. (2004). Leprosy in Toronto: An analysis of 184 imported cases. *Canadian Medical Association Journal*, 170, 55-59.

CDC (2004). Epidemiology of measles–United States, 2001-2003. *Morbidity and Mortality Weekly Report*, 53, 713-716.

Collins, T. (2003). Globalization, global health, and access to healthcare. *International Journal of Health Planning and Management*, 18, 97-104.

DesMeules, M., Gold, J., Kazanjian, A., Manuel, D., Payne, J., Vissandee, B., McDermott, S., & Mao, Y. (2004). New approaches to immigrant health assessment. *Canadian Journal of Public Health*, 95, 122-126.

Fauci, A.S. (2001). Infectious diseases: Considerations for the 21st century. *Clinical Infectious Diseases*, 32, 675-685.

Fidler, D.P. (2003). Emerging trends in international law concerning global infectious disease control. *Emerging Infectious Diseases*, 9, 285-290.

Global Commission on International Migration. (2005). *Migration in an interconnected world: New directions for action*. Report of the Global Commission on International Migration. Geneva, October 2005. http://www.gcim.org/attachements/gcim-complete-report- 2005.pdf

Goodman, N.M. (1971). *International health organizations and their work*, 2nd Ed. London, UK: Churchill Livingstone.

Grein, T.W., Kamara, K.B., Rodier, G., Plant, A.J., Bovier, P., Ryan, M.J., Ohyama, T., & Heymann, D.L. (2000). Rumors of disease in the global village: Outbreak verification. *Emerging Infectious Diseases*, 6, 97-102.

Hardiman, M. (2003). The revised International Health Regulations: A framework for global health security. *International Journal of Antimicrobial Agents*, 21, 207-211.

Harper, M., Ahmadu, F.A., Ogden, J.A., McAdam, K.P., & Lienhardt, C. (2003). Identifying the determinants of tuberculosis control in resource-poor countries: Insights from a qualitative study in The Gambia. *Transacations of the Royal Society of Tropical Medicine and Hygiene*, 97, 506-510.

Keiser, J. & Utzinger, J. (2004). Chemotherapy for major food-borne trematodes: A review. *Expert Opinion on Pharmacotherapy*, 5, 1711-1726.

Krilov, L.R. (2004). Emerging infectious disease issues in international adoptions: severe acute respiratory syndrome (SARS), avian influenza and measles. *Current Opinion in Infectious Diseases*, 17, 391-395.

Lee, K. (2000). The impact of globalization on public health: implications for the UK Faculty of Public Health Medicine. *Journal of Public Health Medicine*, 22, 253-262.

Lee, L.M. & Henderson, D.K. (2001). Emerging viral infections. *Current Opinion in Infectious Diseases*, 14, 467-480.

Levison, J.H. (2003). Beyond quarantine: a history of leprosy in Puerto Rico, 1898-1930s. *Historia, ciencias, saude—Manguinhos*, 10(Suppl 1), 225-245.

Loewenson, R. (2004). Epidemiology in the era of globalization: Skills transfer or new skills? *International Journal of Epidemiology*, May 6 [Epub ahead of print]

MacLean, J.D., Demers, A.M., Ndao, M., Kokoskin, E., Ward, B.J., & Gyorkos, T.W. (2004). Malaria Epidemics and Surveillance Systems in Canada. *Emerging Infectious Diseases*, 10, 1195-1201.

Mayer, J.D. (2000). Geography, ecology and emerging infectious diseases. *Social Science and Medicine*, 50, 937-952.

McMichael, A.J. (2004). Environmental change and food production: Consequences for human nutrition and health. *Asia Pacific Journal of Clinical Nutrition*, 13(Suppl), S19.

Patz, J.A., Daszak, P., Tabor, G.M., Aguirre, A.A., Pearl, M., Epstein, J., Wolfe, N.D., Kilpatrick, A.M., Foufopoulos, J., Molyneux, D., & Bradley, D.J. (2004). Working Group on Land Use Change and Disease Emergence. Unhealthy landscapes: Policy recommendations on land use change and infectious disease emergence. *Environmental Health Perspectives*, 112, 1092-1098.

Rodriguez-Garcia, R. (2001). The health-development link: travel as a public health issue. *Journal of Community Health*, 26, 93-112.

Samaan, G., Patel, M., Spencer, J., & Roberts, L. (2004). Border screening for SARS in Australia: what has been learnt? *Medical Journal of Australia*, 180, 220-223.

Sattar, S.A., Tetro, J., & Springthorpe, V.S. (1999). Impact of changing societal trends on the spread of infections in American and Canadian homes. *American Journal of Infection Control*, 27, S4-S21.

Siem, H. (1997). Migration and health-the international perspective. *Schweizerische Rundschau fur Medizin Praxis*, 86, 788-793.

Speakman, J., Gonzalez-Martin, F., & Perez, T. (2003). Quarantine in severe acute respiratory syndrome (SARS) and other emerging infectious diseases. *Journal of Law Medicine and Ethics*, 31(4 Suppl), 63-64.

US Homeland Security Council (2005). *National Strategy for Pandemic Influenza*. Washington DC. November 2005. http://www.pandemicflu.gov/

WHO (1951). *International Sanitary Regulations. World Health Organization Regulations No. 2.* Geneva, World Health Organization, 1951 (WHO Technical Report Series, No. 41). WHO World Health Assembly adopts new International

Health Regulations. http://www.who.int/mediacentre/news/releases/2005/pr_wha03/en/index.html

Zlotnik, H. (1995). Migration and the family: The female perspective. *Asian and Pacific Migration Journal*, 4, 253-271.

Zuckerman, A. (2004). Plague and contagionism in eighteenth-century England: the role of Richard Mead. *Bulletin of the History of Medicine*, 78, 273-308.

# Index

Printed in the United States
72759LV00001B/172-189

9 780387 476674